BASIC AND CLINICAL SCIENCE COURSE

Glaucoma

Section 10

2004–2005

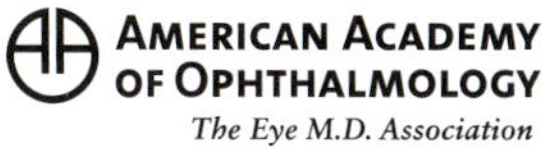

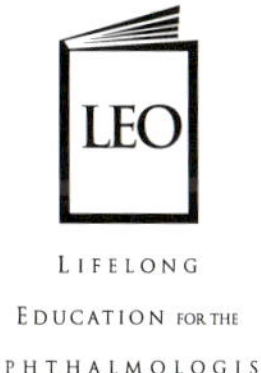

LIFELONG
EDUCATION FOR THE
OPHTHALMOLOGIST®

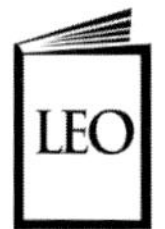

The Basic and Clinical Science Course is one component of the Lifelong Education for the Ophthalmologist (LEO) framework, which assists members in planning their continuing medical education. LEO includes an array of clinical education products that members may select to form individualized, self-directed learning plans for updating their clinical knowledge. Active members or fellows who use LEO components may accumulate sufficient CME credits to earn the LEO Award. Contact the Academy's Clinical Education Division for further information on LEO.

The American Academy of Ophthalmology is accredited by the Accreditation Council for Continuing Medical Education to provide continuing medical education for physicians.

The American Academy of Ophthalmology designates this educational activity for a maximum of 30 category 1 credits toward the AMA Physician's Recognition Award. Each physician should claim only those hours of credit that he/she actually spent in the activity.

The American Medical Association has determined that non-US licensed physicians who participate in this CME activity are eligible for AMA PRA category 1 credit.

The Academy provides this material for educational purposes only. It is not intended to represent the only or best method or procedure in every case, nor to replace a physician's own judgment or give specific advice for case management. Including all indications, contraindications, side effects, and alternative agents for each drug or treatment is beyond the scope of this material. All information and recommendations should be verified, prior to use, with current information included in the manufacturers' package inserts or other independent sources, and considered in light of the patient's condition and history. Reference to certain drugs, instruments, and other products in this publication is made for illustrative purposes only and is not intended to constitute an endorsement of such. Some material may include information on applications that are not considered community standard, that reflect indications not included in approved FDA labeling, or that are approved for use only in restricted research settings. The FDA has stated that it is the responsibility of the physician to determine the FDA status of each drug or device he or she wishes to use, and to use them with appropriate patient consent in compliance with applicable law. The Academy specifically disclaims any and all liability for injury or other damages of any kind, from negligence or otherwise, for any and all claims that may arise from the use of, any recommendations or other information contained herein.

Printed in the United States of America

Basic and Clinical Science Course

Thomas J. Liesegang, MD, Jacksonville, Florida, *Senior Secretary for Clinical Education*
Gregory L. Skuta, MD, Oklahoma City, Oklahoma, *Secretary for Ophthalmic Knowledge*
Louis B. Cantor, MD, Indianapolis, Indiana, *BCSC Course Chair*

Section 10

Faculty Responsible for This Edition

Steven T. Simmons, MD, *Chair*, Slingerlands, New York
George A. Cioffi, MD, Portland, Oregon
Ronald L. Gross, MD, Houston, Texas
Jonathan S. Myers, MD, Philadelphia, Pennsylvania
Peter A. Netland, MD, Memphis, Tennessee
John R. Samples, MD, Portland, Oregon
Martha M. Wright, MD, Minneapolis, Minnesota
Steven V. L. Brown, MD, Evanston, Illinois
Practicing Ophthalmologists Advisory Committee for Education

The authors state the following financial relationships:

Dr. Cioffi: consultant for Alcon, Allergan, Heidelberg Engineering, Humphrey-Zeiss, Merck, and Novartis

Dr. Gross: consultant and lecture honoraria recipient for Alcon, Allergan, and Pfizer

Dr. Myers: research grant recipient from Allergan, Merck, and Pfizer

Dr. Samples: Speakers Bureau honoraria recipient from Alcon and Merck; drug study researcher for Alcon and Allergan

Dr. Simmons: research grant recipient from Alcon, Allergan, and Pfizer; consultant for Allergan

The other authors state that they have no significant financial interest or other relationship with the manufacturer of any commercial product discussed in the chapters that they contributed to this publication or with the manufacturer of any competing commercial product.

Recent Past Faculty

A. Robert Bellows, MD
Michael S. Berlin, MD
Frank G. Berson, MD
Louis B. Cantor, MD
Robert D. Fechtner, MD
Elizabeth A. Hodapp, MD
Michael A. Kass, MD
David A. Lee, MD
Stephen B. Lichtenstein, MD
Andrew J. Michael, MD
Bradford J. Shingleton, MD
Robert L. Stamper, MD
Richard Stone, MD
M. Roy Wilson, MD

In addition, the Academy gratefully acknowledges the contributions of numerous past faculty and advisory committee members who have played an important role in the development of previous editions of the Basic and Clinical Science Course.

American Academy of Ophthalmology Staff

Richard A. Zorab, *Vice President, Ophthalmic Knowledge*
Hal Straus, *Director, Publications Department*
Carol L. Dondrea, *Publications Editor*
Christine Arturo, *Acquisitions Editor*
Maxine Garrett, *Administrative Coordinator*

Cover design: Paula Shuhert Design
Cover photograph: Choroidal folds, by Patrick J. Saine, MEd, CRA, Dartmouth-Hitchcock Medical Center

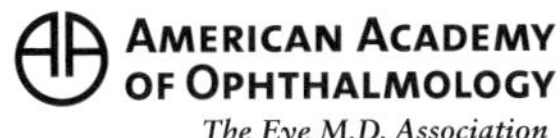

655 Beach Street
Box 7424
San Francisco, CA 94120-7424

Contents

General Introduction xi

Objectives 1

1 Introduction to Glaucoma: Terminology, Epidemiology, and Heredity 3

Definitions 3
Classification 4
  Open-Angle, Angle-Closure, Primary, and Secondary Glaucomas . . . 5
  Combined-Mechanism Glaucoma 5
Epidemiologic Aspects of Glaucoma 7
  Primary Open-Angle Glaucoma. 7
  Primary Angle-Closure Glaucoma 11
Hereditary and Genetic Factors 12
  Open-Angle Glaucoma Genes 14
  Angle-Closure Glaucoma Genes. 15
  Congenital Glaucoma Genes 15
  Other Identified Glaucoma Genes 15
  Environmental Factors 15
  Genetic Testing 15

2 Intraocular Pressure and Aqueous Humor Dynamics 17

Aqueous Humor Formation 17
  Suppression of Aqueous Formation 19
  Rate of Aqueous Formation 20
Aqueous Humor Outflow 20
  Trabecular Outflow (Pressure-dependent Outflow) 20
  Uveoscleral Outflow (Pressure-independent Outflow) 22
  Tonography. 22
Episcleral Venous Pressure 22
Intraocular Pressure 23
  Distribution in the Population and Relation to Glaucoma 23
  Factors Influencing Intraocular Pressure. 24
  Diurnal Variation. 25
  Clinical Measurement of Intraocular Pressure 25
  Infection Control in Clinical Tonometry. 29

3 Clinical Evaluation 31

History and General Examination 31
  History 31

Refraction 31
External Adnexae 32
Pupils 33
Biomicroscopy 33
Gonioscopy 36
Direct and Indirect Gonioscopy 37
Gonioscopic Assessment and Documentation 39
The Optic Nerve 44
Anatomy and Pathology 44
Glaucomatous Optic Neuropathy 49
Theories of Glaucomatous Optic Nerve Damage 50
Examination of the Optic Nerve Head 51
Clinical Evaluation of the Optic Nerve Head 51
The Visual Field 57
Clinical Perimetry 59
Patterns of Glaucomatous Nerve Loss 60
Variables in Perimetry 60
Automated Static Perimetry 65
Interpretation of a Single Field 68
Interpretation of a Series of Fields 72
Manual Perimetry 78
Other Tests 80

4 Open-Angle Glaucoma 83
Primary Open-Angle Glaucoma 83
Clinical Features 83
Associated Disorders 87
Prognosis 91
Open-Angle Glaucoma Without Elevated IOP (Normal-tension Glaucoma) 92
Clinical Features 92
Differential Diagnosis 93
Diagnostic Evaluation 94
Prognosis and Therapy 95
The Glaucoma Suspect 96
Secondary Open-Angle Glaucoma 99
Exfoliation Syndrome (Pseudoexfoliation) 99
Pigmentary Glaucoma 101
Lens-Induced Glaucoma 103
Intraocular Tumors 106
Ocular Inflammation and Secondary Open-Angle Glaucoma 106
Elevated Episcleral Venous Pressure 108
Accidental and Surgical Trauma 109
Drugs and Glaucoma 116

5 Angle-Closure Glaucoma 119
Introduction 119
Pathogenesis and Pathophysiology of Angle Closure 120

Pupillary Block 120
Angle Closure Without Pupillary Block 121
Lens-Induced Angle-Closure Glaucoma 122
Iris-Induced Angle Closure 122
Primary Angle Closure 122
Risk Factors for Developing Primary Angle Closure. 122
Acute Primary Angle Closure 124
Subacute or Intermittent Angle Closure 125
Chronic Angle Closure. 126
The Occludable, or Narrow, Anterior Chamber Angle 127
Plateau Iris 128
Secondary Angle Closure With Pupillary Block 128
Lens-Induced Angle Closure 128
Secondary Angle Closure Without Pupillary Block 132
Neovascular Glaucoma. 132
Iridocorneal Endothelial (ICE) Syndrome 136
Tumors 138
Inflammation 138
Aqueous Misdirection 140
Nonrhegmatogenous Retinal Detachment and Uveal Effusions . . . 141
Epithelial and Fibrous Downgrowth 141
Trauma 143
Retinal Surgery and Retinal Vascular Disease 143
Nanophthalmos 145
Retinopathy of Prematurity/Persistent Hyperplastic
Primary Vitreous. 145
Flat Anterior Chamber. 145
Drug-Induced Secondary Angle-Closure Glaucoma 145

6 Childhood Glaucoma **147**
Definitions and Classification 147
Epidemiology and Genetics 147
Pathophysiology 148
Clinical Features 148
Differential Diagnosis 150
Long-term Prognosis and Follow-up 150
Developmental Glaucomas With Associated
Ocular or Systemic Anomalies 152
Axenfeld-Rieger (A-R) Syndrome 152
Peters Anomaly 152
Aniridia 153
Other Anomalies and Syndromes 154

7 Medical Management of Glaucoma **157**
Medical Agents 159
Beta-Adrenergic Antagonists (Beta Blockers) 159
Parasympathomimetic Agents 166
Carbonic Anhydrase Inhibitors 168

Adrenergic Agonists . . . 169
Hypotensive Lipids (Prostaglandin Analogs, Prostamide, Decosanoid) . . . 171
Combined Medications. . . . 173
Hyperosmotic Agents . . . 173
General Approach to Medical Treatment . . . 174
Open-Angle Glaucoma . . . 174
Angle-Closure Glaucoma . . . 175
Use of Glaucoma Medications During Pregnancy or by Nursing Mothers . . . 176
Compliance. . . . 176
Future Therapy . . . 176

8 Surgical Therapy for Glaucoma . . . 179
Surgery for Open-Angle Glaucoma . . . 180
Laser Trabeculoplasty . . . 180
Incisional Surgery for Open-Angle Glaucomas . . . 183
Full-Thickness Sclerectomy . . . 194
Combined Cataract and Filtering Surgery . . . 195
Surgery for Angle-Closure Glaucoma . . . 197
Laser Iridectomy . . . 197
Laser Gonioplasty, or Peripheral Iridoplasty . . . 199
Incisional Surgery for Angle Closure . . . 200
Other Procedures to Lower IOP . . . 201
Glaucoma Tube Shunt . . . 201
Ciliary Body Ablation Procedures . . . 204
Cyclodialysis . . . 206
Nonpenetrating Glaucoma Surgery . . . 206
Congenital/Infantile Glaucoma . . . 207
Goniotomy and Trabeculotomy . . . 207

Basic Texts . . . 211
Related Academy Materials . . . 213
Credit Reporting Form . . . 217
Study Questions . . . 221
Answers . . . 229
Index . . . 233

General Introduction

The Basic and Clinical Science Course (BCSC) is designed to meet the needs of residents and practitioners for a comprehensive yet concise curriculum of the field of ophthalmology. The BCSC has developed from its original brief outline format, which relied heavily on outside readings, to a more convenient and educationally useful self-contained text. The Academy updates and revises the course annually, with the goals of integrating the basic science and clinical practice of ophthalmology and of keeping ophthalmologists current with new developments in the various subspecialties.

The BCSC incorporates the effort and expertise of more than 80 ophthalmologists, organized into 14 section faculties, working with Academy editorial staff. In addition, the course continues to benefit from many lasting contributions made by the faculties of previous editions. Members of the Academy's Practicing Ophthalmologists Advisory Committee for Education serve on each faculty and, as a group, review every volume before and after major revisions.

Organization of the Course

The Basic and Clinical Science Course comprises 14 volumes, incorporating fundamental ophthalmic knowledge, subspecialty areas, and special topics:

1. Update on General Medicine
2. Fundamentals and Principles of Ophthalmology
3. Optics, Refraction, and Contact Lenses
4. Ophthalmic Pathology and Intraocular Tumors
5. Neuro-Ophthalmology
6. Pediatric Ophthalmology and Strabismus
7. Orbit, Eyelids, and Lacrimal System
8. External Disease and Cornea
9. Intraocular Inflammation and Uveitis
10. Glaucoma
11. Lens and Cataract
12. Retina and Vitreous
13. International Ophthalmology
14. Refractive Surgery

In addition, a comprehensive Master Index allows the reader to easily locate subjects throughout the entire series.

References

Readers who wish to explore specific topics in greater detail may consult the journal references cited within each chapter and the Basic Texts listed at the back of the book.

These references are intended to be selective rather than exhaustive, chosen by the BCSC faculty as being important, current, and readily available to residents and practitioners.

Related Academy educational materials are also listed in the appropriate sections. They include books, audiovisual materials, self-assessment programs, clinical modules, and interactive programs.

Study Questions and CME Credit

Each volume of the BCSC is designed as an independent study activity for ophthalmology residents and practitioners. The learning objectives for this volume are given on page 1. The text, illustrations, and references provide the information necessary to achieve the objectives; the study questions allow readers to test their understanding of the material and their mastery of the objectives. Physicians who wish to claim CME credit for this educational activity may do so by mail, by fax, or online. The necessary forms and instructions are given at the end of the book.

Conclusion

The Basic and Clinical Science Course has expanded greatly over the years, with the addition of much new text and numerous illustrations. Recent editions have sought to place a greater emphasis on clinical applicability, while maintaining a solid foundation in basic science. As with any educational program, it reflects the experience of its authors. As its faculties change and as medicine progresses, new viewpoints are always emerging on controversial subjects and techniques. Not all alternate approaches can be included in this series; as with any educational endeavor, the learner should seek additional sources, including such carefully balanced opinions as the Academy's Preferred Practice Patterns.

The BCSC faculty and staff are continuously striving to improve the educational usefulness of the course; you, the reader, can contribute to this ongoing process. If you have any suggestions or questions about the series, please do not hesitate to contact the faculty or the editors.

The authors, editors, and reviewers hope that your study of the BCSC will be of lasting value and that each section will serve as a practical resource for quality patient care.

Objectives

Upon completion of BCSC Section 10, *Glaucoma,* the reader should be able to:

- Identify the epidemiologic features of glaucoma, including the social and economic impacts of the disease
- Summarize recent advances in the understanding of hereditary and genetic factors in glaucoma
- Outline the physiology of aqueous humor dynamics and the control of intraocular pressure (IOP)
- Review the clinical evaluation of the glaucoma patient, including history and general examination, gonioscopy, optic nerve examination, and visual field
- Describe the clinical features of the patient considered a "glaucoma suspect"
- Summarize the clinical features, evaluation, and therapy of primary open-angle glaucoma and normal-tension glaucoma
- List the various clinical features of and therapeutic approaches for the primary and secondary open-angle glaucomas
- Explain the underlying causes of the increased IOP in various forms of secondary open-angle glaucoma and the impact these underlying causes have on management
- Review the mechanisms and pathophysiology of primary angle-closure glaucoma
- Review the pathophysiology of secondary angle-closure glaucoma, both with and without pupillary block
- Outline the pathophysiology and therapy of infantile and juvenile-onset glaucoma
- Differentiate among the various classes of medical therapy for glaucoma, including efficacy, mechanism of action, and safety
- Compare the indications and techniques of various laser and incisional surgical procedures for glaucoma
- Describe cyclodestructive treatment for refractory glaucoma

CHAPTER 1

Introduction to Glaucoma: Terminology, Epidemiology, and Heredity

Definitions

The term *glaucoma* refers to a group of diseases that have in common a characteristic *optic neuropathy* with associated *visual field loss* for which elevated *intraocular pressure (IOP)* is one of the primary risk factors. The commonly accepted range for normal IOP in the general population is 10–22 mm Hg. Three factors determine the IOP (Fig 1-1):

- the rate of aqueous humor production by the ciliary body
- resistance to aqueous outflow across the trabecular meshwork–Schlemm's canal system; the specific site of resistance is generally thought to be in the juxtacanalicular meshwork
- the level of episcleral venous pressure

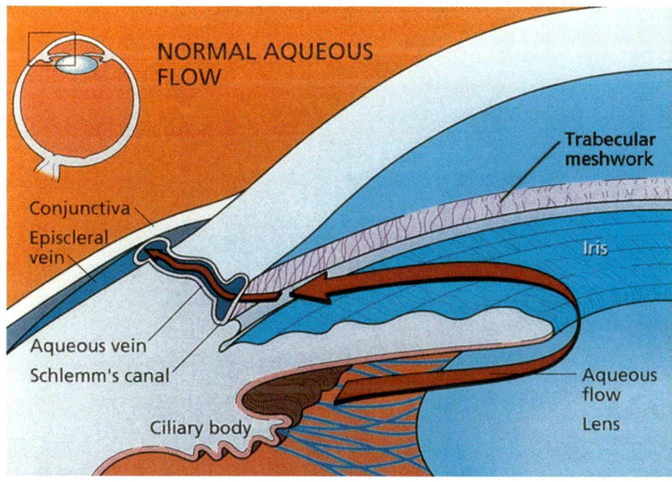

Figure 1-1 Diagrammatic cross section of the anterior segment of the normal eye, showing the site of aqueous production (ciliary body) and sites of resistance to aqueous outflow (trabecular meshwork–Schlemm's canal system and episcleral venous plexus).

Generally, increased IOP is caused by increased resistance to aqueous humor outflow.

In most individuals, the optic nerve and visual field changes seen in glaucoma are determined by both the level of the IOP and the resistance of the optic nerve axons to pressure damage. Other biological factors also predispose the optic nerve axons to damage. Although progressive changes in the visual field and optic nerve are usually related to increased IOP and cupping, in cases of normal-tension glaucoma, the IOP remains within the normal range (see Chapter 4). In most cases of glaucoma, it is presumed that the IOP is too high for proper functioning of the optic nerve axons and that lowering the IOP will stabilize the damage. In cases involving other pathophysiologic mechanisms that may affect the optic nerve, however, progression of optic nerve damage may continue despite lowering of IOP.

Classification

The terms *primary* and *secondary* have been helpful in current definitions of glaucoma, and they are still in widespread use. However, new concepts are emerging that may change this common usage. There are separate anatomic, gonioscopic, biochemical, molecular, and genetic views of the classification of the glaucomas, among others, each with its own individual merit (Table 1-1). For instance, glaucoma can be defined on the basis of genetic terms related to a very specific mutation. Within the next 20 years, knowing the mutation an individual with glaucoma harbors may be the most definitive method by which to understand the disease; however, it is unlikely that all glaucomas will be understood in

Table 1-1 Conceptual Means of Classifying Glaucoma

Anatomic
- Gonioscopic angle appearance
- Gonioscopic pigmentation

Biochemical
- Extracellular matrix abnormalities
- Cellular abnormality
- Inflammatory status or post–inflammatory status
- Presence of cytotoxic phenomena (such as soluble CD44)

Genetic
- Simple: family history
- Complex: known mutations

Classic
- Primary versus secondary

Risk factor–based
- Number of risk factors for primary open-angle glaucoma (POAG) or primary angle-closure glaucoma (PACG)

Intraocular pressure–based
- High or low
- Degree of diurnal fluctuation
- Absolute peak pressure

Optic nerve–based
- Cupping regarded irrespective of pressure
- Cupping in the context of pressure

genetic terms. By definition, the *primary glaucomas* are not associated with known ocular or systemic disorders that cause increased resistance to aqueous outflow or angle closure. The primary glaucomas usually affect both eyes. Conversely, the *secondary glaucomas* are associated with ocular or systemic disorders responsible for decreased aqueous outflow. The diseases that cause secondary glaucoma are often unilateral.

Open-Angle, Angle-Closure, Primary, and Secondary Glaucomas

Traditionally, glaucoma has been classified as open angle or closed angle and as primary or secondary (Table 1-2). Differentiation of open-angle glaucoma from closed-angle glaucoma is essential from a therapeutic standpoint (Figs 1-2, 1-3; see Chapters 4 and 5). The concept of primary and secondary glaucomas is also useful, but it reflects our lack of understanding of the pathophysiologic mechanisms underlying the glaucomatous process. Open-angle glaucoma is classified as primary when no anatomically identifiable underlying cause of the events that led to outflow obstruction and elevation of IOP can be found. The etiology is generally regarded as an abnormality in the trabecular meshwork extracellular matrix in the juxtacanalicular region, although other views exist. Trabecular cells and their surrounding extracellular matrix are now understood in fairly specific terms, and the basic scientific understanding of the outflow structures is constantly increasing. Glaucoma has been classified as secondary when an abnormality is identified and a putative role in the pathogenesis can be ascribed to this abnormality. With the development of a specific understanding of the genetic and biochemical abnormalities in the outflow pathway, the classic division of glaucoma as either primary or secondary breaks down, and it is now recognized that all glaucomas are secondary to some abnormality, whether currently identified or not. As knowledge of the mechanisms underlying the causes of glaucoma continues to expand, the primary/secondary classification has become increasingly artificial. This scheme is particularly inadequate for classifying the angle-closure glaucomas.

Other schemes for classifying glaucoma have been proposed. Classification of the glaucomas based on initial events and on mechanisms of outflow obstruction are 2 schemes that have gained increasing popularity (Table 1-3).

Ritch R, Shields MB, Krupin T, eds. *The Glaucomas.* 2nd ed. St Louis: Mosby; 1996:722.

Combined-Mechanism Glaucoma

Combined-mechanism glaucoma can appear in a patient with open-angle glaucoma who develops secondary angle closure from other causes. Examples include a patient with open-angle glaucoma who develops angle closure as a result of miotic therapy, when the miotic causes a forward shift of the lens-iris diaphragm, or a patient with pseudophakic open-angle glaucoma who develops peripheral anterior synechiae (PAS) after an episode of pupillary block.

IOP elevation in these cases can occur as a result of either or both of the following:

- the intrinsic resistance of the trabecular meshwork to aqueous outflow in open-angle glaucoma
- the direct anatomic obstruction of the filtering meshwork by synechiae in angle-closure glaucoma

Table 1-2 Classification of Glaucoma

Type	Characteristics
Open-angle glaucoma (Fig 1-2)	
Primary open-angle glaucoma (POAG)	Not associated with known ocular or systemic disorders that cause increased resistance to aqueous outflow or damage to optic nerve; usually associated with elevated IOP
Normal-tension glaucoma	Considered in continuum of POAG; terminology often used when IOP is not elevated
Juvenile open-angle glaucoma	Terminology often used when open-angle glaucoma diagnosed at young age (typically 10–30 years of age)
Glaucoma suspect	Normal optic disc and visual field associated with elevated IOP Suspicious optic disc and/or visual field with normal IOP
Secondary open-angle glaucoma	Increased resistance to trabecular meshwork outflow associated with other conditions (eg, pigmentary glaucoma, phacolytic glaucoma, steroid-induced glaucoma) Increased posttrabecular resistance to outflow secondary to elevated episcleral venous pressure (eg, carotid cavernous sinus fistula)
Angle-closure glaucoma (Fig 1-3)	
Primary angle-closure glaucoma with relative pupillary block	Movement of aqueous humor from posterior chamber to anterior chamber restricted; peripheral iris in contact with trabecular meshwork
Acute angle closure	Occurs when IOP rises rapidly as a result of relatively sudden blockage of the trabecular meshwork
Subacute angle closure (intermittent angle closure)	Repeated, brief episodes of angle closure with mild symptoms and elevated IOP, often a prelude to acute angle closure
Chronic angle closure	IOP elevation caused by variable portions of anterior chamber angle being permanently closed by peripheral anterior synechiae
Secondary angle-closure glaucoma with pupillary block	(For example, swollen lens, secluded pupil)
Secondary angle-closure glaucoma without pupillary block	Posterior pushing mechanism: lens–iris diaphragm pushed forward (eg, posterior segment tumor, scleral buckling procedure, uveal effusion) Anterior pulling mechanism: anterior segment process pulling iris forward to form peripheral anterior synechiae (eg, iridocorneal endothelial syndrome, neovascular glaucoma, inflammation)
Plateau iris syndrome	Primary angle closure with or without component of pupillary block, but pupillary block is not predominant mechanism of angle closure
Childhood glaucoma	
Primary congenital/infantile glaucoma	Primary glaucoma present from birth to first few years of life
Glaucoma associated with congenital anomalies	Associated with ocular disorders (eg, anterior segment dysgenesis, aniridia) Associated with systemic disorders (eg, rubella, Lowe syndrome)
Secondary glaucoma in infants and children	(For example, glaucoma secondary to retinoblastoma or trauma)

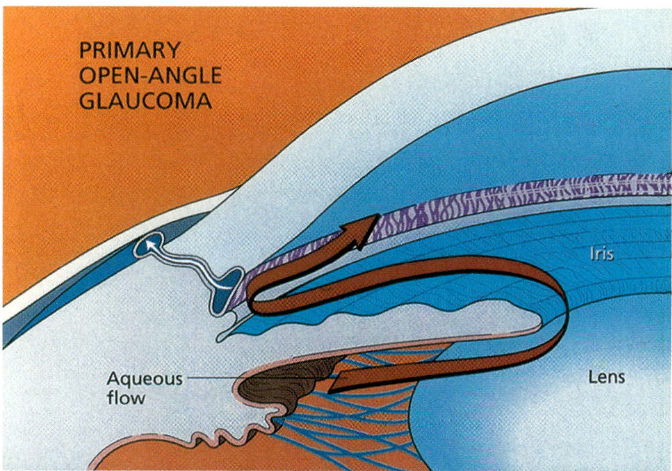

Figure 1-2 Schematic of open-angle glaucoma with resistance to aqueous outflow through the trabecular meshwork–Schlemm's canal system in the absence of gross anatomic obstruction. Small white arrow shows normal path of outflow and indicates that resistance in this illustration is relative, not total.

Treatment is modified based on the proportion of open angle to closed angle and the etiology of the angle-closure component, as well as the status and vulnerability of the optic nerve.

Epidemiologic Aspects of Glaucoma

Primary Open-Angle Glaucoma

Magnitude of the problem

Primary open-angle glaucoma (POAG) represents a significant public health problem. At least 2.25 million individuals in the United States 45 years of age or older are estimated to have this disease. Estimates based on the available data indicate that between 84,000 and 116,000 of them have become bilaterally blind (best-corrected visual acuity ≤20/200 or visual field <20°). POAG is thus an important cause of blindness in the United States and the most frequent cause of nonreversible blindness in blacks.

The World Health Organization (WHO) has undertaken an extensive analysis of the literature to estimate the prevalence, incidence, and severity of the different types of glaucoma on a worldwide basis. Using data collected predominantly in the late 1980s and early 1990s, WHO estimated the global population of people with high IOP (>21 mm Hg) at 104.5 million. The incidence of POAG was estimated at 2.4 million people per year. Blindness prevalence for all types of glaucoma was estimated at more than 8 million people, with 4 million cases caused by POAG. The different types of glaucoma were theoretically calculated to be responsible for 15% of blindness, placing glaucoma as the third leading cause of blindness worldwide, following cataract.

Despite these staggering statistics, the impact of glaucoma from a public health perspective has not been fully appreciated. Relatively little information is currently available

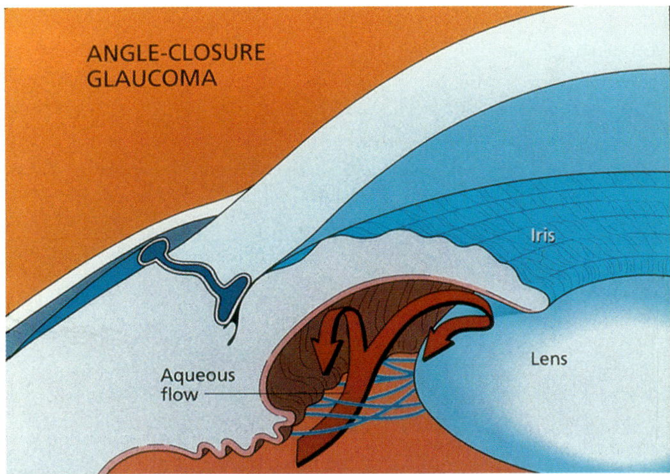

Figure 1-3 Schematic of angle-closure glaucoma with pupillary block leading to peripheral iris obstruction of the trabecular meshwork.

regarding the individual burden associated with the psychological effects of having a potentially blinding chronic disease, the debilitating side effects of treatment, and the qualitative functional loss associated with diminished visual fields. Nor does reliable information exist on the societal costs associated with the detection, treatment, and rehabilitation of this disease.

Prevalence

The prevalence of POAG shows a strong racial disparity. Among whites 40 years of age and older, a prevalence of between 1.1% and 2.1% has been consistently obtained by population-based studies performed throughout the world. The prevalence among blacks is 3 to 4 times higher. The prevalence of POAG increases with age, and estimates for people in their 70s have generally been 3 to 8 times higher than for people in their 40s.

Risk factors

Identifying risk factors is important because this information may lead to development of strategies for disease screening and prevention and may be useful in identifying persons for whom close medical supervision is indicated. Strictly defined, a factor can be considered a risk factor only if it predates disease occurrence. From a clinical perspective, it is often difficult to differentiate very early disease from normal. In fact, this determination often depends on how the disease is defined.

Glaucoma is usually defined by the presence of characteristic visual field defects and sometimes, in the absence of visual field defects, by the appearance of optic nerve damage. How often this diagnosis is made in marginal cases is influenced by the sensitivity of available diagnostic tests. Thus, it may be difficult to determine whether abnormalities in certain parameters—for example, optic nerve parameters such as nerve fiber layer loss—are indicative of increased susceptibility to developing glaucoma or are signs of early disease. From a practical standpoint, the distinction is unimportant. Individuals

Table 1-3 Classification of the Glaucomas Based on Mechanisms of Outflow Obstruction*

Open-Angle Glaucoma Mechanisms			Angle-Closure Glaucoma Mechanisms		
Pretrabecular (Membrane Overgrowth)	**Trabecular**	**Posttrabecular**	**Anterior ("Pulling")**	**Posterior ("Pushing")**	**Developmental Anomalies of Anterior Chamber Angle**
Fibrovascular membrane (neovascular glaucoma) Endothelial layer, often with Descemet-like membrane Iridocorneal endothelial syndrome Posterior polymorphous dystrophy Penetrating and non-penentrating trauma Epithelial downgrowth Fibrous ingrowth Inflammatory membrane Fuchs heterochromic iridocyclitis Luetic interstitial keratitis	Idiopathic Chronic open-angle glaucoma Juvenile open-angle glaucoma "Clogging" of trabecular meshwork Red blood cells Hemorrhagic glaucoma Ghost cell glaucoma Sickled red blood cells Macrophages Hemolytic glaucoma Phacolytic glaucoma Melanomalytic glaucoma Neoplastic cells Primary ocular tumors Neoplastic tumors Juvenile xanthogranuloma Pigment particles Pigmentary glaucoma Exfoliation syndrome (glaucoma capsulare) Malignant melanoma Protein Uveitis Lens-induced glaucoma Viscoelastic agents α-chymotrypsin–induced glaucoma Alterations of the trabecular meshwork Steroid-induced glaucoma Edema Uveitis (trabeculitis) Scleritis and episcleritis Alkali burns Trauma (angle recession) Intraocular foreign bodies (hemosiderosis, chalcosis)	Obstruction of Schlemm's canal, eg, collapse at canal Elevated episclera venous pressure Carotid cavernous fistula Cavernous sinus thrombosis Retrobulbar tumors Thyroid ophthal-mopathy Superior vena cava obstruction Mediastinal tumors Sturge-Weber syndrome Familial episcleral venous pressure elevation	Contracture of membranes Neovascular glaucoma Iridocorneal endothelial syndrome Posterior polymorphous dystrophy Penetrating and non-penetrating trauma Consolidation of inflammatory products	With pupillary block Pupillary-block glaucoma Lens-induced mechanisms Phacomorphic lens Ectopia lentis Posterior synechiae Iris–vitreous block Pseudophakia Uveitis Without pupillary block Ciliary block (malignant) glaucoma Lens-induced mechanisms Phacomorphic lens Ectopia lentis Following lens extraction (forward vitreous shift) Anterior rotation of ciliary body Following scleral buckling Following panretinal photocoagulation Central retinal vein occlusion Intraocular tumors Malignant melanoma Retinoblastoma Cysts of the iris and ciliary body Retrolenticular tissue contracture Retinopathy of prematurity (retrolental fibroplasia) Persistent hyperplastic primary vitreous	Incomplete development of trabecular meshwork–Schlemm's canal Congenital (infantile) glaucoma Axenfeld-Rieger syndrome Peters anomaly Glaucomas associated with other developmental anomalies Iridocorneal adhesions Broad strands (Axenfeld-Rieger syndrome) Fine strands that contract to close angle (aniridia)
			Plateau Iris Syndrome		

* Clinical examples cited in this table do not represent an inclusive list of the glaucomas.

(Modified with permission from Ritch R, Shields MB, Krupin T, eds. *The Glaucomas.* 2nd ed. St Louis; Mosby; 1996:722.)

manifesting such abnormalities must be closely monitored for signs of clinically significant disease development or progression.

Several risk factors—and not all risk factors are known—increase the likelihood of the development of POAG. Besides increased IOP, factors known to be associated with an increased risk for the development of glaucoma include advanced age, decreased corneal thickness, racial background, and a positive family history. The importance of decreased corneal thickness has only recently been appreciated and may be more than just an artifact that causes underreading of true IOP. Thinner corneas may be correlated with underlying factors. African Americans have thinner corneas on average, but initial interpretation of data suggests that this is a separate risk factor from race.

In terms of assessing risk factors, the importance of the diurnal variation in IOP has been increasingly recognized. Commonly, IOP is elevated upon awakening and decreases throughout the day, but many factors influence it. In addition, other patterns are known—in one group of individuals, IOP peaks in the late afternoon. It has been suggested by a number of authors that fluctuation in the pressure per se is a risk factor for optic nerve damage. Clinicians record the time of day that IOP is checked because variations occur throughout the day and are impacted by medications. The relative degree to which peak pressures constitute a risk factor versus overall elevation of pressure is not known for glaucoma and seems likely to vary based on the status and structure of the optic nerve.

The quality of available data regarding potential risk factors for the development of POAG varies greatly. Evidence that IOP, age, race, and positive family history are risk factors for POAG is considerable and reliable. Data also support diabetes and myopia as risk factors, but these data are generally less convincing. The relevance of sex and of various systemic factors, such as systemic hypertension and arteriosclerotic and ischemic vascular disease, to glaucoma risk has been widely debated, and currently available data are inconclusive.

Demographic risk factors for POAG include age. It is clear that as an individual gets older, the risk of POAG increases. In the Baltimore Eye Survey, the prevalence of glaucoma among whites was 3.5 times higher for individuals in their 70s than for those in their 40s. Among blacks, the ratio was 7.4. The demographic view on gender is mixed. In the Framingham and Barbados eye studies, males had a higher rate of POAG, whereas the Sweden, St. Lucia, and Blue Mountains studies reported higher numbers in females. In the Wales, Baltimore, Beaver Dam, and Melbourne studies, no statistical associations were found. As a result of these mixed findings, gender is not usually regarded as a risk factor for glaucoma.

Racial studies have generally shown that blacks are at increased risk of developing POAG. In the Baltimore Eye Survey, blacks were more than 3 times more likely than whites to have glaucoma. The risk among Hispanics living in Arizona appears to be intermediate between the reported values for whites and blacks. The cause of the higher prevalence of glaucoma among blacks is not known. Blacks do have larger discs and more nerve fibers. It has been hypothesized that the increased disc size is associated with increased mechanical stress in the region of the optic nerve

Adult-onset diabetes has been demonstrated to be associated with POAG, although debate persists. People with diabetes undergo frequent detailed eye examinations to rule out diabetic retinopathy, and this may mean that there is a greater opportunity to diagnose POAG.

Primary Angle-Closure Glaucoma

Compared with POAG, the epidemiology of primary angle-closure glaucoma (PACG) has received much less attention. Most of the available information is derived from hospital-based surveys or from population screenings of small high-risk subpopulations.

Race

The prevalence of PACG varies among different racial and ethnic groups. Among white populations in the United States and Europe, it is estimated at approximately 0.1%. Inuit populations from Arctic regions have the highest known prevalence of PACG—20–40 times higher than that for whites. The relative prevalences of PACG and POAG among Inuits are also the reverse of what is noted in white populations, with POAG being uncommon.

Estimates of the prevalence of PACG in Asian populations have varied considerably. Some of this variability may be the result of differences in the definition used and in the design of the studies from which the estimates were derived. Another factor, however, is that Asian populations are not one homogeneous group, and substantial differences in PACG prevalence are likely between Asian groups. Available data suggest that most Asian population groups have a prevalence rate of PACG between that of whites and Inuits.

Acute angle-closure glaucoma is relatively uncommon among blacks. However, chronic angle-closure glaucoma is much more common than initially believed. Some studies have suggested that the prevalence of PACG among blacks is similar to that among whites, with most cases among blacks being of the chronic variety. Several population surveys demonstrate that women are at increased risk for angle-closure glaucoma. Although most attention in the field of glaucoma genetics has gone to POAG and congenital glaucoma, a positive family history is also a risk factor for PACG. For example, among Eskimos, the prevalence of PACG in first-degree relatives of patients with this disorder may be 3.5 times higher than in the general population. A population-based survey in China suggested that a family history of glaucoma increased by sixfold the risk of PACG.

Gender

Women of all races develop acute angle-closure glaucoma 3 to 4 times more often than do men. Studies of normal eyes have shown that women have shallower anterior chambers than men.

Age

The anterior chamber decreases in depth and volume with age. These changes predispose to pupillary block, and the prevalence of pupillary-block–induced angle-closure glaucoma thus increases with age. Acute angle-closure glaucoma is most common between the ages of 55 and 65 years, but it can occur in young adults and has been reported in children.

Refraction

The anterior chamber depth and volume are smaller in hyperopic eyes. Although PACG may occur in eyes with any type of refractive error, it is thus typically associated with hyperopia.

Inheritance

Some of the anatomic features of the eye that predispose to pupillary block, such as more forward position of the lens and greater than average lens thickness, are inherited. Thus, relatives of subjects with angle-closure glaucoma are at greater risk of developing angle closure than the general population. However, estimates of the exact risk vary greatly.

Epstein DL, Allingham RR, Schuman JS, eds. *Chandler and Grant's Glaucoma.* 4th ed. Baltimore: Williams & Wilkins; 1997:641–646.

Ritch RM, Shields MB, Krupin T, eds. *The Glaucomas.* 2nd ed. St Louis: Mosby; 1996: 753–765.

Hereditary and Genetic Factors

The recent explosion of knowledge regarding the genetic basis for many diseases has had a profound impact, including in the field of glaucoma. In glaucoma mapping techniques, the localization of several genes and the understanding of the mutations within the genes have significantly changed our knowledge of the disease. In the near future, early diagnosis of specific forms of glaucoma may have a genetic basis. Eventually, this information will lead to the development of new drugs or specific types of gene therapy, with replacement of deoxyribonucleic acid (DNA), modification of messenger ribonucleic acid (mRNA), or replacement of the defective proteins providing long-term lowering of IOP or improving optic neuropathy.

Kass and Becker were among the first to observe a strong correlation between family history and glaucoma, particularly in terms of elevated pressure, cup–disc ratio, and the glucocorticoid response. Based on their observations, the researchers suggested that the most effective method of glaucoma detection would be to check family members. However, in the early study of glaucoma, the disease seemed to defy the simple classification as either autosomal dominant or autosomal recessive. Becker, and later Armaly, found that glucocorticoid treatment elevated IOP more often in glaucoma patients than in individuals without glaucoma. Testing of family members showed that this response was usually inherited as an autosomal recessive trait. Subsequently, Polansky hypothesized that mutations of the trabecular meshwork glucocorticoid genes could cause elevated IOP. He identified a specific protein, the TIGR protein (also termed myocilin) produced by trabecular meshwork cells. Initially, the TIGR protein was identified in juvenile glaucoma families; later it was reported to affect up to 3% of the general open-angle glaucoma population. In the mid-1990s, *GLC1A*, the gene responsible for mutations in the TIGR protein, was mapped to chromosome 1. Since then, 5 additional open-angle glaucoma genes have been mapped. Although major gene defects cause glaucoma in specific individuals, the proportion of all glaucoma patients affected by 1 or several major genes is unknown. This is likely due to the complex nature of glaucoma and to complex interactions between genetic and environmental factors. The relative contributions of environmental factors versus genetic factors remain unknown for glaucoma. In 2003, known genes accounted for only a small percentage of glaucoma (Table 1-4).

The prevalence of glaucoma, enlarged cup–disc ratio, and elevated IOP are all much higher in siblings and offspring of patients with glaucoma than in the general population. A positive family history is a major risk factor for the development of POAG. The prevalence of glaucoma among siblings of patients is approximately 10%, and the lifetime absolute risk of glaucoma at age 89 years is 10 times higher for relatives of glaucoma patients than for relatives of unaffected persons.

The precise mechanism of inheritance is not always clear. Complicated genetic interactions may involve the presence of both causal and susceptibility genes. To date, many of the glaucomas appear to have an autosomal dominant inheritance that may involve more that 1 gene (polygenic), have a late or variable age of onset, demonstrate incomplete penetrance (the disease may not develop even when the causative gene has been inherited), and may be substantially influenced by environmental factors. See also BCSC Section 2, *Fundamentals and Principles of Ophthalmology,* Part III, Genetics.

Kass MA, Becker B. Genetics of primary open-angle glaucoma. *Sight Sav Rev.* 1978;48:21–28.

Wolfs RC, Klaver CC, Ramrattan RS, et al. Genetic risk of primary open-angle glaucoma: population-based familial aggregation study. *Arch Ophthalmol.* 1998;116:1640–1645.

The discipline of genetic therapy is evolving very rapidly. Several potential approaches to transferring genetic material to trabecular meshwork cells exist, each with its own advantages and disadvantages. These genetic therapeutic methods include replacing the actual DNA of the gene, modifying mRNA, or replacing a protein. Of these, replacing DNA is most likely to have a permanent effect. The prospect exists of improving aqueous humor outflow through the trabecular meshwork, where the primary defect appears to reside in the majority of patients with POAG. Both the trabecular meshwork and the ciliary epithelium are relatively accessible to treatment and have been successfully infected

Table 1-4 Currently Mapped Glaucoma Genes

Locus	Location (Reference)	Phenotype	Inheritance	Age at Onset	Gene
GLC1A	1q23-q25 (7)	JOAG	Dominant	5–45	*TIGR/MYOC*
GLC1B	2cen-q13 (16)	POAG	Dominant	>40	—
GLC1C	3q21-24 (12)	POAG	Dominant	56 (38–80)	—
GLC1D	8q23 (15)	POAG	Dominant	>30	—
GLC1E	10P15-14 (14, 24)	POAG	Dominant	44 (23–65)	*OPTN*
GLC1F	7q35 (13)	POAG	Dominant	53 (22–70)	—
GLC3A	2p21 (30, 32)	Congenital	Recessive	<3	*CYP1B1*
GLC3B	1p36 (29)	Congenital	Recessive	<3	—
NNOS	11 (27)	Angle-closure	Dominant	28.3 (7–77)	—
RIEG1	4q25 (33)	Rieger syndrome	Dominant	<3	*PITX2*
RIEG2	13q14 (57)	Rieger syndrome	Dominant	<3	—
IRID1	6p25 (33)	Iridogoniodysgenesis	Dominant	<3	*FKHL7*
	7q35 (24)	Pigment dispersion	Dominant	20s	—
NPS	9q34 (34)	Nail-patella syndrome	Dominant	32 (18–41)	*LMX1B*

POAG = primary open-angle glaucoma; JOAG = juvenile open-angle glaucoma.

by adenovirus vectors as a means of adding a corrective DNA. Conceptually, it is important to realize that identifying causal genes in specific forms of glaucoma may ultimately allow researchers to design recombinant proteins to correct the defects using an array of possible strategies. Although viral vector therapies with retrovirus, adenovirus, or herpesvirus are logical considerations, other, nonvector approaches include the use of liposomes, oligonucleotide antisense, recombinant proteins, and human artificial chromosomes.

Open-Angle Glaucoma Genes

GLC1A, the first open-angle glaucoma gene, was initially mapped in a large juvenile glaucoma family and localized to chromosome 1. The mutations in this gene, which are suspected to be responsible for open-angle glaucoma, produce a protein, myocilin, that is also induced in trabecular meshwork cells by treatment with dexamethasone (TIGR). Because of this protein, the *TIGR/myocilin* gene has been given the gene symbol *TIGR/MYOC*. The mutations in *TIGR/MYOC* are not limited to juvenile glaucoma and have been reported in 3% of individuals with adult-onset POAG. Although corticosteroids may increase IOP in a high percentage of glaucoma patients, it is hypothesized that a *TIGR/MYOC*-related protein could be responsible. However, the *TIGR/MYOC* protein is also expressed in the retina, especially in retinoblastomas, skeletal muscle, and fetal heart.

Other researchers have identified 2 loci for the normal-tension forms of open-angle glaucoma: *GLC1B* maps to chromosome 2 and *GLC1E* maps to chromesome 10. Because the majority of individuals with the *GLC1B* and *GLC1E* genes appear to develop a type of glaucoma with lower pressure, these mutations may render the optic nerve abnormally sensitive to IOP or otherwise facilitate optic nerve damage independent of IOP. Recently, mutations in *OPTN*, the gene that encodes the optineurin protein, has been identified in patients with the *GLC1E* gene. The characterization of the protein(s) governed by these genes may potentially lead to greater insight.

In contrast to *GLC1A* and *GLC1B*, *GLC1C*, located on chromosome 3, appears to produce a glaucoma characterized by high pressure, late onset, and moderate response to glaucoma medications. Although relatively rare, its phenotypic similarity to POAG suggests that this gene may provide valuable insight into the mechanism of many other types of adult-onset open-angle glaucoma. The glaucoma associated with *GLC1D* also resembles high-pressure POAG and may provide further insights into POAG. *GLC1D* has been mapped to band 23 on the long arm of chromosome 8.

GLC1F and *GLC1G*, additional loci for POAG, have been mapped. In another family, pigment dispersion syndrome has been mapped to a chromosome distal to *GLC1F*.

Each of these gene locations represents only a small fraction of the total open-angle glaucoma population. Their identification indicates the diversity of glaucoma genetics. Given this diversity and the many families that do not map to any of these regions, it is likely that many other regions exist.

Angle-Closure Glaucoma Genes

One angle-closure gene has been mapped. Autosomal dominant nanophthalmos (*NNO1*) is associated with angle-closure glaucoma due to the distortion of the anterior segment and maps to chromosome 11.

Congenital Glaucoma Genes

Three congenital glaucoma genes have been mapped. The majority of congenital glaucoma families map to *GLC3A* on chromosome 2p21. In addition, several *GLC3A* genes appear to be associated with a mutation of cytochrome P4501B1. As a second locus for congenital glaucoma, *GLC3B,* which probably affects fewer cases, has been mapped to chromosome 1p36. The third congenital glaucoma locus has been identified on chromosome 14.

Other Identified Glaucoma Genes

Other genetic discoveries are directly relevant to glaucoma. For instance, *RIEG,* a homeobox gene, is associated with Rieger anomaly and forkhead transcription factor (congenital glaucoma, Rieger anomaly, Axenfeld anomaly, and iris hypoplasia).

Environmental Factors

Evidence that environmental factors can also affect glaucoma arises from studies of twins, analysis of the season of birth of patients with glaucoma, and light exposure in animal models. Theoretically, if glaucoma is genetically determined, identical twins should share this trait more often than fraternal twins. In the Finnish Twin Cohort Study, 3 of 29 monozygotic twin pairs were concordant for POAG compared with 1 of 79 dizygotic twin pairs. Although a higher percentage of monozygotic twins were concordant for glaucoma, most were not. These data suggest that although genetic factors contribute to the etiology of glaucoma, other factors such as environmental influences are important.

Genetic Testing

A genetic test is presently available for human testing. It tests 3 of more than 40 mutations for *GLC1A,* in addition to testing for a mutation of special interest, the MT1 promoter. Whether this mutation is associated with severity or prognosis for glaucoma is controversial and awaits further data.

CHAPTER 2

Intraocular Pressure and Aqueous Humor Dynamics

The clinical approach to glaucoma begins with an understanding of *aqueous humor*, which flows from the posterior chamber through the pupil into the anterior chamber and exits the eye by passing through the *trabecular meshwork* into *Schlemm's canal* and then draining into the venous system through a plexus of collector channels, as shown in Figure 1-1. The formation and outflow of aqueous humor are discussed in detail in this chapter. The *Goldmann equation* summarizes the relationship between these factors and the IOP in the undisturbed eye:

$$P_0 = (F/C) + P_v$$

where P_0 is the IOP in millimeters of mercury (mm Hg), F is the rate of aqueous formation in microliters per minute (µL/min), C is the facility of outflow in microliters per minute per millimeter of mercury (µL/min/mm Hg), and P_v is the episcleral venous pressure in millimeters of mercury. Resistance to outflow (R) is the inverse of facility (C) and may replace C in rearrangements of the Goldmann equation.

Impaired outflow (reduced C value) in open portions of the angle, and various amounts of angle closure, may result in elevated IOP, as shown in Table 2-1.

Aqueous Humor Formation

Aqueous humor formation is a biological process that is subject to circadian rhythms. Aqueous humor is formed by the *ciliary processes*, each of which is composed of a double layer of epithelium over a core of stroma and a rich supply of fenestrated capillaries (Fig 2-1). Each of the 80 or so processes contains a large number of capillaries, which are supplied mainly by branches of the major arterial circle of the iris. The apical surfaces of both the outer pigmented and the inner nonpigmented layers of epithelium face each other and are joined by tight junctions, which are probably an important part of the blood–aqueous barrier. The inner nonpigmented epithelial cells, which protrude into the posterior chamber, contain numerous mitochondria and microvilli; these cells are thought to be the actual site of aqueous production. The ciliary processes provide a large surface area for secretion.

Table 2-1 Examples of Difference in the Degree to Which the Intraocular Pressure *(P)* is Calculated to Be Affected by Changes in Flow *(F)* and Facility of Outflow *(C)* in Different Types of Eyes, Assuming Constant Episcleral Venous Pressure (P_e [or P_v])

	(mm Hg) P_e	+	(μL/min) *(F*	÷	(μL/min/mm Hg) *C)*	=	(mm Hg) *P*
Normal =	9		1.5		0.25		15
	9		1 to 2		0.25		13 to 17
	9		1.5		0.30		14
Glaucoma =	9		1.5		0.05		39
	9		1 to 2		0.05		29 to 49
	9		1.5		0.10		24
Good normal =	9		1.5		0.30		14
½ angle closed =	9		1.5		0.15		19
¾ angle closed =	9		1.5		0.075		29
Poor normal =	9		1.5		0.15		19
½ angle closed =	9		1.5		0.075		29
¾ angle closed =	9		1.5		0.0375		49

(Used with permission from Epstein DL, Allingham RR, Schuman JS. *Chandler and Grant's Glaucoma.* 4th ed. Baltimore: Williams & Wilkins; 1997;21.)

The aqueous humor is produced by 3 processes:

- active secretion, which takes place in the double-layered ciliary epithelium
- ultrafiltration
- simple diffusion

Active secretion, or transport, consumes energy to move substances against an electrochemical gradient and is independent of pressure. The identity of the precise ion or ions transported is not known, but sodium, chloride, and bicarbonate are involved. Active secretion accounts for the majority of aqueous production and involves, at least in part, activity of the enzyme carbonic anhydrase II. *Ultrafiltration* refers to a pressure-dependent movement along a pressure gradient. In the ciliary processes, the hydrostatic pressure difference between capillary pressure and IOP favors fluid movement into the eye, whereas the oncotic gradient between the two resists fluid movement. The relationship between secretion and ultrafiltration is not known. *Diffusion* is the passive movement of ions across a membrane related to charge and concentration.

The aqueous humor in humans has an excess of hydrogen and chloride ions, an excess of ascorbate, and a deficit of bicarbonate. Aqueous humor is essentially protein free (1/200–1/500 of the protein found in plasma), which allows for optical clarity. Albumin accounts for about half of the total protein. Other components include growth factors; several enzymes, such as carbonic anhydrase, lysozyme, diamine oxidase, plasminogen activator, dopamine β-hydroxylase, and phospholipase A_2; and prostaglandins, cyclic adenosine monophosphate (cAMP), catecholamines, steroid hormones, and hyaluronic acid. Aqueous humor is produced at an average rate of 2.0 μL/min, and its composition is altered as it flows from the posterior chamber through the pupil and into the anterior chamber. This alteration occurs across the hyaloid face of the vitreous, the

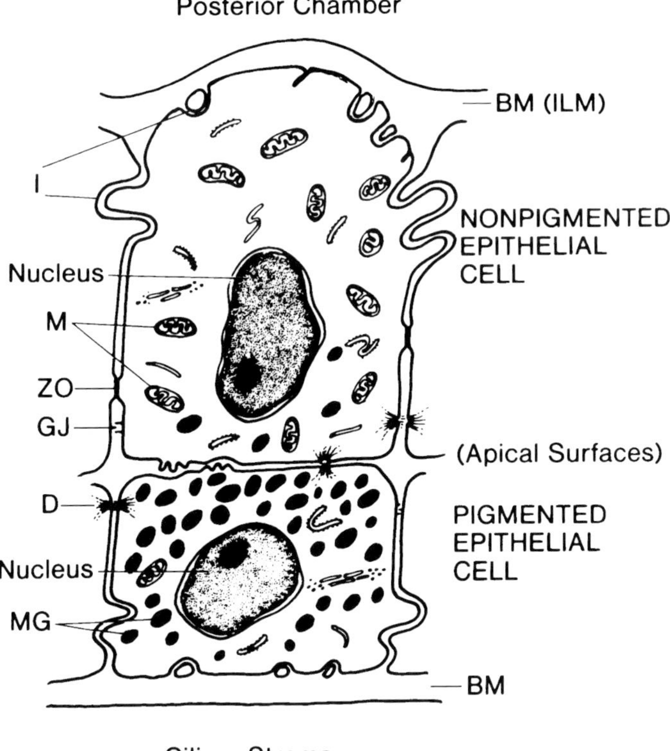

Figure 2-1 The two layers of the ciliary epithelium showing apical surfaces in apposition to each other. Basement membrane *(BM)* lines the double layer and constitutes the internal limiting membrane *(ILM)* on the inner surface. The nonpigmented epithelium is characterized by mitochondria *(M)*, zonula occludens *(ZO)*, and lateral and surface interdigitations *(I)*. The pigmented epithelium contains numerous melanin granules *(MG)*. Additional intercellular junctions include desmosomes *(D)* and gap junctions *(GJ)*. *(Reproduced with permission from Shields MB.* Textbook of Glaucoma. *3rd ed. Baltimore: Williams & Wilkins; 1992.)*

blood vessels of the iris, and the corneal endothelium and is secondary to other dilutional exchanges and active processes. BCSC Section 2, *Fundamentals and Principles of Ophthalmology,* discusses aqueous humor composition and production in detail in Part IV, Biochemistry and Metabolism.

Suppression of Aqueous Formation

The mechanisms of action of the classes of drugs that suppress aqueous formation—the *carbonic anhydrase inhibitors, beta-adrenergic antagonists (beta blockers),* and *alpha$_2$ agonists*—are also not precisely understood. The role of the enzyme carbonic anhydrase has been debated vigorously. Evidence suggests that the bicarbonate ion is actively secreted in human eyes; thus, the function of the enzyme may be to provide this ion. Carbonic anhydrase may also provide bicarbonate or hydrogen ions for an intracellular buffering system.

Current evidence indicates that beta$_2$ receptors are the most prevalent adrenergic receptors in the ciliary epithelium. The significance of this finding is unclear, but beta-adrenergic antagonists may affect active transport by causing a decrease either in the efficiency of the Na^+/K^+ pump or in the number of pump sites. For a detailed discussion and illustration of the sodium pump and pump–leak mechanism, see BCSC Section 2, *Fundamentals and Principles of Ophthalmology.*

Rate of Aqueous Formation

The most common method used to measure the rate of aqueous formation is *fluorophotometry.* Fluorescein is administered systemically or topically, and the subsequent decline in its anterior chamber concentration is measured optically and used to calculate aqueous flow. Normal flow is an average 2 μL/min, or a 1% turnover in aqueous volume per minute.

Aqueous formation varies diurnally and drops during sleep. It also decreases with age, as does outflow facility. The rate of aqueous formation is affected by a variety of factors:

- integrity of the blood–aqueous barrier
- blood flow to the ciliary body
- neurohumoral regulation of vascular tissue and the ciliary epithelium

Aqueous inflow falls when the eye is injured or inflamed and following the administration of certain drugs such as general anesthetics and some systemic hypotensive agents. Carotid occlusive disease may also decrease aqueous humor production.

Aqueous Humor Outflow

Aqueous humor outflow occurs by 2 major mechanisms: pressure-dependent outflow and pressure-independent outflow. The facility of outflow (*C* in the Goldmann equation; see the beginning of the chapter) varies widely in normal eyes. The mean value reported ranges from 0.22 to 0.28 μL/min/mm Hg. Outflow facility decreases with age and is affected by surgery, trauma, medications, and endocrine factors. Patients with glaucoma and elevated IOP have decreased outflow facility.

Trabecular Outflow (Pressure-dependent Outflow)

Most of the aqueous humor exits the eye by way of the trabecular meshwork–Schlemm's canal–venous system. The meshwork is classically divided into 3 parts (Fig 2-2). The uveal part is adjacent to the anterior chamber and is arranged in bands that extend from the iris root and the ciliary body to the peripheral cornea. The corneascleral meshwork is sheets of trabeculum that extend from the scleral spur to the lateral wall of the scleral sulcus. The juxtacanalicular meshwork, which is thought to be the major site of outflow resistance, is adjacent to Schlemm's canal and actually forms the inner wall of Schelmm's canal. Aqueous moves both across and between the endothelial cells lining the inner wall of Schlemm's canal.

The trabecular meshwork is composed of multiple layers, each of which consists of a collagenous connective tissue core covered by a continuous endothelial layer covering. It is the site of pressure-dependent outflow. The trabecular meshwork functions as a one-

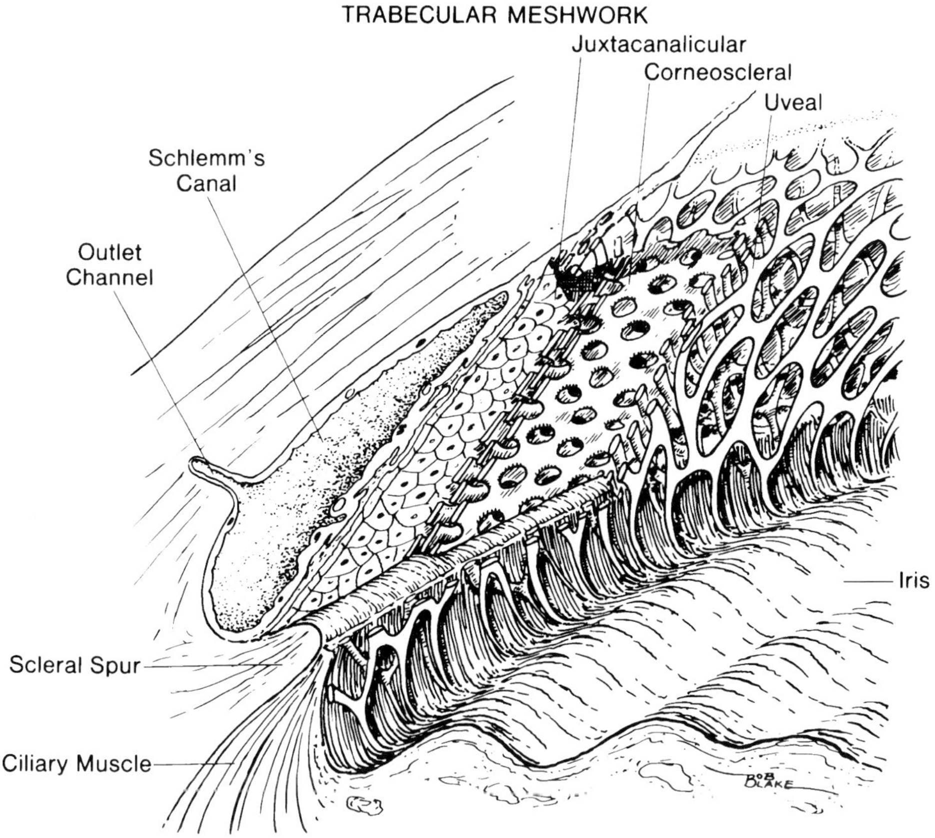

Figure 2-2 Three layers of trabecular meshwork (shown in cutaway views): uveal, corneoscleral, and juxtacanalicular. *(Reproduced with permission from Shields MB.* Textbook of Glaucoma. *3rd ed. Baltimore: Williams & Wilkins; 1992.)*

way valve that permits aqueous to leave the eye by bulk flow but limits flow in the other direction independently of energy. Its cells are phagocytic, a response they may sustain in the presence of inflammation and after laser treatment.

In older eyes, trabecular cells contain a large number of pigment granules within their cytoplasm that give the entire meshwork a brown or muddy appearance. In addition, the number of trabecular cells decreases with age, and the basement membrane beneath them thickens. There are relatively few trabecular cells—approximately 200,000–300,000 cells per eye. An interesting effect of laser trabeculoplasty is to induce trabecular cell division and cause a change in the production of cytokines and other structurally important elements of extracellular matrix. The extracellular matrix material is found through the dense portions of the trabecular meshwork.

Schlemm's canal is lined with endothelium and transversed by tubules. The canal is a single channel, with an average diameter of about 370 μm. The inner wall contains giant vacuoles that have direct communication with the intertrabecular spaces. Schlemm's canal has a complete endothelial lining that does not rest on a continuous basement membrane. The outer wall is actually a single layer of endothelial cells that do not contain pores. A complex system of vessels connects Schlemm's canal to the episcleral veins, which subsequently drain into the anterior ciliary and superior ophthalmic veins. These, in turn, drain into the cavernous sinus.

When IOP is low, the trabecular meshwork may collapse, or blood may reflux into Schlemm's canal and be visible on gonioscopy.

Uveoscleral Outflow (Pressure-independent Outflow)

In the normal eye, any nontrabecular outflow is termed *uveoscleral outflow.* Uveoscleral outflow is also termed *pressure-independent outflow.* A variety of mechanisms are involved, predominantly aqueous passage from the anterior chamber into the ciliary muscle and then into the supraciliary and suprachoroidal spaces. The fluid then exits the eye through the intact sclera or along the nerves and the vessels that penetrate it. As noted, uveoscleral outflow is pressure-independent and is believed to be influenced by age. There is evidence that humans, like primates, have a clinically significant outflow through the uveoscleral pathway. Uveoscleral outflow has been estimated to account for 5%–15% of total aqueous outflow, but recent studies indicate it may be a higher percentage of total outflow in the normal eyes of young people. It is increased by cycloplegia, adrenergic agents, prostaglandin analogs, and certain forms of surgery (eg, cyclodialysis) and is decreased by miotics.

Tonography

The ease with which aqueous can leave the eye—the facility of outflow—is measured by tonography. The measurement can be taken using a Schiøtz tonometer of known weight, which is placed on the cornea, suddenly elevating IOP. The rate at which the pressure declines with time is related to the ease with which the aqueous leaves the eye. The decline in IOP over time can be used to determine outflow facility in μL/min/mm Hg through a series of mathematical calculations.

Unfortunately, tonography depends on a number of assumptions (concerning, for example, the elastic properties of the eye, stability of aqueous formation, constancy of ocular blood volume) and is subject to many sources of error (eg, calibration problems, patient fixation, eyelid squeezing, technician errors). These problems reduce the accuracy and reproducibility of tonography for an individual patient. At present, tonography is best used as a research tool for the investigation of pharmacokinetics. It is rarely used clinically.

Episcleral Venous Pressure

Episcleral venous pressure is relatively stable, except when alterations in body position and certain diseases of the orbit, head, and neck obstruct venous return to the heart or shunt blood from the arterial to the venous system. The usual range of values is 8–10 mm Hg. The pressure in the episcleral veins can be measured with specialized equipment. In acute conditions, according to the Goldmann equation, IOP rises approximately 1 mm Hg for every 1 mm Hg increase in episcleral venous pressure. The relationship is more complex and less well understood, however, in chronic conditions. Chronic elevations of episcleral venous pressure may be accompanied by changes in IOP that are of greater, lesser, or the same magnitude predicted by the Goldmann equation and may not vary directly with the episcleral venous pressure. Abnormal elevated episcleral venous pressure can cause the collapse of Schlemm's canal and an increase in aqueous humor resistance. Episcleral venous pressure is often increased in facial hemangiomas and thyroid ophthalmopathy and is partially responsible for the elevated IOP seen in thyroid eye disease.

Intraocular Pressure

Distribution in the Population and Relation to Glaucoma

Pooled data from large epidemiologic studies indicate that the mean IOP is approximately 16 mm Hg, with a standard deviation of 3 mm Hg. IOP, however, has a nongaussian distribution with a skew toward higher pressures, especially in individuals over age 40 (Fig 2-3). The value 22 mm Hg has been used in the past both to separate normal and abnormal pressures and to define which patients required ocular hypotensive therapy. This division was based largely on the erroneous assumptions that glaucomatous damage is caused exclusively by pressures that are higher than normal and that normal pressures do not cause damage. Screening for glaucoma based solely on IOP >21 mm Hg may miss up to half of the people with glaucoma in the screened population.

General agreement has now been reached that, for the population as a whole, no clear line exists between safe and unsafe IOP: some eyes undergo damage at IOPs of 18 mm Hg or less, whereas others tolerate IOPs in the 30s. However, IOP is still seen as a

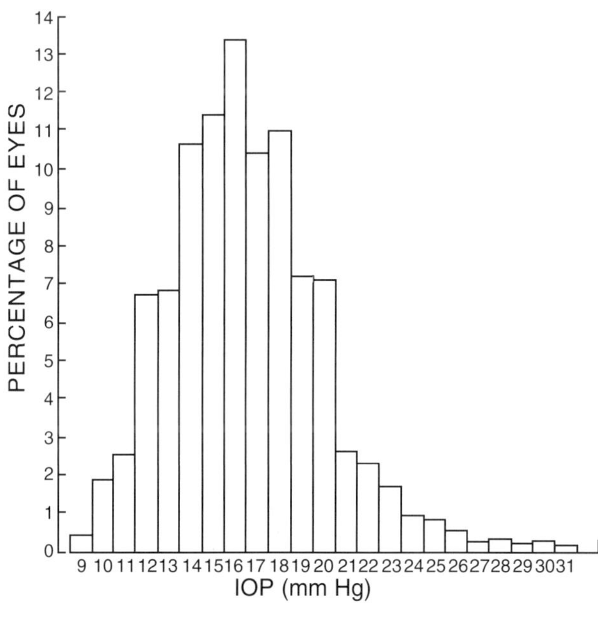

Figure 2-3 Frequency distribution of intraocular pressure: 5220 eyes in the Framingham Eye Study. *(Reproduced from Colton T, Ederer F. The distribution of intraocular pressures in the general population.* Surv Ophthalmol. *1980;25:123–129.)*

very important risk factor for the development of glaucomatous damage. Although other risk factors affect an individual's susceptibility to glaucomatous damage, IOP is the only one that can be altered at this time.

Factors Influencing Intraocular Pressure

IOP varies with a number of factors, including the following (Table 2-2):

- time of day
- heartbeat
- respiration
- exercise
- fluid intake
- systemic medications
- topical drugs

Alcohol consumption results in a transient decrease in IOP. In most studies, caffeine has not shown an appreciable effect on IOP. Cannabis decreases IOP but has not been proven clinically useful. IOP is higher when the patient is recumbent rather than upright. Some people have an exaggerated rise in IOP when they lie down, and this tendency may be important in the pathogenesis of some forms of glaucoma. IOP usually increases with

Table 2-2 Factors That Affect Intraocular Pressure

- Elevated venous pressure
  - Valsalva maneuver
  - Musical instruments
  - Tight collar
  - Bending over
  - Elevated central venous pressure
  - Intubation
- Pressure on the eye
  - Blepharospasm
  - Squeezing and crying, especially in young children
- Chronic exercise: lowers intraocular pressure
- Elevated body temperature: associated with increased aqueous humor production
- Anesthetic drugs
  - Ketamine
  - Depolarizing muscle relaxants such as succinylcholine
- Metabolic or respiratory acidosis: decreases aqueous humor production
- Hormonal influences
  - IOP lower during pregnancy
  - IOP higher with hypothyroidism
  - Thyroid ophthalmitis
- Drugs unrelated to therapy that lower intraocular pressure
  - Alcohol
  - Heroin
  - Marijuana
- Drugs unrelated to therapy that increase intraocular pressure
  - LSD
  - Corticosteroids: cause an open-angle glaucoma
  - Anticholinergics: precipitate angle closure in some patients

age and is genetically influenced: higher pressures are more common in relatives of patients with POAG than in the general population.

Diurnal Variation

In normal individuals, IOP varies 2–6 mm Hg over a 24-hour period, as aqueous humor production changes. Higher IOP is associated with greater fluctuation, and a diurnal fluctuation of greater than 10 mm Hg is suggestive of glaucoma. Many people reach their peak pressures in the morning hours, but others do so in the afternoon, in the evening, or during sleep; still others follow no reproducible pattern. To detect such fluctuations, ocular pressure is measured at multiple times around the clock. These measurements can sometimes be useful in evaluating patients with suspected normal-tension glaucoma, assessing the effects of therapy, and determining why optic nerve damage might occur despite apparently adequately controlled pressure. The relationship between blood pressure and IOP may be important in optic nerve damage: systemic hypotension, especially while sleeping, has been suggested as a possible cause of decreased optic nerve perfusion resulting in damage.

Clinical Measurement of Intraocular Pressure

Measurement of IOP in a clinical setting requires a force that indents or flattens the eye. *Applanation tonometry* is the method used most widely. It is based on the Imbert-Fick principle, which states that the pressure inside an ideal dry, thin-walled sphere equals the force necessary to flatten its surface divided by the area of the flattening:

$$P = F/A$$

where P = pressure, F = force, and A = area. In applanation tonometry, the cornea is flattened, and IOP is determined by measuring the applanating force and the area flattened (Fig 2-4).

The *Goldmann applanation tonometer* measures the force necessary to flatten an area of the cornea of 3.06 mm diameter. At this diameter, the resistance of the cornea to flattening is counterbalanced by the capillary attraction of the tear film meniscus for the tonometer head. Furthermore, the IOP (in mm Hg) equals the flattening force (in grams) multiplied by 10. A split-image prism allows the examiner to determine the flattened area with great accuracy. Fluorescein in the tear film is used to outline the area of flattening. The semicircles move with the ocular pulse, and the endpoint is reached when the inner edges of the semicircles touch each other at the midpoint of their excursion (Fig 2-5).

Applanation measurements are safe, easy to perform, and relatively accurate in most clinical situations. Of the currently available devices, the Goldmann applanation tonometer is the most valid and reliable. Because applanation does not displace much fluid (approximately 0.5 μL) or substantially increase the pressure in the eye, this method is relatively unaffected by ocular rigidity. Table 2-3 lists possible sources of error in tonometry.

Excessive fluorescein results in wide mires and an inaccurately high reading, whereas inadequate fluorescein leads to low readings.

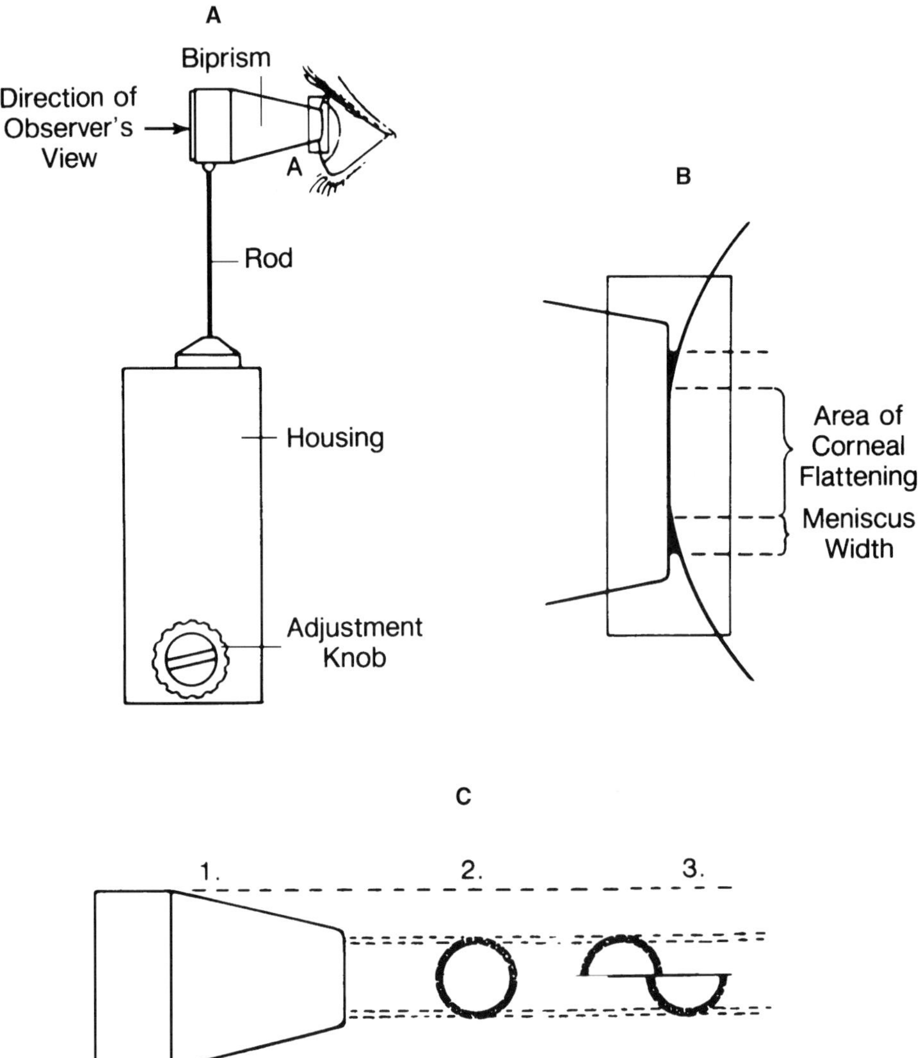

Figure 2-4 Goldmann-type applanation tonometry. **A,** Basic features of tonometer, shown in contact with patient's cornea. **B,** Enlargement shows tear film meniscus created by contact of biprism and cornea. **C,** View through biprism *(1)* reveals circular meniscus *(2),* which is converted into semicircle *(3)* by prisms. *(Reproduced with permission from Shields MB.* Textbook of Glaucoma. *3rd ed. Baltimore: Williams & Wilkins; 1992.)*

Marked corneal astigmatism causes an elliptical fluorescein pattern. To obtain an accurate reading, the clinician should rotate the prism so the red mark on the prism holder is set at the least curved meridian of the cornea (along the negative axis). Alternately, 2 pressure readings taken 90° apart can be averaged.

The accuracy of applanation tonometry is reduced in certain situations. Corneal edema predisposes to inaccurately low readings, whereas pressure measurements taken over a corneal scar will be falsely high. Tonometry performed over a soft contact lens

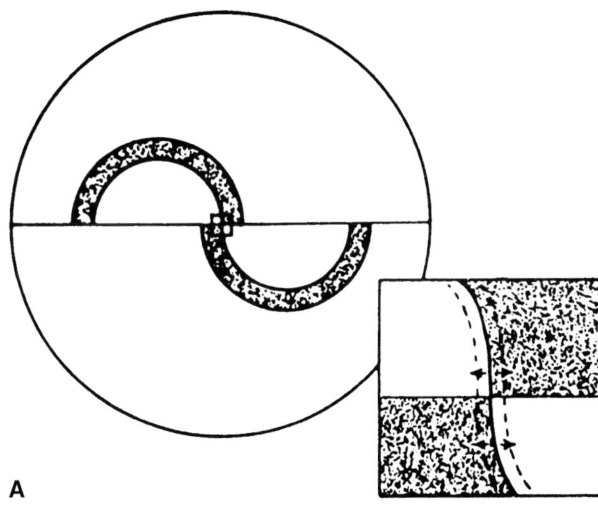

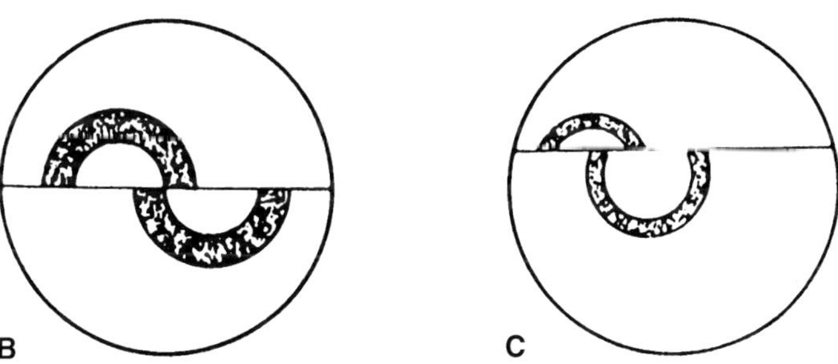

Figure 2-5 Semicircles of Goldmann-type applanation tonometer. **A,** Proper width and position. Enlargement depicts excursions of semicircles caused by ocular pulsations. **B,** Semicircles are too wide. **C,** Improper vertical and horizontal alignment. *(Reproduced with permission from Shields MB.* Textbook of Glaucoma. *3rd ed. Baltimore: Williams & Wilkins; 1992.)*

gives falsely low values. Alterations in scleral rigidity may compromise the accuracy of measurements; for example, applanation readings that follow scleral buckling procedures may be inaccurately low.

Applanation tonometry measurements are also affected by the central corneal thickness (CCT). Recently, the importance of CCT and its effect on the accuracy of IOP meansurement has become better understood. The Goldmann tonometer is most accurate, with a CCT of 520 μm; however, population studies have shown a wide range of normal, with mean CCT between 537 and 554 μm.

Increased CCT may give an artificially high, and decreased CCT may give an artificially low, IOP measurement. IOP measured after photorefractive keratectomy (PRK) and laser in situ keratomileusis (LASIK) may be reduced because of changes in the corneal

Table 2-3 Possible Sources of Error in Tonometry

Squeezing of the eyelids
Breath holding or Valsalva maneuver
Pressure on the globe
Extraocular muscle force applied to a restricted globe
Tight collar or tight necktie
Obesity or straining to reach slit lamp
An inaccurately calibrated tonometer
Excessive or inadequate fluorescein
High corneal astigmatism
Corneal thickness greater or less than normal
Corneal scarring or band keratopathy
Corneal irregularity
Technician errors

thickness induced by these and other refractive procedures. As a rough guide, using an overview of published studies, it can be estimated that for every 10-µm difference in CCT from the population mean (approximately 542 µm), there is a 0.5 mm Hg difference between actual IOP and the IOP measured with a Goldmann tonometer. However, because the relationship of measured IOP and CCT is not linear, it is important to remember that such correction factors as this are only estimates at best. The Goldmann tonometer, Perkins tonometer, pneumatonometer, noncontact tonometer, and Tonopen are all affected by CCT.

The Ocular Hypertension Treatment Study (OHTS) found that a thinner central cornea was a strong predictive factor for the development of glaucoma in subjects with ocular hypertension. Subjects with a corneal thickness of 555 µm or less had a threefold greater risk of developing POAG compared with participants who had a corneal thickness of more than 588 µm. Whether this increased risk of glaucoma is due to underestimating actual IOP in patients with thinner corneas or whether thin corneas are a risk factor independent of IOP measurement has not been completely determined, but the OHTS found CCT to be a risk factor for progression independent of IOP level.

The *Perkins tonometer* is a counterbalanced tonometer that is portable and can be used with the patient either upright or supine. It is similar to the Goldmann tonometer in using a split-image device and fluorescein staining of the tears.

Methods other than Goldmann-type applanation tonometry

Noncontact (air-puff) tonometers measure IOP without touching the eye, by measuring the time necessary for a given force of air to flatten a given area of the cornea. Readings obtained with these instruments vary widely, and they often overestimate IOP. The instruments are often used in large-scale glaucoma-screening programs or by nonmedical health care providers.

The group of *portable electronic applanation* devices (eg, Tonopen) that applanate a very small area of the cornea are particularly useful in the presence of corneal scars or edema. The *pneumatic tonometer,* or *pneumatonometer,* has a pressure-sensing device that consists of a gas-filled chamber covered by a Silastic diaphragm. The gas in the chamber escapes through an exhaust vent. As the diaphragm touches the cornea, the gas vent is reduced in size and the pressure in the chamber rises. Because this instrument, too, applanates only a small area of the cornea, it is especially useful in the presence of corneal scars or edema.

Schiøtz tonometry determines IOP by measuring the indentation of the cornea produced by a known weight. The indentation is read on a linear scale on the instrument and is converted to mm Hg by a calibration table. Because of a number of practical and theoretical problems, however, Schiøtz tonometry is now rarely used.

It is possible to estimate IOP by *digital pressure* on the globe. This test may be used with uncooperative patients, but it may be inaccurate even in very experienced hands. In general, tactile tensions are only useful for detecting large differences between 2 eyes.

Infection Control in Clinical Tonometry

Many infectious agents, including the viruses responsible for acquired immunodeficiency syndrome (AIDS), hepatitis, and epidemic keratoconjunctivitis, can be recovered from tears. To prevent transfer of such agents, tonometers must be cleaned after each use:

- The prism head of both Goldmann-type tonometers and the Perkins tonometer should be cleaned immediately after use. The prisms should either be soaked in a 1:10 sodium hypochlorite solution (household bleach), 3% hydrogen peroxide, or 70% isopropyl alcohol for 5 minutes, or be thoroughly wiped with an alcohol sponge. If a soaking solution is used, the prism should be rinsed and dried before reuse. If alcohol is employed, it should be allowed to evaporate, or the prism head should be dried before reuse, to prevent damage to the epithelium.
- The front surface of the air-puff tonometer should be wiped with alcohol between uses because tears from the patient may contaminate the instrument.
- Portable electronic applanation devices employ a disposable cover, which should be replaced immediately after each use.
- The Schiøtz tonometer requires disassembly to clean both the plunger and the footplate. Unless the plunger is clean (as opposed to sterile), the measurements may be falsely elevated because of increased friction between the plunger and the footplate. The inside of the footplate can be cleaned of tears and any tear film debris with a pipe cleaner. The same solutions used for cleaning prism heads may then be employed to sterilize the instrument.

For other tonometers, consult the manufacturer's recommendations.

Brandt JD. The influence of corneal thickness on the diagnosis and management of glaucoma. *J Glaucoma.* 2001;10(5 Suppl 1):S65–S67.

Brubaker RF. Measurement of uveoscleral outflow in humans. *J Glaucoma.* 2001;10(5 Suppl 1): S45–S48.

Doherty MJ, Zaman ML. Human corneal thickness and its impact on intraocular pressure measures: a review and meta-analysis approach. *Surv Ophthalmol.* 2000;44:367–408.

Gordon MA, Beiser JA, Brandt JA, et al. The Ocular Hypertension Treatment Study: baseline factors that predict the onset of primary open-angle glaucoma. *Arch Ophthalmol.* 2002; 120:714–720.

Mills RP. If intraocular pressure measurement is only an estimate—then what? *Ophthalmology.* 2000;107:1807–1808.

Shah S. Accurate intraocular pressure measurement—the myth of modern ophthalmology? *Ophthalmology.* 2000;107:1805–1807.

Sommer A, Tielsch JM, Katz J, et al. Relationship between intraocular pressure and primary open angle glaucoma among white and black Americans. The Baltimore Eye Survey. *Arch Ophthalmol.* 1991;109:1090–1095.

CHAPTER 3

Clinical Evaluation

History and General Examination

Appropriate management of glaucoma depends on the clinician's ability to diagnose the specific form of glaucoma in a given patient, to determine the severity of the condition, and to detect progression in that patient's disease status. The most important aspects of the clinical evaluation of a glaucoma patient are presented in the following discussion.

History

The history should include the following:

- patient's current complaint
- symptoms, onset, duration, severity, location
- ocular history
- history of present illness
- past ocular, medical, and surgical history
- general medical history
- past systemic medical history (including medications and allergies)
- review of systems
- social history
- history of alcohol and tobacco use
- occupation, avocation, interests
- family history

It is often useful to question the patient specifically regarding symptoms and conditions associated with glaucoma, such as pain, redness, halos around lights, alteration of vision, and loss of vision. Similarly, the general medical history should include specific inquiry regarding diseases that may have ocular manifestations or may affect the patient's ability to tolerate medications. Such conditions include diabetes, cardiac and pulmonary disease, hypertension, hemodynamic shock, migraine and other neurologic diseases, and renal stones. In addition to identifying present medications and medication allergies, the clinician should take note of a history of corticosteroid use. See also BCSC Section 1, *Update on General Medicine,* for further discussion of these conditions and medications.

Refraction

Neutralizing any refractive error is crucial for accurate perimetry with most perimeters, and the clinician should understand how the patient's refractive state affects the diagnosis.

Hyperopic eyes are at increased risk of angle-closure glaucoma and generally have smaller discs. Myopia is associated with disc morphologies that can be clinically confused with glaucoma, and myopic eyes are at increased risk for pigment dispersion. Whether myopic eyes have increased risk of open-angle glaucoma remains a controversial issue.

External Adnexae

Examination and assessment of the external ocular adnexae is useful in determining the presence of a variety of conditions associated with secondary glaucomas as well as external ocular manifestations of glaucoma therapy. The entities described in this section are discussed in greater depth and illustrated in other volumes of the BCSC series; consult the *Master Index.*

An example of an association between adenexal changes and systemic disease is *tuberous sclerosis (Bourneville syndrome),* in which glaucoma may occur secondary to vitreous hemorrhage, anterior segment neovascularization, or retinal detachment. Typical external and cutaneous signs of tuberous sclerosis include a hypopigmented lesion termed the "ash-leaf sign" and a red-brown papular rash (adenoma sebaceum) that is often found on the face and chin.

Glaucoma is commonly associated with *neurofibromatosis (von Recklinghausen disease),* likely secondary to developmental abnormalities of the anterior chamber angle. Subcutaneous plexiform neuromas are a hallmark of the type 1 variant of neurofibromatosis. When found in the upper eyelid, the plexiform neuroma can produce a classic S-shaped upper eyelid deformity strongly associated with risk of glaucoma.

In *juvenile xanthogranuloma,* yellow and/or orange papules are commonly found on the skin of the head and neck. Secondary glaucoma may cause acute pain and photophobia and ultimately significant visual loss. *Oculodermal melanocytosis (nevus of Ota)* presents with the key finding of hyperpigmentation of periocular skin. Intraocular pigmentation is also increased, which contributes to a higher incidence of glaucoma and may possibly increase the risk of malignant melanoma. *Axenfeld-Rieger syndrome,* an autosomal dominant disorder with variable penetrance, is associated with microdontia (small, peglike incisors), hypodontia (decreased number of teeth), and anodontia (focal absence of teeth). Maxillary hypoplasia may also be present. Glaucoma occurs in 50% of cases in late childhood or adulthood.

A number of entities are associated with signs of increased episcleral venous pressure. The presence of a facial cutaneous angioma (nevus flammeus, or port-wine stain) can indicate *encephalofacial angiomatosis (Sturge-Weber syndrome).* Hemifacial hypertrophy may also be observed. The cutaneous hemangiomas of the *Klippel-Trénaunay-Weber syndrome* extend over an affected, secondarily hypertrophied limb and may also involve the face.

Orbital varices are associated with secondary glaucoma. Intermittent unilateral proptosis and dilated eyelid veins are key external signs of orbital varices. Carotid cavernous, dural cavernous, and other *arteriovenous fistulae* can produce orbital bruits, restricted ocular motility, proptosis, and pulsating exophthalmos. *Superior vena cava syndrome* can cause proptosis and facial and eyelid edema, as well as conjunctival chemosis. *Thyroid ophthalmopathy* and its associated glaucoma are associated with exophthalmos, eyelid retraction, and motility disorders.

Use of topical hypotensive lipids such as prostaglandin analogs, prostamides, and decosanoids may result in trichiasis, distichiasis, and growth of facial hair around the eyes, as well as increased skin pigmentation involving the eyelids. Use of glaucoma hypotensive agents may also result in an allergic contact dermatitis. Chapter 7, Medical Management of Glaucoma, discusses these agents in detail.

Pupils

Pupil size may be affected by glaucoma therapy, and pupillary responses are one measure of compliance in patients who are on miotic therapy. Testing for a relative afferent pupillary defect may detect asymmetric optic nerve damage, a common and important finding in glaucoma. Corectopia, ectropion uveae, and pupillary abnormalities may also be observed in some forms of secondary open-angle glaucoma and angle-closure glaucoma. In some clinical situations, it is not possible to assess the pupils objectively for the presence of a relative afferent defect. Under those circumstances, it can be useful to ask the patient to make a subjective comparison between the eyes of the perceived brightness of a test light.

Biomicroscopy

Biomicroscopy of the anterior segment is performed for signs of underlying or associated ocular disease. BCSC Section 8, *External Disease and Cornea,* discusses slit-lamp technique and the examination of the external eye in greater depth.

Conjunctiva

Eyes with acutely elevated IOP may show conjunctival hyperemia. The chronic elevation of IOP that can occur with arteriovenous fistulae may produce massive episcleral venous dilation. Chronic use of sympathomimetics and hypotensive lipids may also cause conjunctival injection, and chronic use of epinephrine derivatives may result in black adrenochrome deposits in the conjunctiva. The use of topical antiglaucoma medication can also cause decreased tear production, allergic and hypersensitivity reactions (papillary and follicular conjunctivitis), foreshortening of the conjunctival fornices, and scarring. The presence or absence of any filtering bleb should be noted. If a bleb is present, its size, height, degree of vascularization, and integrity should be noted.

Episclera and sclera

Dilation of the episcleral vessels may indicate elevated episcleral venous pressure, a finding that can be seen in the secondary glaucomas associated with Sturge-Weber syndrome, arteriovenous fistulae, or thyroid ophthalmopathy. Sentinel vessels may be seen in eyes harboring an intraocular tumor. Any thinning or staphylomatous areas should be noted.

Cornea

Enlargement of the cornea associated with breaks in Descemet's membrane (Haab's striae) is commonly found in developmental glaucoma patients. Glaucomas associated with other anterior segment anomalies are described in the following discussions. Punctate epithelial defects, especially in the inferonasal interpalpebral region, are often indicative of medication toxicity. Microcystic epithelial edema is commonly associated with elevated IOP, particularly when the pressure rise is acute. Corneal endothelial abnormalities, such as the following, can be important clues to the presence of an underlying associated secondary glaucoma:

- Krukenberg spindle in pigmentary glaucoma
- deposition of exfoliation material in exfoliation syndrome
- keratic precipitates in uveitic glaucoma
- guttatae in Fuchs endothelial dystrophy
- irregular and vesicular lesions in posterior polymorphous dystrophy
- a "beaten bronze" appearance in the iridocorneal endothelial syndrome

An anteriorly displaced Schwalbe's line is found in Axenfeld-Rieger syndrome. The presence of traumatic or surgical corneal scars should be noted. The central corneal thickness (CCT) of all patients suspected of glaucoma should be assessed (corneal pachymetry) because of the effect of CCT on the accuracy of applanation tonometry and its possible implication as a risk factor in some types of glaucomas. (See Chapters 2 and 4.)

Anterior chamber

To estimate the width of the chamber angle, the examiner directs a narrow slit beam at an angle of 60° onto the cornea just anterior to the limbus (Van Herick method). If the distance from the anterior iris surface to the posterior surface of the cornea is less than one fourth the thickness of the cornea, the angle may be narrow. This test should alert the examiner to narrow angles, but it is not a substitute for gonioscopy, which is discussed in detail in the following major section (Figs 3-1, 3-2, Table 3-1).

The uniformity of depth of the anterior chamber should be noted. Iris bombé can result in an anterior chamber that is deep centrally and shallow or flat peripherally. Iris masses can produce an irregular iris surface contour and nonuniformity in anterior

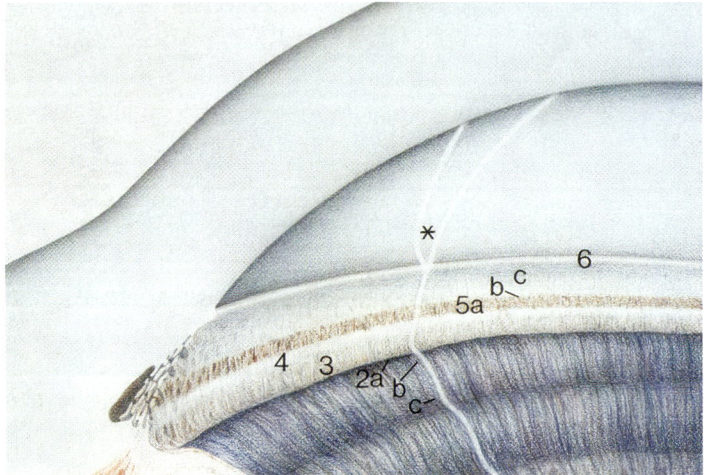

Figure 3-1 Gonioscopic appearance of a normal anterior chamber angle. *2,* Peripheral iris: *a,* insertion; *b,* curvature; *c,* angular approach. *3,* Ciliary body band. *4,* Scleral spur. *5,* Trabecular meshwork: *a,* posterior; *b,* mid; *c,* anterior. *6,* Schwalbe's line. *Asterisk,* Corneal optical wedge.

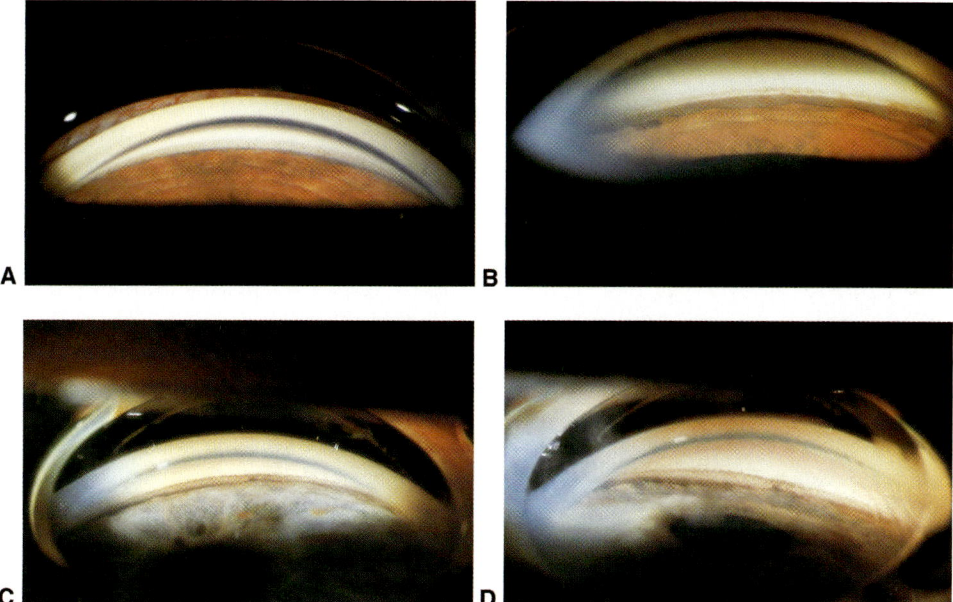

Figure 3-2 **A,** Normal open angle. Gonioscopic photograph shows trace pigmentation of the posterior trabecular meshwork and normal insertion of the iris into a narrow ciliary body band. The Goldmann lens was used. **B,** Normal open angle. This gonioscopic view using the Goldmann lens shows mild pigmentation of the posterior trabecular meshwork. A wide ciliary body band with posterior insertion of the iris can also be seen. **C,** Narrow angle. This gonioscopic view using the Zeiss lens without indentation shows pigment in inferior angle but poor visualization of angle anatomy. **D,** Narrow angle. Gonioscopy with a Zeiss lens with indentation shows peripheral anterior synechiae in the posterior trabecular meshwork. Pigment deposits on Schwalbe's line can also be seen. This is the same angle as shown in **C**. *(Photographs courtesy of Elizabeth A. Hodapp, MD.)*

Table 3-1 Gonioscopic Examination

Tissue	Features
Posterior cornea	Pigmentation, guttata
Schwalbe's line	Thickening, anterior displacement
Trabecular meshwork	Pigmentation, peripheral anterior synechiae (PAS), inflammatory or neovascular membranes, keratic precipitates
Scleral spur	Iris processes, presence or absence
Ciliary body band	Width, regularity, cyclodialysis cleft
Iris	Contour, rubeosis, atrophy, cysts, iridodonesis
Pupil and lens	Exfoliation syndrome, posterior synechiae, position and regularity, sphincter rupture, ectropion uveae
Zonular fibers	Pigmentation, rupture

chamber depth. In many circumstances, especially in the assessment of narrow-angle glaucoma, comparison of chamber depth between eyes is of significant value. The presence of inflammatory cells, red blood cells, ghost cells, fibrin, vitreous, or other findings should be noted. The degree of inflammation (flare and cell) should be determined prior to instillation of eyedrops.

Iris

Examination should be performed prior to dilation. Heterochromia, iris atrophy, transillumination defects, ectropion uveae, corectopia, nevi, nodules, and exfoliative material should be noted. Early stages of neovascularization of the anterior segment may appear as either fine tufts around the pupillary margin or as a fine network of vessels on the surface of the iris. Visualization of neovascular tufts with biomicroscopy may require increased magnification. The iris should also be examined for evidence of trauma, such as sphincter tears or iridodonesis. The degree of baseline iris pigmentation should be noted, especially in patients being considered for treatment with a hypotensive lipid.

Lens

The lens is generally best examined after dilation. Material associated with pseudoexfoliation, phacodonesis, subluxation, and dislocation should be noted, along with lens size, shape, and clarity. A posterior subcapsular cataract may be indicative of chronic corticosteroid use. An intraocular foreign body with siderosis and glaucoma may also result in characteristic lens changes. The presence, type, and position of an intraocular lens should be recorded, along with the status of the posterior capsule.

Fundus

Careful assessment of the optic disc is an essential part of the clinical examination for glaucoma, and this is covered in detail later in the chapter. In addition, fundus examination may reveal posterior segment pathology such as hemorrhages, effusions, masses, inflammatory lesions, retinovascular occlusions, diabetic retinopathy, or retinal detachments that can be associated with the glaucomas. Funduscopy is best performed with a dilated pupil.

Gonioscopy

Gonioscopy is an essential diagnostic tool and examination technique used to visualize the structures of the anterior chamber angle. Mastering the various techniques of gonioscopy is crucial in the evaluation of glaucoma patients. Figures 3-1 and 3-2 give schematic and clinical views of the angle as seen with gonioscopy. Gonioscopy is required to visualize the chamber angle because under normal conditions light reflected from the angle structures undergoes total internal reflection at the tear–air interface. At the tear–air interface, the critical angle (approximately 46°) is reached and light is totally reflected back into the corneal stroma. This prevents direct visualization of the angle structures. All gonioscopy lenses eliminate the tear–air interface by placing a plastic or glass surface adjacent to the front surface of the eye. The small space between the lens and cornea is filled by the patient's tears, saline solution, or a clear viscous substance. Depending on the type of lens employed, the angle can be examined with a direct system (eg, Koeppe) or a mirrored indirect (Goldmann-type or Zeiss-type) system (Fig 3-3).

Direct and Indirect Gonioscopy

Gonioscopy techniques fall into 1 of 2 broad categories: direct and indirect (see Fig 3-3) To diagnose the various types of outflow obstruction, it is critical to master several gonioscopic techniques. Direct gonioscopy is performed with a binocular microscope, a fiberoptic illuminator or slit-pen light, and a direct goniolens, such as the Koeppe, Barkan, Wurst, Swan-Jacob, or Richardson. These lenses are placed on the eye, and saline solution is used to fill the space between the cornea and the lens. The saline acts as an optical coupler between the 2 surfaces. The lenses provide direct visualization of the chamber

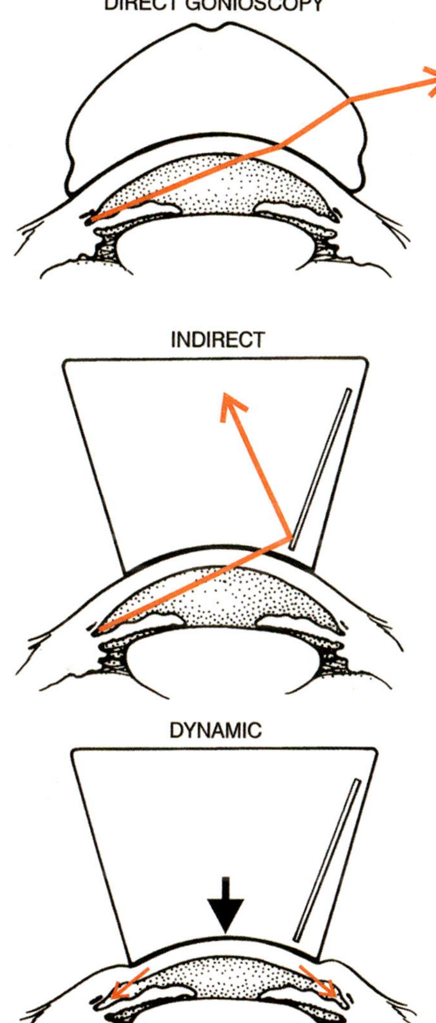

Figure 3-3 Direct and indirect gonioscopy. Gonioscopic lenses eliminate the tear–air interface and total internal reflection. With direct lenses, the light ray reflected from the anterior chamber angle is observed directly, whereas with indirect lenses the light ray is reflected by a mirror within the lens. Posterior pressure with an indirect lens forces open an appositionally closed or narrow anterior chamber angle (dynamic gonioscopy). *(Reprinted with permission from Wright KW, ed.* Textbook of Ophthalmology. *Baltimore: Williams and Wilkins; 1997.)*

angle (ie, light reflected directly from the chamber angle is visualized). With direct gonioscopy lenses, the physician has an erect view of the angle structures. Because it provides an erect orientation of the chamber angle, direct gonioscopy is essential when performing goniotomies. Direct gonioscopy is most easily performed with the patient in a supine position and is commonly used in the operating room for examining the eyes of infants under anesthesia.

Koeppe-type lenses are also quite useful in performing funduscopy. When used with a direct ophthalmoscope and high-plus-power lens, they can provide a good view of the fundus, even through a very small pupil. These lenses are especially helpful in individuals with nystagmus or irregular corneas. Inconvenience is the major disadvantage of the direct gonioscopy systems.

Indirect gonioscopy is more frequently used in the clinician's office. Indirect gonioscopy also eliminates the total internal reflection at the surface of the cornea. Light reflected from the chamber angle passes into the indirect gonioscopy lens and is reflected by a mirror within the lens. These lenses are commonly referred to as "gonioprisms," and a large variety has been developed. Many gonioprisms, such as the Goldmann lens, require a viscous optical coupler between the lens and the cornea to fill the domed space over the cornea. These lenses provide the clearest visualization of the anterior chamber angle structures and may be modified with antireflective coatings for use during laser procedures. Because an internal mirror is present in all indirect gonioscopy lenses, the image seen by the observer is inverted, while the right–left orientation in the horizontal mirror and the up–down orientation in the vertical mirror remain unchanged. Indirect gonioscopy may be used with the patient in an upright position, with illumination and magnification provided by a slit lamp. The Sussman and Zeiss 4-mirror gonioprisms allow all 4 quadrants of the chamber angle to be visualized without manipulating the lens. These lenses also allow the examiner to use the patient's tear film as the optical coupler between the cornea and the lens. Many clinicians prefer these lenses because of their ease of use, as well as their ability to perform dynamic gonioscopy.

With dynamic gonioscopy (compression or indentation gonioscopy), gentle pressure is placed on the cornea, and aqueous humor is forced into the chamber angle (see Fig 3-3). The posterior diameter of these gonioprisms is smaller than the corneal diameter, and posterior pressure can be used to force open a narrowed angle. In inexperienced hands, dynamic gonioscopy may be misleading, as undue pressure on the anterior surface of the cornea may distort the chamber angle or may give the observer the false impression of an open angle. The examiner can detect this pressure by noting the induced folds in Descemet's membrane. With all indirect gonioscopy techniques, the observer may manipulate the chamber angle by positioning the patient's eye (having the patient look toward the mirror) or by applying pressure with the posterior surface of the lens to provide more complete evaluation of the chamber angle. However, caution must be used not to induce artificial opening or closing of the anterior chamber angle with these techniques.

A *goniolens,* which contains a mirror or mirrors, yields an inverted and slightly foreshortened image of the opposite angle. Although the image is inverted with an indirect goniolens, the right–left orientation of a horizontal mirror and the up–down orientation of a vertical mirror remain unchanged. The foreshortening, combined with the upright position of the patient, makes the angle appear a little shallower than it does with direct gonioscopy systems.

The Goldmann-type goniolens requires a viscous fluid such as methylcellulose for optical coupling with the cornea. In lenses with only 1 mirror, the lens must be rotated to view the entire angle. Posterior pressure on the lens, especially if tilted, indents the sclera and may falsely narrow the angle. The combination of the lens manipulation and use of viscous fluid often temporarily reduces the clarity of the cornea and may make subsequent fundus examination, visual field testing, and photography more difficult.

The Zeiss-type lens and similar goniolenses or gonioprisms with a smaller area of contact than the Goldmann-type lens have about the same radius of curvature as the cornea and are optically coupled by the patient's tears. Because the Zeiss-type lens has 4 mirrors, the entire angle is visible without rotation during examination. The diameter of the lens is smaller than the diameter of the cornea, and pressure on the cornea may distort the chamber angle. The examiner can detect this pressure by noting the induced Descemet's membrane folds. Although pressure may falsely open the angle, the technique of indentation gonioscopy (dynamic gonioscopy) is sometimes essential in distinguishing iridocorneal apposition from synechial closure.

Gonioscopic Assessment and Documentation

In performing both direct and indirect gonioscopy, the clinician must recognize the angle landmarks. The scleral spur and Schwalbe's line are the most consistent; a convenient gonioscopic technique to determine the exact position of Schwalbe's line is the parallelopiped technique. The parallelopiped, or corneal light wedge, technique allows the observer to determine the exact junction of the cornea and the trabecular meshwork. Using a narrow slit beam and sharp focus, the examiner sees 2 linear reflections, one from the external surface of the cornea and its junction with the sclera and the other from the internal surface of the cornea. The 2 reflections meet at Schwalbe's line (see Fig 3-1). The scleral spur is a thin, pale stripe between the ciliary face and the pigmented zone of the trabecular meshwork. The inferior portion of the angle is generally wider and is the easiest place in which to locate the landmarks. After verifying the landmarks, the clinician should examine the entire angle in an orderly manner (see Table 3-1).

Proper management of glaucoma requires that the clinician determine not only whether the angle is open or closed, but also whether other pathologic findings, such as angle recession or low peripheral anterior synechiae (PAS), are present. In angle closure, the peripheral iris obstructs the trabecular meshwork—that is, the meshwork is not visible on gonioscopy. The width of the angle is determined by the site of insertion of the iris on the ciliary face, the convexity of the iris, and the prominence of the peripheral iris roll. In many cases, the angle appears open but very narrow. It is often difficult to distinguish a narrow but open angle from an angle with partial closure; indentation gonioscopy is useful in this situation (see Figs 3-2 and 3-3).

The best method for describing the angle is to use a standardized grading system or draw the iris contour, the location of the iris insertion, and the angle between the iris and the trabecular meshwork. A variety of gonioscopic grading systems has been developed. All grading systems facilitate standardized description of angle structures and abbreviate that description. Keep in mind that, by abbreviating, some details of the angle structure will be eliminated. The most commonly used gonioscopic grading systems are the Shaffer and Spaeth systems. A quadrant-by-quadrant narrative description of the chamber angle noting localized findings such as neovascular tufts, angle recession, or PAS is also helpful and descriptive and may also be used to document serial gonioscopic findings. If a grading system is used, the clinician should specify which system is being used.

The *Shaffer system* describes the angle between the trabecular meshwork and the iris as follows:

- *Grade 4:* The angle between the iris and the surface of the trabecular meshwork is 45°.
- *Grade 3:* The angle between the iris and the surface of the trabecular meshwork is greater than 20° but less than 45°.
- *Grade 2:* The angle between the iris and the surface of the trabecular meshwork is 20°. Angle closure is possible.
- *Grade 1:* The angle between the iris and the surface of the trabecular meshwork is 10°. Angle closure is probable in time.
- *Slit:* The angle between the iris and the surface of the trabecular meshwork is less than 10°. Angle closure is very likely.
- *O:* The iris is against the trabecular meshwork. Angle closure is present.

The *Spaeth gonioscopic grading system* expands this system to include a description of the peripheral iris contour, the insertion of the iris root, and the effects of indentation gonioscopy on the angle configuration (Fig 3-4).

Ordinarily, Schlemm's canal is invisible by gonioscopy. Occasionally during gonioscopy in normal eyes, blood refluxes into Schlemm's canal, where it is seen as a faint red line in the posterior portion of the trabecular meshwork (Fig 3-5). Blood enters Schlemm's canal when episcleral venous pressure exceeds IOP, most commonly because of compression of the episcleral veins by the lip of the goniolens. Pathologic causes include hypotony and elevated episcleral venous pressure, as in carotid cavernous fistula or Sturge-Weber syndrome.

Normal blood vessels in the angle include radial iris vessels, portions of the arterial circle of the ciliary body, and vertical branches of the anterior ciliary arteries. Normal vessels are oriented either radially along the iris or circumferentially (in a serpentine manner) in the ciliary body face. Vessels that cross the scleral spur to reach the trabecular meshwork are usually abnormal (Fig 3-6). The vessels seen in Fuchs heterochromic iridocyclitis are fine, branching, unsheathed, and meandering. Patients with neovascular glaucoma have trunklike vessels crossing the ciliary body and scleral spur and arborizing over the trabecular meshwork. Contraction of the myofibroblasts accompanying these vessels leads to PAS formation.

It is important to distinguish PAS from iris processes (uveal meshwork), which are open and lacy and follow the normal curve of the angle. The angle structures are visible in the open spaces between the processes. Synechiae are more solid or sheetlike (Fig 3-7). They are composed of iris stroma and obliterate the angle recess.

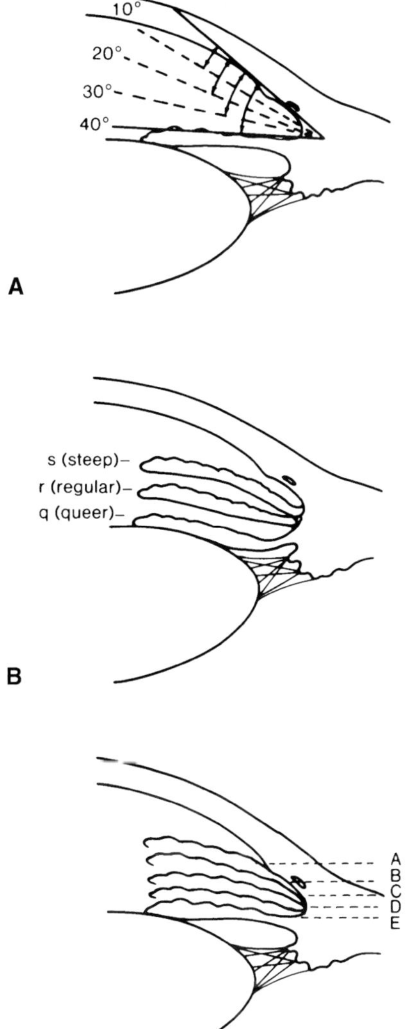

Figure 3-4 Spaeth's gonioscopic classification of the anterior chamber angle, based on 3 variables: **A,** angular width of the angle recess; **B,** configuration of the peripheral iris; and **C,** apparent insertion of the iris root. *(Reproduced with permission from Shields MB.* Textbook of Glaucoma. *3rd ed. Baltimore: Williams & Wilkins; 1992.)*

Pigmentation of the trabecular meshwork increases with age, and tends to be more marked in individuals with darkly pigmented irides. Pigmentation can be segmental and is usually most marked in the inferior angle. The pigmentation pattern of an individual angle is dynamic over time, especially in conditions such as pigment dispersion syndrome. Heavy pigmentation of the trabecular meshwork should suggest pigment dispersion or exfoliation syndrome. Exfoliation syndrome may appear clinically similar to pigmentary dispersion syndrome, with pigment granules on the anterior surface of the iris, increased pigment in the anterior chamber angle, and secondary open-angle glaucoma. Pigmentation of the angle structures is usually patchy in exfoliation syndrome, as compared to the more uniform pigment distribution seen in pigmentary dispersion sysndrome. In addition, a line of pigment deposition anterior to Schwalbe's line is often present in

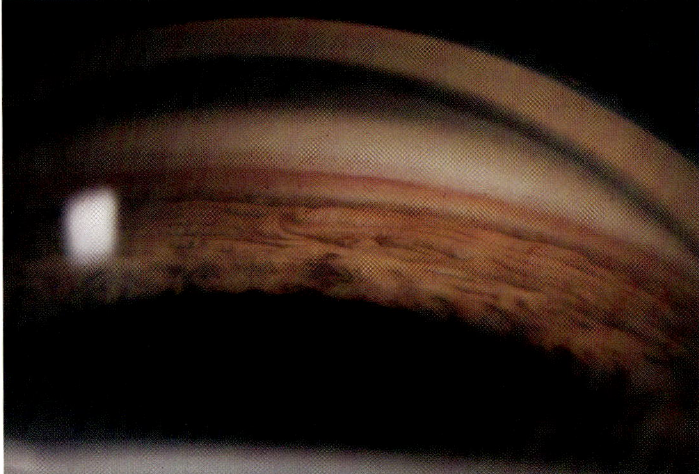

Figure 3-5 Blood in Schlemm's canal. Note the red line posterior to the trabecular meshwork in the indivividual with elevated episcleral venous pressure resulting in blood reflux into Schlemm's canal. *(Photograph courtesy of G. A. Cioffi, MD.)*

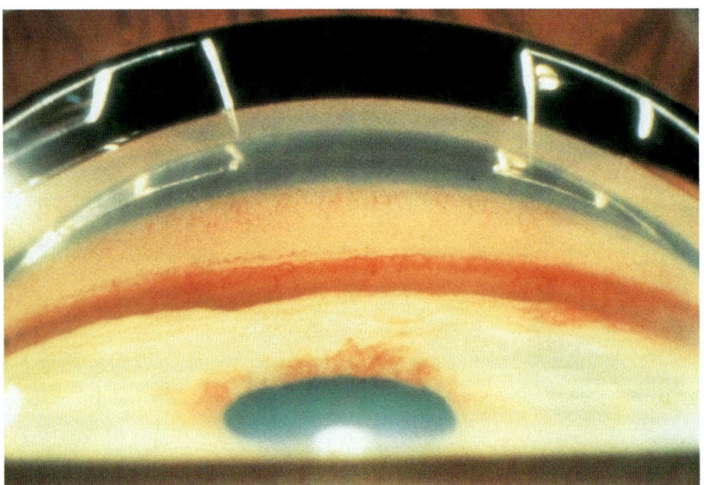

Figure 3-6 Goniophoto of an eye with neovascularization of the angle. *(Photograph courtesy of Tom Richardson, MD.)*

exfoliation syndrome (Sampaolesi's line). Other conditions that cause increased anterior chamber angle pigmentation include malignant melanoma, trauma, surgery, inflammation, angle closure, and hyphema.

Posttraumatic angle recession may be associated with monocular open-angle glaucoma. The gonioscopic criteria for diagnosing angle recession include

- an abnormally wide ciliary body band (Fig 3-8)
- increased prominence of the scleral spur
- torn iris processes

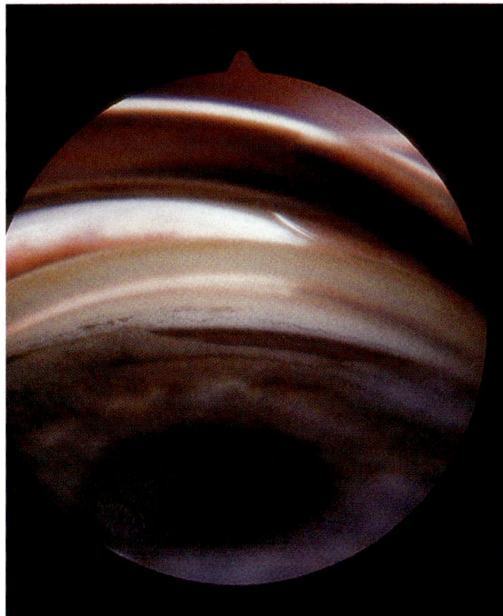

Figure 3-7 Goniophoto showing both an area of sheetlike PAS (left) and open angle (right). *(Photograph courtesy of Louis B. Cantor, MD.)*

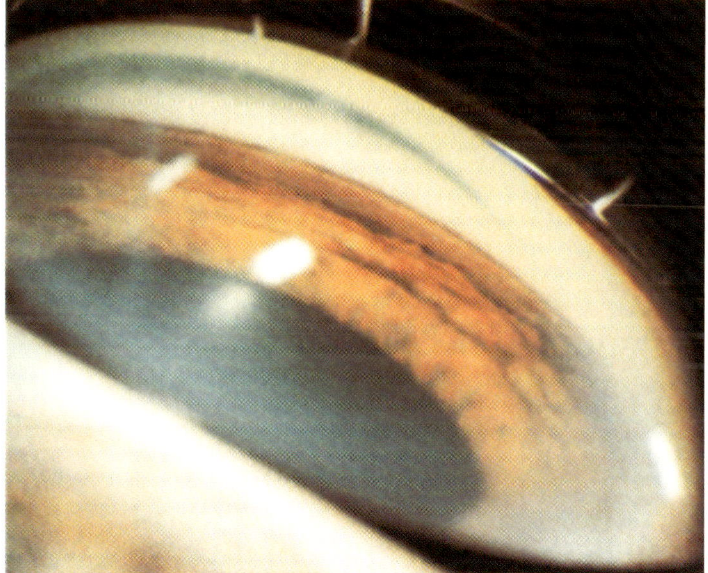

Figure 3-8 Angle recession. Note the widening of the ciliary body band. *(Reprinted with permission from Wright KW, ed.* Textbook of Ophthalmology. *Baltimore: Williams & Wilkins; 1997.)*

- marked variation of ciliary face width and angle depth in different quadrants of the same eye

In evaluating for angle recession, it is helpful to compare 1 part of the angle to other areas in the same eye or to the same area in the fellow eye.

Figure 3-9 illustrates the variety of gonioscopic findings caused by blunt trauma. If the ciliary body separates from the scleral spur (cyclodialysis), it will appear gonioscopically as a deep angle recess with a gap between the scleral spur and the ciliary body. Detection of a very small cleft may require ultrasound biomicroscopy. Other findings that may be visible gonioscopically are

- microhyphema or hypopyon
- retained anterior chamber foreign body
- iridodialysis
- angle precipitates suggestive of glaucomatocyclitic crisis
- pigmentation of the lens equator
- other peripheral lens abnormalities
- intraocular lens haptics
- ciliary body tumors

Campbell DG. A comparison of diagnostic techniques in angle-closure glaucoma. *Am J Ophthalmol.* 1979;88:197–204.

Fellman RL, Spaeth GL, Starita RJ. Gonioscopy: key to successful management of glaucoma. *Focal Points: Clinical Modules for Ophthalmologists.* San Francisco: American Academy of Ophthalmology; 1984, module 7.

The Optic Nerve

The entire visual pathway is described and illustrated in BCSC Section 5, *Neuro-Ophthalmology.* For further discussion of retinal involvement in the visual process, see Section 12, *Retina and Vitreous.*

Anatomy and Pathology

The optic nerve is the neural connection between the neurosensory retina and the lateral geniculate body. An understanding of the normal and pathologic appearance of the optic nerve allows clinicians to detect glaucoma, as well as follow glaucoma patients. The optic nerve is composed of neural tissue, glial tissue, extracellular matrix, and blood vessels. The human optic nerve consists of approximately 1.2–1.5 million axons of retinal ganglion cells (RGCs), although there is significant individual variability. The RGC cell bodies lie in the ganglion cell layer of the retina. The intraorbital optic nerve is divided into 2 components: the anterior optic nerve and the posterior optic nerve. The anterior optic nerve extends from the retinal surface to the retrolaminar region, just where the nerve exits the posterior aspect of the globe. The diameter of the optic nerve head and the intraocular portion of the optic nerve is approximately 1.5 mm; it expands to approximately 3–4 mm immediately upon exiting the globe. The increase in size is accounted for by axonal myelination, glial tissue, and the beginning of the leptomeninges (optic nerve sheath). The axons are separated into fascicles within the optic nerve, with the intervening spaces occupied by astrocytes.

In primates, 2 main subpopulations of RGCs are recognized: *magnocellular neurons (M cells)* and *parvocellular neurons (P cells).* Approximately 10% of RGCs are large M

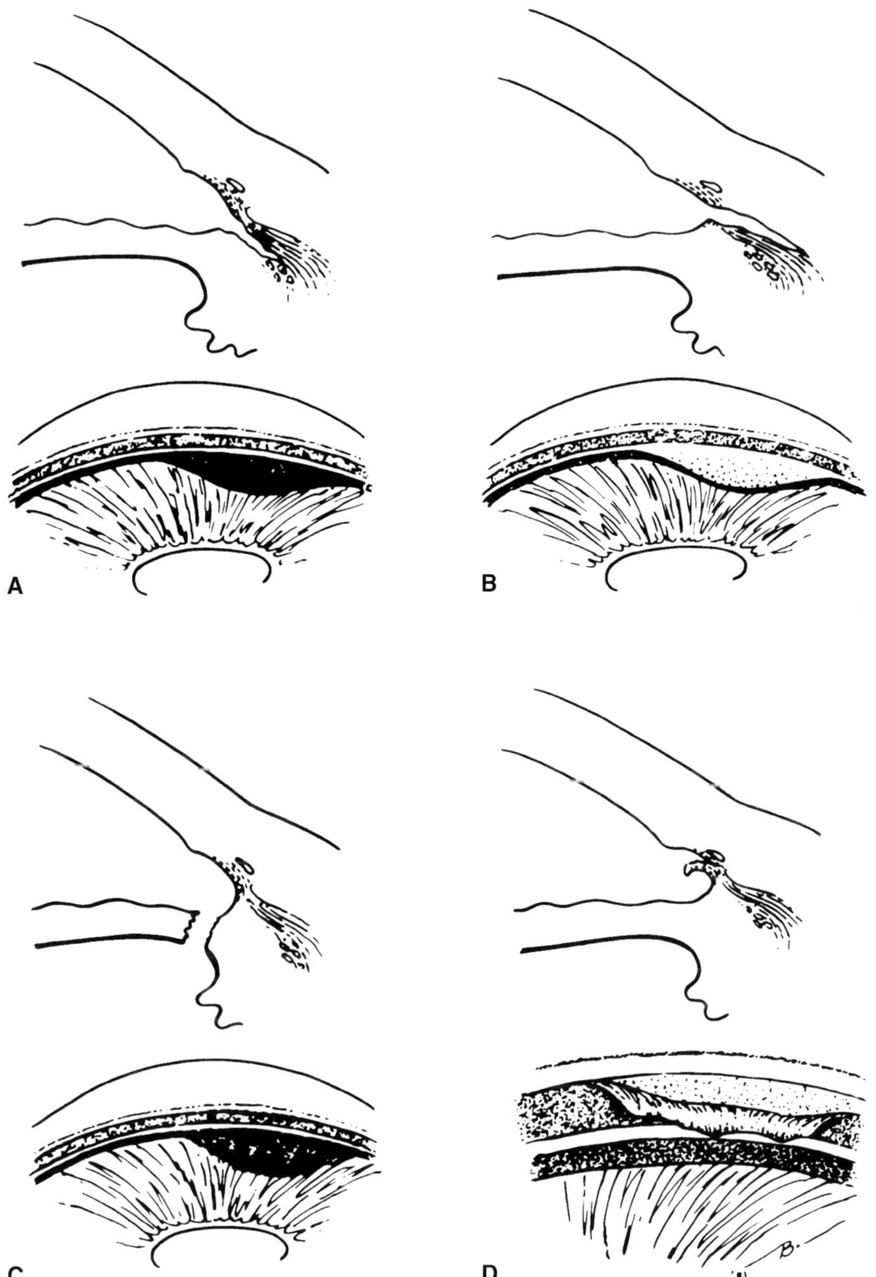

Figure 3-9 Forms of anterior chamber angle injury associated with blunt trauma, showing cross-sectional and corresponding gonioscopic appearance. **A,** Angle recession (tear between longitudinal and circular muscles of ciliary body). **B,** Cyclodialysis (separation of ciliary body from scleral spur) with widening of suprachoroidal space. **C,** Iridodialysis (tear in root of iris). **D,** Trabecular damage (tear in anterior portion of meshwork, creating a flap that is hinged at the scleral spur). *(Reproduced with permission from Shields MB.* Textbook of Glaucoma. *3rd ed. Baltimore: Williams & Wilkins; 1992.)*

cells. They have large-diameter axons, synapse in the magnocellular layer of the lateral geniculate body, and are sensitive to luminance changes in dim illumination (scotopic conditions). The smaller P cells account for approximately 90% of all ganglion cells. In comparison to the M cells, the P cells have smaller-diameter axons, smaller receptive fields, and slower conduction velocity. They synapse in the parvocellular layers of the lateral geniculate body. P cells subserve color vision, are most active under higher luminance conditions, and discriminate fine detail.

The distribution of nerve fibers as they enter the optic nerve head is shown in Figure 3-10. The arcuate nerve fibers entering the superior and inferior poles of the disc seem to be more susceptible to glaucomatous damage. This susceptibility explains the frequent occurrence of arcuate nerve fiber bundle visual field defects in glaucoma. The arrangement of the axons in the optic nerve head and their differential susceptibility to damage determines the patterns of visual field loss seen in glaucoma, which are described and illustrated later in this chapter.

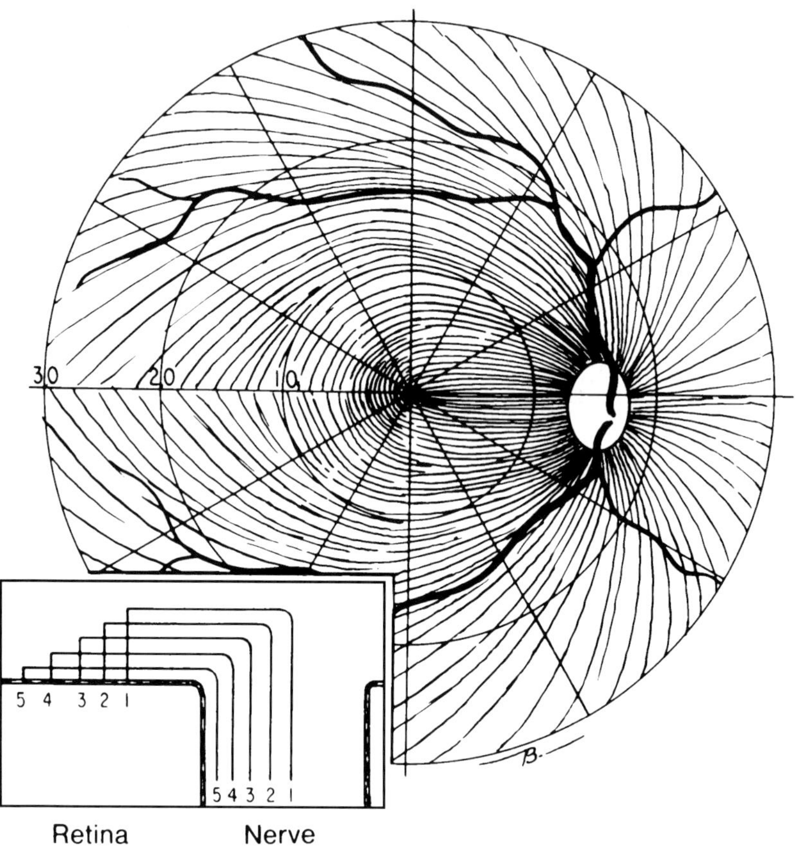

Figure 3-10 Anatomy of retinal nerve fiber distribution. Inset depicts cross-sectional view of axonal arrangement. Peripheral fibers run closer to choroid and exit in periphery of optic nerve, while fibers originating closer to the nerve head are situated closer to the vitreous and occupy a more central portion of the nerve. *(Reproduced with permission from Shields MB.* Textbook of Glaucoma. *3rd ed. Baltimore: Williams & Wilkins; 1992.)*

The anterior optic nerve can be divided into 4 layers (Fig 3-11):

- nerve fiber
- prelaminar
- laminar
- retrolaminar

The most anterior zone is the superficial nerve fiber layer region, which is continuous with the *nerve fiber layer* of the retina. This region is primarily composed of the axons of the RGCs in transition from the superficial retina to the neuronal component of the optic nerve. The nerve fiber layer can be viewed with the ophthalmoscope using the red-free (green) filter (red-free ophthalmoscopy). Immediately posterior to the nerve fiber

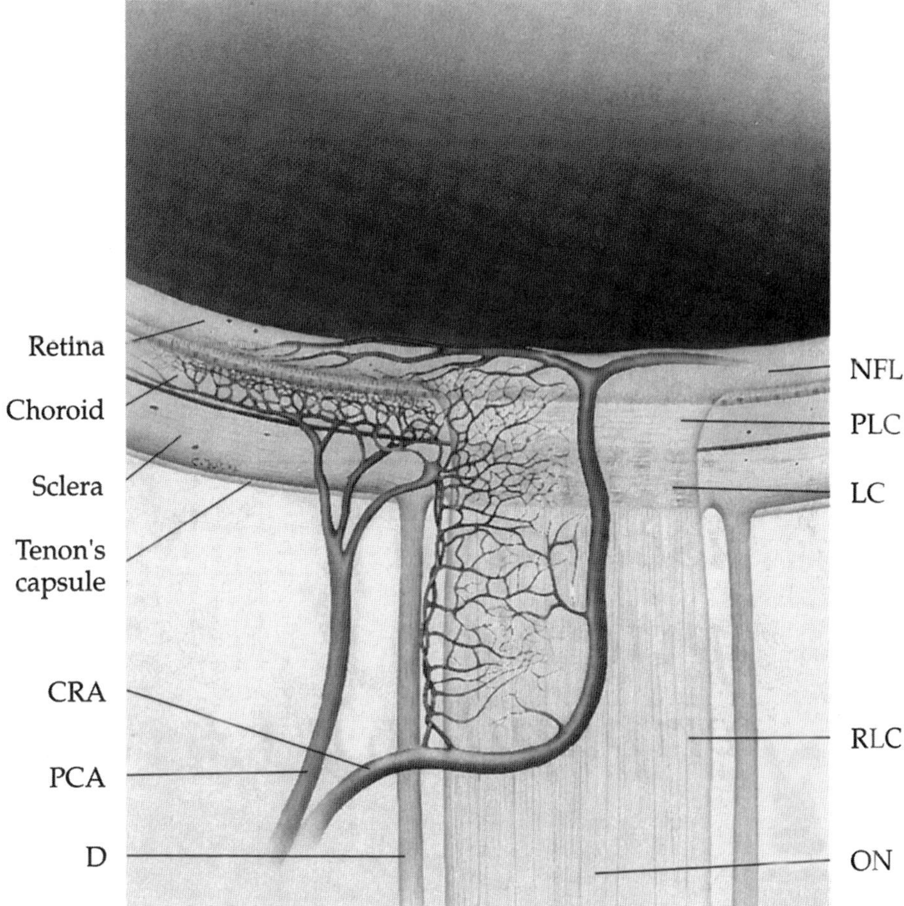

Figure 3-11 Anterior optic nerve vasculature. Arterial supply to the anterior optic nerve and peripapillay choroids. Lamina cribosa (LC), superficial nerve fiber layer (NFL), prelamina (PL), retrolamina (RL), cranial retinal artery (CRA), optic nerve (ON), choroid (C), posterior ciliary artery (PCA), retina (R), sclera (S). *(Reprinted with permission from Wright KW, ed.* Textbook of Ophthalmology. *Baltimore: Williams & Wilkins; 1997. Originally from Ritch R, Shields MB, Krupin T, eds.* The Glaucomas. *2nd ed. St. Louis: Mosby; 1996:178, Fig 8-2. Used with permission.)*

layer is the *prelaminar region,* which lies adjacent to the peripapillary choroid. More posteriorly, the *laminar region* is continuous with the sclera and is composed of the lamina cribrosa, a structure consisting of fenestrated, connective tissue lamellae that allow the transit of neural fibers through the scleral coat. Finally, the *retrolaminar region* lies posterior to the lamina cribrosa, is marked by the beginning of axonal myelination, and is surrounded by the leptomeninges of the central nervous system.

The laminar cribrosa is composed of a series of fenestrated sheets of connective tissue and elastic fibers. This layer provides the main support for the optic nerve as it exits the eye, penetrating the scleral coat. The beams of connective tissue are composed primarily of collagen; other extracellular matrix components include elastin, laminin, and fibronectin. These connective tissue beams are perforated by various-sized fenestrations through which the neural component of the optic nerve passes. In addition, larger, central fenestrations allow transit of the central retinal artery and central retinal vein. The fenestrations within the lamina have been described histologically as larger superiorly and inferiorly as compared to the temporal and nasal aspects of the optic nerve. It has been suggested that these differences play a role in the development of glaucomatous optic neuropathy. The fenestrations of the laminar cribrosa may often be seen, by ophthalmoscopy, at the base of the optic nerve head cup. Between the optic nerve and the adjacent choroidal and scleral tissue lies a rim of connective tissue, the ring of Elschnig. The connective tissue beams of the lamina cribrosa extend from this surrounding connective tissue border and are arranged in a series of parallel, stacked plates.

The vascular anatomy of the anterior optic nerve and peripapillary region has been extensively studied (see Fig 3-11). The arterial supply of the anterior optic nerve is derived entirely from branches of the ophthalmic artery via 1 to 5 posterior ciliary arteries. Typically, between 2 and 4 posterior ciliary arteries course anteriorly before dividing into approximately 10–20 short posterior ciliary arteries prior to entering the posterior globe. Often, the posterior ciliary arteries separate into a medial and a lateral group before branching into the short posterior ciliary arteries. The short posterior ciliary arteries penetrate the perineural sclera of the posterior globe to supply the peripapillary choroid, as well as most of the anterior optic nerve. Some short posterior ciliary arteries course, without branching, through the sclera directly into the choroid; others divide within the sclera to provide branches to both the choroid and the optic nerve. Often a noncontinuous, arterial circle exists within the perineural sclera, the circle of Zinn-Haller. The central retinal artery, also a posterior orbital branch of the ophthalmic artery, penetrates the optic nerve approximately 10–15 mm behind the globe. The central retinal artery has few if any intraneural branches, the exception being an occasional small branch within the retrolaminar region, which may anastomose with the pial system. The central retinal artery courses adjacent to the central retinal vein within the central portion of the optic nerve.

The superficial nerve fiber layer is supplied principally by recurrent retinal arterioles branching from the central retinal artery. These small vessels, originating in the peripapillary nerve fiber layer, run toward the center of the optic nerve head and have been referred to as "epipapillary vessels." The capillary branches from these vessels are continuous with the retinal capillaries at the disc margin, but they also have posterior anastomoses with the prelaminar capillaries of the optic nerve. The temporal nerve fiber layer may have an arterial contribution from the cilioretinal artery, when it is present.

The prelaminar region is principally supplied by direct branches of the short posterior ciliary arteries and by branches of the circle of Zinn-Haller, when it is present. In eyes with a well-developed circle of Zinn-Haller, arterial branches emerge to supply both the prelaminar and laminar regions. The lamina cribrosa region also receives its blood supply from branches of the short posterior ciliary arteries or from branches of the circle of Zinn-Haller; this is similar to the prelaminar region. These precapillary branches perforate the outer aspects of the lamina cribrosa before branching into an intraseptal capillary network. Arterioles also branch from the short posterior ciliary arteries and the circle of Zinn-Haller and course posteriorly to supply the pial arteries. These pial arteries often contribute to the laminar region. As in the prelaminar region, the larger vessels of the peripapillary choroid may contribute occasional small arterioles to this region, although there is no connection between the peripapillary choriocapillaris and the capillaries of the optic nerve.

The retrolaminar region is also supplied by branches from the short posterior ciliary arteries, as well as by the pial arterial branches coursing adjacent to the retrolaminar optic nerve region. The pial arteries originate from both the central retinal artery, before it pierces the retrobulbar optic nerve, and branches of the short posterior ciliary arteries more anteriorly. The central retinal artery may supply several small intraneural branches in the retrolaminar region.

The rich capillary beds of each of the 4 anatomic regions within the anterior optic nerve are anatomically confluent. The venous drainage of the anterior optic nerve is almost exclusively via a single vein, the central retinal vein. In the nerve fiber layer, blood is drained directly into the retinal veins, which then join to form the central retinal vein. In the prelaminar, laminar, and retrolaminar regions, venous drainage also occurs via the central retinal vein or axial tributaries to the central retinal vein.

Glaucomatous Optic Neuropathy

Glaucomatous optic neuropathy is the sine qua non of all forms of glaucoma (Fig 3-12). On a histologic level, early glaucomatous cupping consists of loss of axons, blood vessels, and glial cells. The loss of tissue seems to start at the level of the lamina cribrosa and is associated with compaction and fusion of the laminar plates. It is most pronounced at the superior and inferior poles of the disc. Structural optic nerve changes usually may precede detectable functional loss.Tissue destruction in more advanced glaucoma extends behind the cribriform plate, and the lamina bows backward. The optic nerve head takes on an excavated and undermined appearance that has been likened to a bean pot.

Glaucomatous cupping in infants and children is accompanied by an expansion of the entire scleral ring, which may explain why cupping seems to occur earlier in children and why reversibility of cupping is more prominent with successful treatment in these cases. Cupping may be reversed in adults as well, but such reversal is less frequent and more subtle.

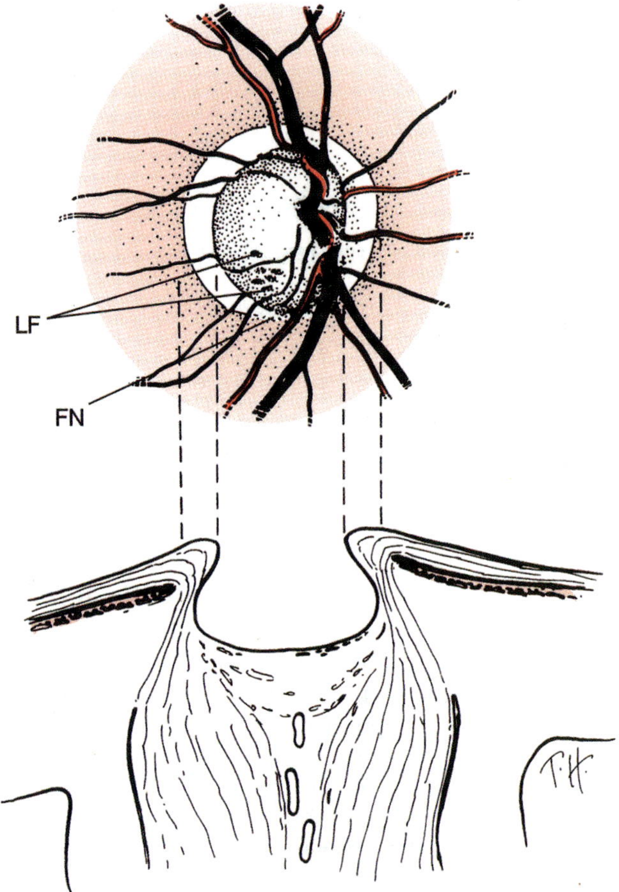

Figure 3-12 Glaucomatous optic nerve (anterior optic nerve head and transverse view, right eye). Note the thinning and undermining of inferior neuroretinal rim and focal notching (FN) of inferior neuroretinal rim, enlarged central cup with visible laminar fenestrations (LF), nasal shift of retinal vessels, and peripapillary atrophy. *(Reprinted with permission from Wright KW, ed.* Textbook of Ophthalmology. *Baltimore: Williams & Wilkins; 1997.)*

Theories of Glaucomatous Optic Nerve Damage

The development of glaucomatous optic neuropathy likely results from a variety of factors, both intrinsic and extrinsic to the optic nerve. Elevated IOP plays a major role in the development of glaucomatous optic neuropathy in most individuals and is considered the most significant risk factor. Unilateral secondary glaucoma, experimental models of glaucoma, and observations of the effect of lowering IOP in patients all point to this conclusion. But it is also clear that factors other than pressure contribute to a given individual's susceptibility to glaucomatous damage.

Two hypotheses have emerged to explain the development of glaucomatous optic neuropathy, the mechanical and ischemic theories. The *mechanical theory* stresses the importance of direct compression of the axonal fibers and support structures of the anterior optic nerve, with distortion of the lamina cribrosa plates and interruption of axoplasmic flow resulting in the death of the RGCs. The *ischemic theory* focuses on the potential development of intraneural ischemia resulting from decreased optic nerve perfusion. This perfusion may result from the stress of IOP on the blood supply to the nerve or from processes intrinsic to the optic nerve.

Disturbance of vascular *autoregulation* may contribute to decreased perfusion and nerve damage. The optic nerve vessels normally increase or decrease their tone to maintain a constant blood flow independent of IOP and blood pressure variations. A disturbance in vascular autoregulation may result in decreased optic nerve blood flow from increased IOP. Alternatively, changes in systemic hemodynamics may result in perfusion deficits, even at normal IOP. Such hypothetical derangement could be related to abnormal vessels or to circulating vasoactive substances, for example.

Current thinking regarding glaucomatous optic neuropathy recognizes that both vascular and mechanical factors probably contribute to damage. The glaucomas are likely a heterogeneous family of disorders, and the ganglion cell death seen in glaucomatous optic neuropathy may be mediated by many factors. Active investigations continue to examine the potential role in glaucomatous optic neuropathy of processes such as excitotoxicity, apoptosis, neurotrophin deprivation, ischemia, and autoimmunity.

Examination of the Optic Nerve Head

The optic disc can be examined clinically with a direct ophthalmoscope, an indirect ophthalmoscope, or a slit-lamp biomicroscope using a posterior pole lens. The direct ophthalmoscope provides a view of the optic disc through a small pupil. In addition, when used with a red-free filter, it enhances detection of the nerve fiber layer of the posterior pole. However, the direct ophthalmoscope does not provide sufficient stereoscopic detail to detect subtle changes in optic disc topography.

The *indirect ophthalmoscope* is used for examining the optic disc in young children, uncooperative patients, individuals with high myopia, and individuals with substantial opacities of the media. With the indirect ophthalmoscope, cupping of the optic nerve can be detected, but, in general, optic nerve cupping and pallor appear less than with slit-lamp methods, and the magnification is often inadequate for detecting subtle or localized details important in the evaluation of glaucoma. Thus, the indirect ophthalmoscope is not recommended for routine use in examining the optic disc.

The best method of examination for the diagnosis of glaucoma is the *slit lamp* combined with a Hruby lens; a posterior pole contact lens; or a 60, 78, or 90 D lens. The slit beam, rather than diffuse illumination, is useful for determining subtle changes in the contour of the nerve head. This system provides high magnification, excellent illumination, and a stereoscopic view of the disc. Slit-lamp techniques require some patient cooperation and moderate pupil size for adequate visibility of the disc.

Clinical Evaluation of the Optic Nerve Head

The *optic nerve head,* or *optic disc,* is usually round or slightly oval in shape and contains a central *cup.* The tissue between the cup and the disc margin is called the *neural rim* or *neuroretinal rim.* The rim in normal patients has a relatively uniform width and a color that ranges from orange to pink. The size of the physiologic cup is developmentally determined and is related to the size of the disc. For a given number of nerve fibers, the larger the overall disc area, the larger the cup. The cup–disc ratio may increase slightly with age. Nonglaucomatous black individuals, on average, have larger disc areas and larger cup–disc ratios than do whites, although a substantial overlap exists. On average, people with myopia have larger eyes and larger discs and cups than do those with normal vision and those with hyperopia.

Differentiating physiologic or normal cupping from acquired *glaucomatous cupping* of the optic disc can be difficult. The early changes of glaucomatous optic neuropathy are very subtle (Table 3-2):

- generalized enlargement of the cup
- focal enlargement of the cup
- superficial splinter hemorrhage
- loss of nerve fiber layer
- translucency of the neuroretinal rim
- development of vessel overpass
- asymmetry of cupping between the patient's eyes
- peripapillary atrophy

Generalized enlargement of the cup may be the earliest change detected in glaucoma. This enlargement can be difficult to appreciate unless previous photographs or diagrams are available. It is useful to compare one eye to the fellow eye because disc asymmetry is unusual in normal individuals (Fig 3-13). The vertical cup–disc ratio is normally between 0.1 and 0.4, although as many as 5% of normal individuals will have cup–disc ratios larger than 0.6. Asymmetry of the cup–disc ratio of more than 0.2 occurs in less than 1% of normal individuals. This asymmetry may be related to disc size asymmetry. Increased size of the physiologic cup may be a familial trait and it is also seen with high myopia. An oblong insertion of the optic nerve into the globe of individuals with high myopia may also cause a tilted appearance to the optic nerve head. Examination of other family members may clarify whether a large cup is inherited or acquired.

Focal enlargement of the cup appears as localized notching or narrowing of the rim. Focal atrophy most typically occurs at the inferior and superior temporal poles of the optic nerve in early glaucomatous optic neuropathy. Thinning of the neuroretinal rim with development of a focal notch or extension of the cup into the neuroretinal rim may be seen. Deep localized notching, where the lamina cribrosa is visible at the disc margin, is sometimes termed an *acquired optic disc pit.* If notching or acquired pit formation

Table 3-2 Ophthalmoscopic Signs of Glaucoma

Generalized	Focal	Less Specific
Large optic cup	Narrowing (notching) of the rim	Exposed lamina cribrosa
Asymmetry of the cups	Vertical elongation of the cup	Nasal displacement of vessels
Progressive enlargement of the cup	Cupping to the rim margin	Baring of circumlinear vessels
	Regional pallor	Peripapillary crescent
	Splinter hemorrhage	
	Nerve fiber layer loss	

occurs at either (or both) the superior or inferior pole of the disc, the cup becomes vertically oval (Fig 3-14). Even in the normal eye, laminar trabeculations or pores may be seen as grayish dots in the base of the physiologic cup. With glaucomatous optic neuropathy, neural atrophy results in more extensive exposure of the underlying lamina and may reveal more laminar pores in the optic nerve cup. Nasalization of the central retinal artery and central retinal vein is often seen as the cup enlarges.

Splinter, or nerve fiber layer, hemorrhages usually appear as a linear red streak on or near the disc surface (Fig 3-15). Nerve fiber layer hemorrhages may occur at the neural retinal rim or in the peripapillary area in as many as one third of glaucoma patients at some time during the course of their disease. Hemorrhages typically clear over several weeks to months but are often followed by localized notching of the rim and visual field loss. Some glaucoma patients have repeated episodes of optic disc hemorrhage; others have none. Individuals with normal-tension glaucoma are more likely to have disc

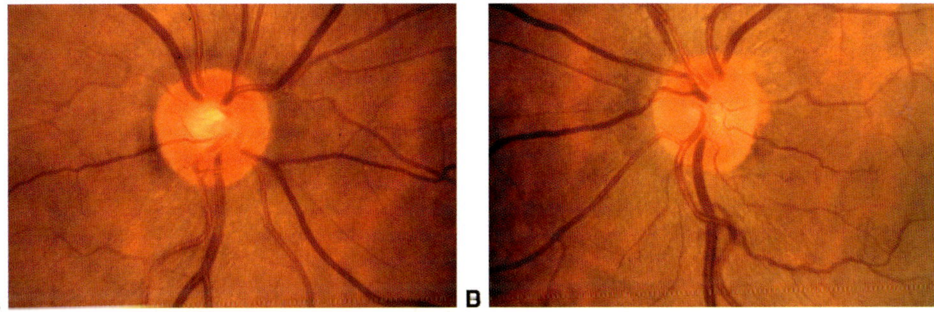

Figure 3-13 Asymmetry of optic nerve cupping. Note the generalized enlargement of the cup in the right eye **(A)** as compared to the left eye **(B).** Asymmetry of the cup–disc ratio of more than 0.2 occurs in less than 1% of normal individuals. *(Photograph courtesy G. A. Cioffi, MD.)*

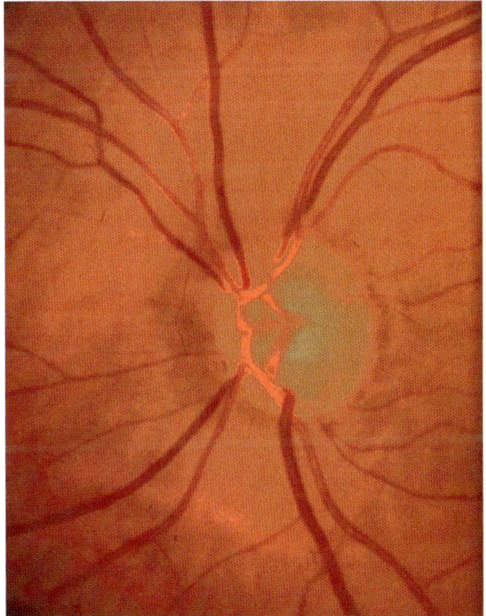

Figure 3-14 Vertical elongation of the cup with localized thinning of the inferior temporal neural retinal rim in the left eye of a patient with moderately advanced glaucoma. *(Photograph courtesy of G. A. Cioffi, MD.)*

hemorrhages. Optic disc hemorrhage is an important prognostic sign for the development or progression of visual field loss, and any patient with a splinter hemorrhage requires detailed evaluation and follow-up. Splinter disc hemorrhages may be caused by posterior vitreous detachments, diabetes mellitus, branch retinal vein occlusions, and anticoagulation.

Axons in the nerve fiber layer of the normal eye may best be visualized with red-free illumination. The nerve fiber layer extending from the neuroretinal rim to the surrounding peripapillary retina appears as fine striations created by the bundles of axons. In the healthy eye, the nerve fiber layer bundles have a plush, refractile appearance. With progressing glaucomatous optic neuropathy, the nerve fiber layer thins and becomes less visible. The loss may be diffuse (generalized) or localized to specific bundles (Fig 3-16). *Focal abnormalities* can consist of slitlike grooves or wedge defects. Slitlike defects can be seen in normal retinal nerve fiber layer anatomy, although they usually do not extend to

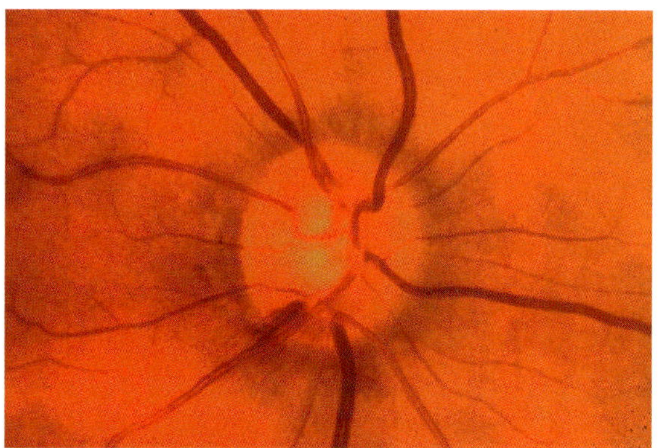

Figure 3-15 Splinter hemorrhage of the right optic nerve at the 7 o'clock position in a patient with early open-angle glaucoma. *(Photograph courtesy of G. A. Cioffi, MD.)*

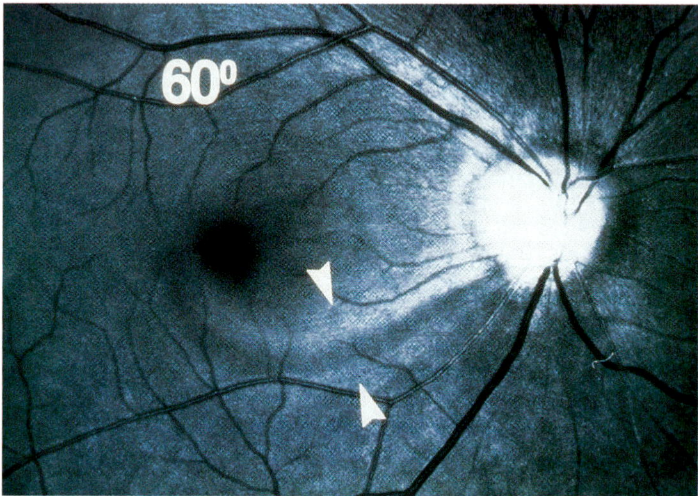

Figure 3-16 Nerve fiber layer photograph shows a nerve fiber bundle defect *(arrowheads)*. *(Photograph courtesy of Louis B. Cantor, MD.)*

the disc margin. Early wedge defects are sometimes visible only at a distance from the optic disc margin. *Diffuse nerve fiber loss* is more common in glaucoma than focal loss but also more difficult to observe. The nerve fiber layer can be visualized clearly in high-contrast black-and-white photographs, and experienced observers can recognize even early disease if good-quality photographs are available. Direct ophthalmoscopy and slit-lamp techniques can both be successfully employed to observe the retinal nerve fiber layer. The combination of red-free filter, wide slit beam, and posterior pole lens at the slit lamp affords the best view.

In the early stages of nerve fiber loss, often before enlargement of the cup, existing neuroretinal rim tissue can be observed to become more translucent. The clinician can best observe this rim translucency by using a lens at the slit-lamp biomicroscope, employing a thin slit beam and confining the beam to the disc surface.

As the nerve fiber loss continues, the cup may begin to enlarge by progressive posterior collapse and compaction of the remaining viable nerve fibers. In circumstances where the neuroretinal tissue—but not the overlying nerve head vasculature—has collapsed, vessel overpass can often be observed. The blood vessels overlying the collapsed neural rim tissue look like a highway overpass suspended over—but not in contact with—the underlying tissue.

Peripapillary atrophy is often observed in glaucomatous eyes. It is seen with greater frequency and is more extensive in eyes with glaucoma than in unaffected eyes. The location of the atrophy often correlates with the position of visual field defects. Other less specific signs of glaucomatous damage include nasal displacement of the vessels, narrowing of peripapillary retinal vessels, and baring of the circumlinear vessels. With advanced damage, the cup becomes pale and markedly excavated.

Quantitative measurement of the optic nerve head and retinal nerve fiber layer

Since the 1850s, the appearance of the optic nerve head has been recognized as critical in assessing the disease status of glaucoma. However, optic disc assessment can be quite subjective, and inter- and intraobserver variation is greater than desirable, given the importance of accurate assessments. Thus, the need for reliable and objective measures of optic disc and associated retinal nerve fiber layer morphology is clear. A number of sophisticated image analysis systems have been developed in recent years to evaluate the optic disc and retinal nerve fiber layer. These instruments give quantitative measurements of various anatomic parameters.

Confocal scanning laser ophthalmoscopy can be used to create a 3-dimensional image of the optic nerve head. The optical design of instruments using confocal scanning laser technology allows for a series of tomographic "slices," or optical sections, of the structure being imaged. The images acquired by this method are stored as a computer data file and manipulated to reconstruct the 3-dimensional structure, display the image, and perform data analysis. Parameters such as cup area, cup volume, rim volume, cup–disc ratio, and peripapillary nerve fiber layer thickness are then calculated.

Techniques such as scanning laser polarimetry and optical coherence tomography have been used to acquire images of the retinal nerve fiber layer. The *scanning laser polarimeter* is essentially a scanning laser ophthalmoscope outfitted with a polarization modulator and detector to take advantage of the birefringent properties of the retinal nerve fiber layer arising from the predominantly parallel nature of its microtubule substructure. As light passes through the nerve fiber layer, the polarization state changes. The deeper layers of retinal tissue reflect the light back to the detector, where the degree to which the polarization has been changed is recorded. The acquired data can then be stored, displayed, and manipulated by computer programs, as with the unmodified confocal scanning laser ophthalmoscope. The fundamental parameter being measured with this instrumentation is *relative* (not absolute) retinal nerve fiber layer thickness.

Optical coherence tomography (OCT) uses interferometry and low coherence light to obtain a high-resolution cross section of biological structures. The resolution of OCT instrumentation in the eye is approximately 10 μm, and OCT has the potential to yield an absolute measurement of nerve fiber layer thickness. In vivo OCT measurements appear to correlate with histologic measurements of the same tissues.

Quantitative measurement of the optic disc and retinal nerve fiber layer is a promising nascent science. The instrumentation and techniques used to acquire quantitative imaging and analysis of nerve head and nerve fiber layer anatomic parameters are rapidly evolving. Both for single measurements directed at detecting the presence of glaucoma and, especially, for serial measurements necessary to determine clinical progression of glaucoma, these technologies have great potential. The clinician must remember that no system of measurement and observation is currently more useful or has proven more reliable than good-quality stereophotographs combined with detailed and careful clinical examination.

Chen YY, Chen PP, Xu L, et al. Correlation of peripapillary nerve fiber layer thickness by scanning laser polarimetry with visual field defects in patients with glaucoma. *J Glaucoma.* 1998;7:312–316.

Wollstein G, Garway-Heath DF, Hitchings RA. Identification of early glaucoma cases with the scanning laser ophthalmoscope. *Ophthalmology.* 1998;105:1557–1563.

Recording of optic nerve findings

It is common practice to grade an optic disc by comparing the diameter of the cup to the diameter of the disc. This ratio is usually expressed as a decimal such as 0.2, but such a description poorly conveys the appearance of the nerve head. To avoid confusion, the examiner must specify whether the cup is being defined by the change in *color* or in *contour* between the central area of the disc and the surrounding rim. Furthermore, the examiner must specify what is being measured: the horizontal diameter, the vertical diameter, or the longest diameter of the disc. If cup–disc ratios are to be used, the description should include the dimensions of the cup specified by both color and contour criteria in both the vertical and horizontal meridians. The rim, which contains the neural elements, should also be described in detail: color, width, focal thinning or pallor, and slope.

A detailed, annotated diagram of the optic disc topography is preferable to the recording of a simple cup–disc ratio. The diagram must be of adequate size to allow depiction of important topographic landmarks and morphologic features. With annotation, the diagram can convey the cup–disc ratio along all dimensions and serves to document the presence or absence of regions of rim thinning, notching, hemorrhage, rim translucency, vessel overpass, and other findings.

Photography, particularly simultaneous stereophotography, is an excellent method for recording the appearance of the optic nerve for detailed examination and sequential follow-up. This record allows the examiner to compare the present status of the patient to baseline status without resorting to memory or grading systems. Moreover, photographs allow better evaluation when a patient has changed doctors. Sometimes subtle optic disc changes become apparent when the clinician compares 1 set of photographs to a previous set. Careful diagrams of the optic nerve head are useful when photography is not possible or available.

The Visual Field

The ultimate goal of glaucoma management is the preservation of the patient's visual function and quality of life. Visual function is a very complex concept that can be measured in a variety of ways. For many years, the standard measurement has been clinical perimetry, which measures differential light sensitivity, or the ability of the subject to distinguish a stimulus light from background illumination. As usually performed in glaucoma examinations, the test uses white light and measures what is conventionally referred to as the *visual field.* The classic description of the visual field given by Harry Moss Traquair (1875–1954) is "an island hill of vision in a sea of darkness." The island of vision is usually described as a 3-dimensional graphic representation of differential light sensitivity at different positions in space (Fig 3-17).

Perimetry refers to the clinical assessment of the visual field. Perimetry has traditionally served 2 major purposes in the management of glaucoma:

1. identification of abnormal fields
2. quantitative assessment of normal or abnormal fields to guide follow-up care

Quantification of visual field sensitivity enables detection of initial loss by comparison with normative data. Regular visual field testing in known cases of disease provides valuable information in helping differentiate between stability and progressive loss. It is likely that in individual patients, different tests will show abnormalities at different times. Some methods may be better for identification than for following the progression of defects, and vice versa.

Over the last 2 decades, automated static perimetry has become the standard for assessing visual function in glaucoma. With this procedure, threshold sensitivity measurements are usually performed at a number of test locations using white stimuli on a white background; this is known as standard automated perimetry (SAP), or achromatic automated perimetry. Assessment of threshold sensitivity by SAP traditionally uses simple staircase algorithms that employ a bracketing approach to estimate threshold. Recently, other technologies have become available that may be useful in evaluating the visual field. Evidence from detailed investigations using these newer perimetric tests, such as short-wavelength automated perimetry, high-pass resolution perimetry, and frequency-doubling technology perimetry, strongly suggest that they may provide beneficial clinical information.

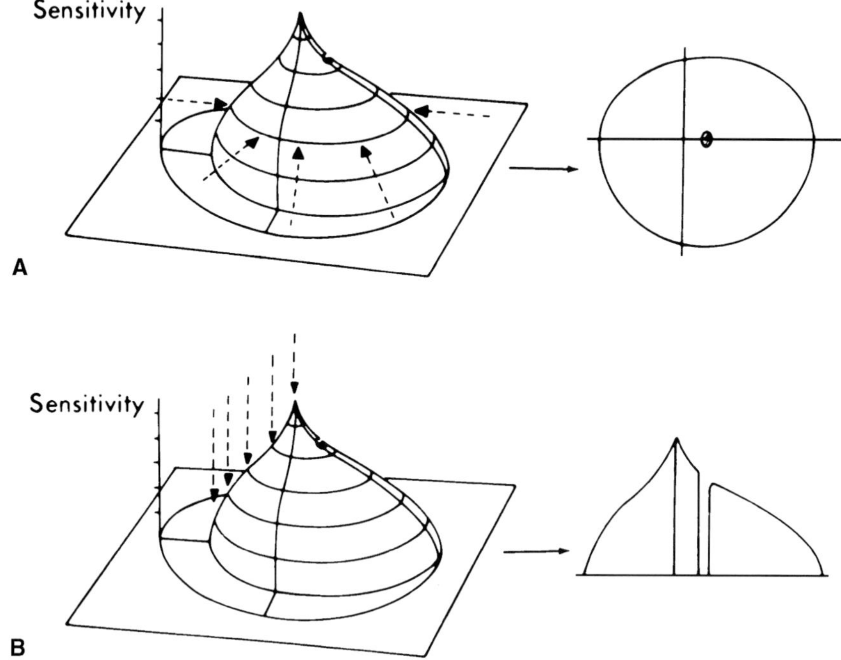

Figure 3-17 **A,** Isopter (kinetic) perimetry. Test object of fixed intensity is moved along several meridians toward fixation. Points where the object is first perceived are plotted in a circle. **B,** Static perimetry. Stationary test object is increased in intensity from below threshold until perceived by patient. Threshold values yield a graphic profile section. *(Reproduced with permission from Kolker AE, Hetherington J, eds.* Becker-Shaffer's Diagnosis and Therapy of the Glaucomas. *5th ed. St Louis: Mosby; 1983. Modified from Aulhorn E, Harms H. In: Leydhecker W.* Glaucoma. *Tutzing Symposium. Basel: S Karger; 1967.)*

A description of these newer perimetric tests follows:

- *short-wavelength automated perimetry (SWAP)*; also known as blue-yellow perimetry. Standard perimeters are available that can project a blue stimulus onto a yellow background. This method is sensitive in the early identification of glaucomatous damage. Several studies suggest that the rate of development of perimetric defects in early glaucoma may be higher with blue on yellow (short-wavelength) testing than with conventional (achromatic) white-on-white visual fields.
- *high-pass resolution perimetry.* The stimulus used to test the visual field is a ring-shaped target that varies in size. It is made up of a dark annulus with bright center and dark borders. The average luminance of this target is the same as the background. Thus, the test stimulus is designed to determine spatial resolution thresholds. Test times using high-pass resolution perimetry are shorter than those used in conventional perimetry.
- *frequency-doubling technology (FDT) perimetry.* This visual field testing paradigm uses a low spatial frequency sinusoidal grating undergoing rapid phase-reversal flicker. Commercially available instruments employ a 0.25 cycle per degree grating, phase-reversed at a rapid 25 Hz. When a low spatial frequency grating is presented in this manner, it appears to have twice as many alternating light and dark bars than are actually present—hence the term *frequency doubling.* It is believed that

the stimuli employed in this test preferentially activate the M cells and may be more sensitive in the detection of early glaucomatous loss.

Other measures of visual field include:

- *contrast sensitivity.* This test measures a subject's ability to detect a pattern of alternating light and dark bands presented at varying frequencies and degrees of contrast.
- *flicker sensitivity.* This test measures the ability of the subject to recognize the difference between a flickering light and one that is constantly on. The contrast can be varied.
- *visually evoked cortical potentials (VECP,* also *VEP* or *VER)* and *electroretinography (ERG).* Cortical (VECP) or retinal (ERG) electrical responses to a stimulus, such as a reversing pattern of light and dark squares or a flickering light, are recorded. The multifocal ERG and multifocal VEP may be a useful objective test for assessing RGC function. Although these tests require visual attention, they do not require a subjective response.

Several of these tests are discussed in greater detail in BCSC Section 12, *Retina and Vitreous.*

Clinical Perimetry

Two major types of perimetry are in general use today:

- automated static perimetry using a bowl perimeter or video monitor
- manual kinetic and static perimetry using a Goldmann-type bowl perimeter

In the United States, the predominant automated static perimeters are currently the Humphrey Visual Field Analyzers I and II. Most of the clinical examples given are from Humphrey perimeters, and the descriptions apply most directly to these instruments. However, many of the principles apply to a number of other perimeters.

The following are brief definitions of some of the major perimetric terms:

- *threshold:* The differential light sensitivity at which a stimulus of given size and duration of presentation is seen 50% of the time—in practice, the dimmest spot detected during testing.
- *suprathreshold:* Above the threshold; generally used to mean brighter than the threshold stimulus. A stimulus may also be made suprathreshold by increasing the size or duration of presentation. This is generally used for screening paradigms.
- *kinetic testing:* Perimetry in which a target is moved from an area where it is not seen toward an area where it is just seen. This is usually performed manually by a perimetrist who chooses the target, moves it, and records the results.
- *static testing:* A stationary stimulus is presented at various locations. In theory, the brightness, size, and duration of the stimulus can be varied at each location to determine the threshold. In practice, in a given automated test session, only the brightness is varied. Although static perimetry may be done manually—and is often combined with manual kinetic perimetry—in current practice the term usually refers to automated perimetry.

- *isopter:* A line on a visual field representation—usually on a 2-dimensional sheet of paper—connecting points with the same threshold.
- *depression:* A decrease in retinal sensitivity.
- *scotoma:* An area of decreased retinal sensitivity within the visual field surrounded by an area of greater sensitivity.
- *decibel (dB):* A 0.1 log unit. This is a relative term used in both kinetic and static perimetry that has no absolute value. Its value depends on the maximum illumination of the perimeter. As usually used, it refers to log units of attenuation of the maximum light intensity available in the perimeter being used.

Patterns of Glaucomatous Nerve Loss

The hallmark defect of glaucoma is the nerve fiber bundle defect that results from damage at the optic nerve head. The pattern of nerve fibers in the retinal area served by the damaged nerve fiber bundle will correspond to the specific defect. The common names for the classic visual field defects are derived from their appearance as plotted on a kinetic visual field chart. In static perimetry, however, the sample points are in a grid pattern, and the representation of visual field defects on a static perimetry chart generally lacks the smooth contours suggested by such terms as *arcuate.*

Glaucomatous visual field defects include the following:

- generalized depression
- paracentral scotoma (Fig 3-18)
- arcuate or Bjerrum scotoma (Fig 3-19)
- nasal step (Fig 3-20)
- altitudinal defect (Fig 3-21)
- temporal wedge

The superior and inferior poles of the optic nerve appear to be most susceptible to glaucomatous damage. However, damage to small, scattered bundles of optic nerve axons commonly produces a generalized decrease in sensitivity, which is harder to recognize than focal defects. Combinations of superior and inferior visual field loss, such as double arcuate scotomata, may occur, resulting in profound peripheral vision loss. Typically, the central island of vision and inferior temporal visual field are retained until late in the course of glaucomatous optic nerve damage (Fig 3-22).

Variables in Perimetry

Whether automated or manual, perimetry is subject to many variables, including the human elements involving the patient and the perimetrist.

Patient

People vary in their attentiveness and response time from moment to moment and from day to day. Longer tests are more likely to produce fatigue and diminish the ability of the patient to maintain peak performance.

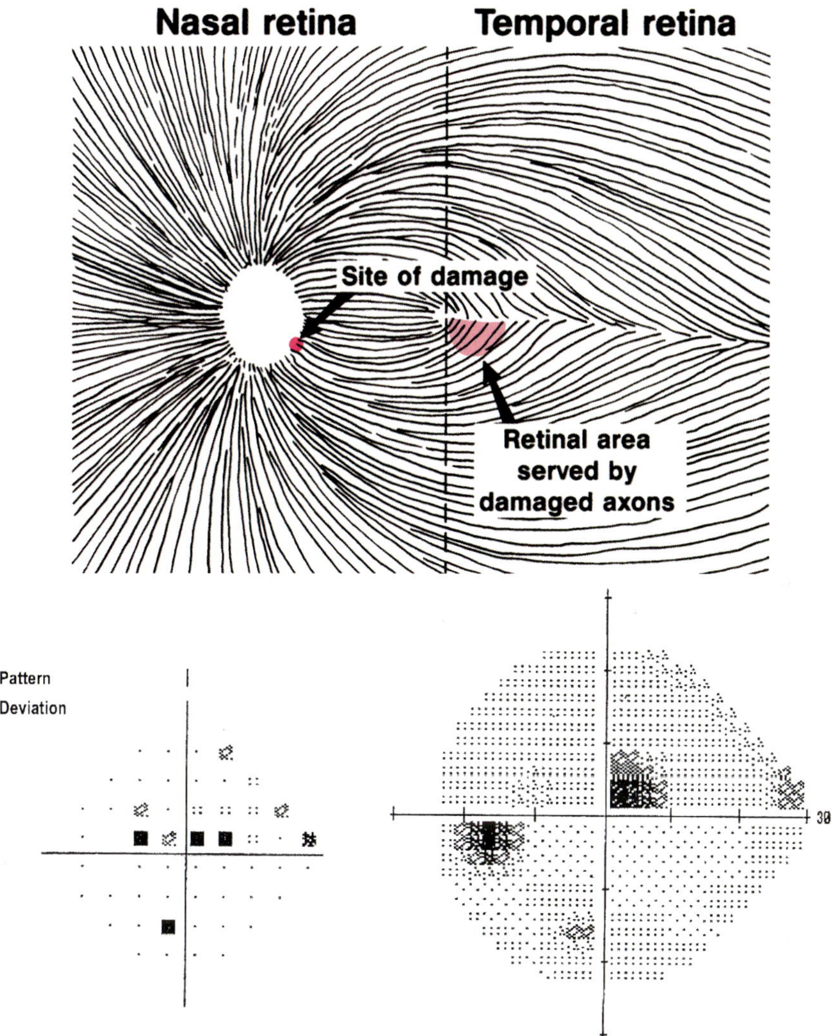

Figure 3-18 A *paracentral scotoma* is an island of relative or absolute visual loss within 10° of fixation. Loss of nerve fibers from the inferior pole, originating from the inferotemporal retina, resulted in the superonasal scotoma shown. Paracentral scotomata may be single, as in this case, or multiple, and they may occur as isolated findings or may be associated with other early defects (Humphrey 30-2 program). *(Visual field courtesy of G. A. Cioffi, MD.)*

Perimetrist

The individual performing manual perimetry can administer the test slightly differently each time. Different technicians or physicians also vary from one another. Perimetrist bias is markedly diminished with automated testing. However, the perimetrist can have an effect on test outcome even in automated testing, by monitoring the patient for proper performance and positioning. Most automated instruments can be paused during the test by perimetrist intervention, thereby allowing repositioning or other adjustments to enhance test reliability.

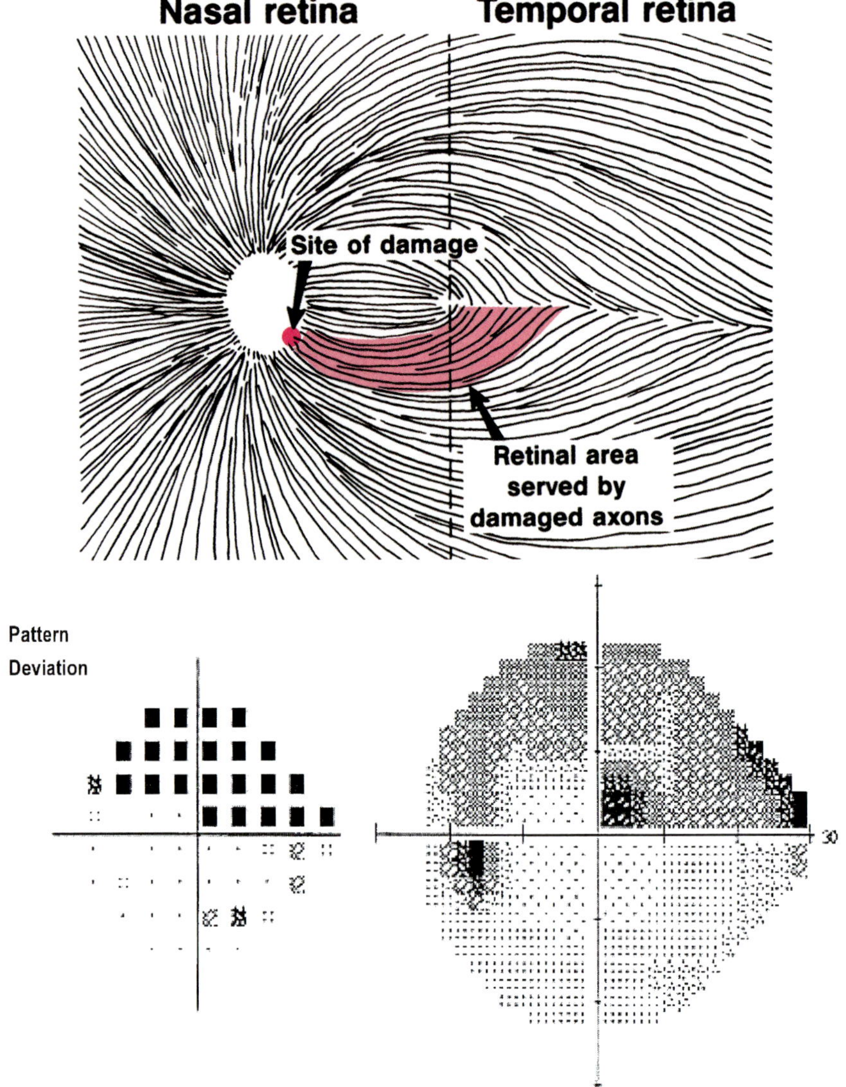

Figure 3-19 An *arcuate scotoma* occurs in the area 10°–20° from fixation. Glaucomatous damage to a nerve fiber bundle that contains axons from both inferonasal and inferotemporal retina resulted in the arcuate defect shown. The scotoma often begins as a single area of relative loss, which then becomes larger, deeper, and multifocal. In its full form an arcuate scotoma arches from the blind spot and ends at the nasal raphe, becoming wider and closer to fixation on the nasal side (Octopus 32 program). *(Visual field courtesy of G. A. Cioffi, MD.)*

Other variables

Other variables of importance include the following:

- *fixation:* If the eye is slightly cyclotorted relative to the test bowl, or if the patient's point of fixation is off center, defects may shift locations. Especially in automated

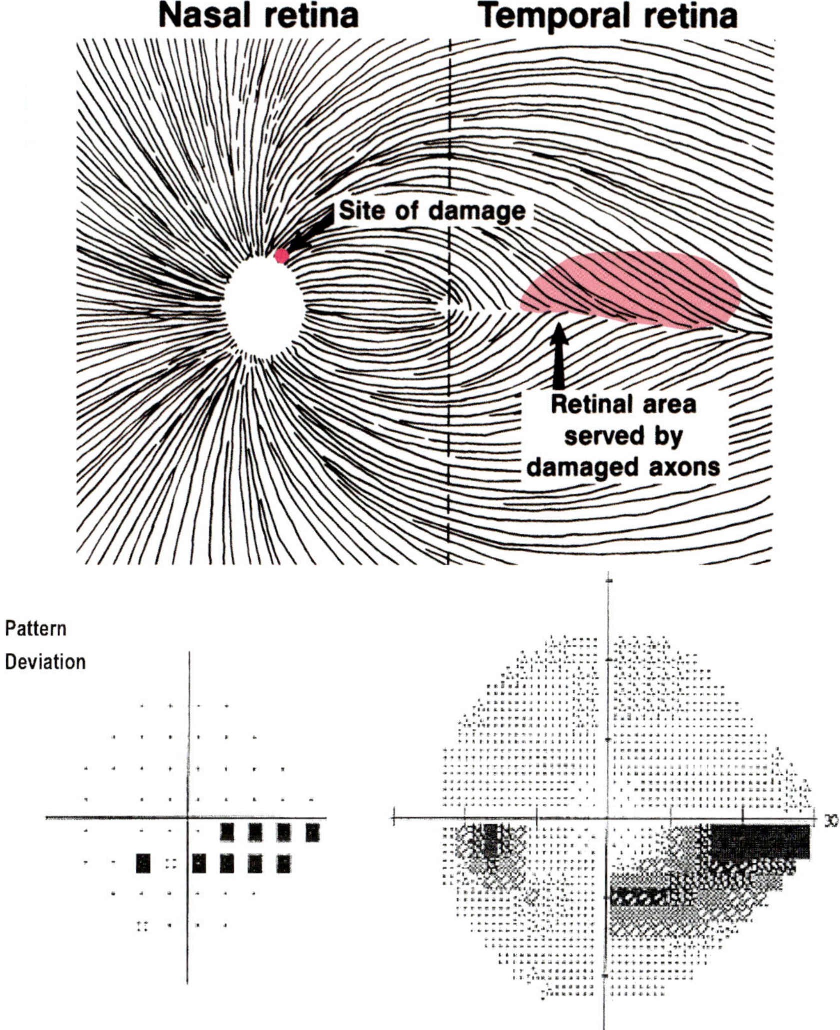

Figure 3-20 A *nasal step* is a relative depression of one horizontal hemifield compared to the other. Damage to superior nerve fibers serving the superotemporal retina beyond the paracentral area resulted in this nasal step. In kinetic perimetry the nasal step is defined as a discontinuity or depression in one or more nasal isopters near the horizontal raphe (Humphrey 30-2 program). *(Visual field courtesy of G. A. Cioffi, MD.)*

static tests (because the test logic does not change), a defect may thus appear and disappear.

- *background luminance:* The luminance of the surface onto which the perimetric stimulus is projected affects retinal sensitivity and thus the hill of vision. Clinical perimetry is usually done with a background luminance of 4.0–31.5 apostilbs. Retinal sensitivity is greatest at fixation and falls steadily toward the periphery.
- *stimulus luminance:* For a given stimulus size and presentation time, the brighter the stimulus, the more visible.

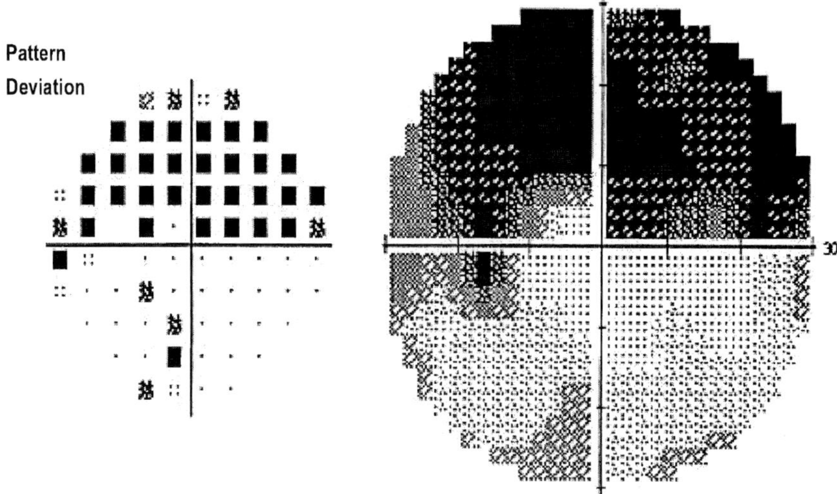

Figure 3-21 Altitudinal defect with near complete loss of the superior visual field, characteristic of moderate to advanced glaucomatous optic neuropathy (left eye). *(Visual field courtesy of G. A. Cioffi, MD.)*

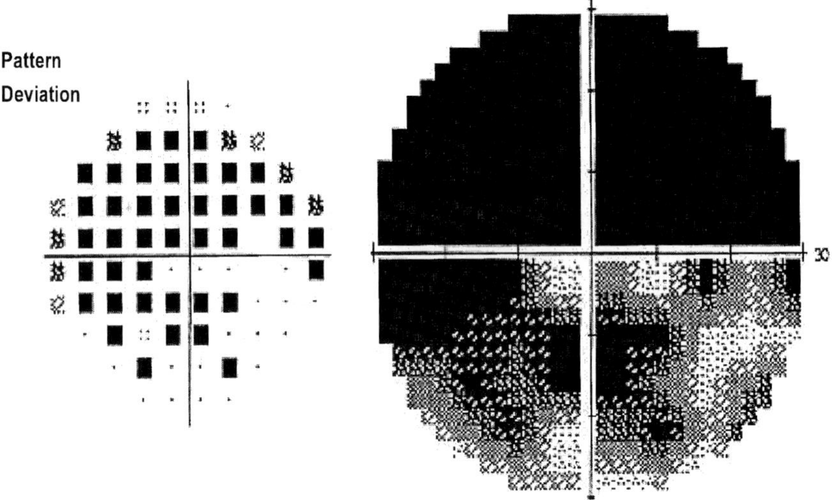

Figure 3-22 Advanced glaucomatous visual field loss with retention of a small central island of vision (foveal threshold: 33 dB) and retention of inferior temporal visual field. *(Courtesy of G. A. Cioffi, MD.)*

- *size of stimulus:* For a given brightness and duration of presentation, the larger the stimulus, the more likely it is to be perceived. The sizes of standard stimuli are: 0 = 1/16 mm^2, I = 1/4 mm^2, II = 1 mm^2, III = 4 mm^2, IV = 16 mm^2, V = 64 mm^2.
- *presentation time:* Fixed on individual automated perimeters. Up to about 0.5 second, temporal summation occurs. In other words, the longer the presentation

time, the more visible a given stimulus. Commercially available static perimeters generally employ a stimulus duration of 0.2 second or less. Comparison of perimetric thresholds between instruments is difficult because different manufacturers use different stimulus durations and background luminances.

- *patient refraction:* Uncorrected refractive errors cause blurring on the retina and decrease the visibility of stimuli. Thus, proper neutralization of refractive errors is essential for accurate perimetry. In addition, presbyopic and many prepresbyopic patients must have a refractive compensation that focuses fixation at the depth of the perimeter bowl. Care needs to be taken to center the patient close to the correcting lens to avoid a lens rim artifact (see Fig 3-28).
- *pupil size:* Pupil size affects the amount of light entering the eye, and it should be recorded on each field. Testing with pupils smaller than 3 mm in diameter may induce artifacts. Pupil size should be kept constant from test to test.
- *wavelength of background and stimulus:* As noted, color perimetry may yield different results from white-on-white perimetry.
- *speed of stimulus movement:* Because temporal summation occurs over a time period as long as 0.5 second, the area of retina stimulated by a test object is affected by the speed of the stimulus movement. If a kinetic target is moved quickly, by the time the patient responds, the target may have gone well beyond the location at which it was first seen. This period of time between visualization and response is termed the *latency period* or *visual reaction time.*

Automated Static Perimetry

A computerized perimeter must be able to determine threshold sensitivity at multiple points in the visual field, to perform an adequate test in a reasonable amount of time, and to present results in a comprehensible form. The objective perimeter should provide valid, reliable information describing visual sensitivity from an adequate sample of locations, obtained over a reasonable time period. The intensity of the stimulus is varied by a system of filters that attenuate the stimulus, usually allowing measurement to approximately 1 dB. Automated static perimeters have traditionally used staircase algorithms, which produce more reliable and efficient threshold estimates compared to previous psychophysical test strategies. Any staircase strategy yields threshold estimates that are a compromise between reliability (accuracy and precision) and efficiency (test duration). Threshold estimates from strategies that cross the threshold (reversal) more often or use smaller staircase intervals are more reliable, but at the expense of longer test times. The "standard" staircase strategy used by both Octopus perimeters and the Humphrey Field Analyzer (HFA) employs an initial 4-dB step size that reduces to 2 dB on first reversal and continues until a second reversal occurs (Figs 3-23 and 3-24).

Four general categories of testing strategy are currently in common use:

1. *Suprathreshold testing:* A stimulus, usually one expected to be a little brighter than threshold, is presented at various locations and recorded as seen or not seen. Sometimes, if it is not seen, it is presented again, and if not seen a second time, it is recorded as not seen. Then the stimulus may be presented at maximum

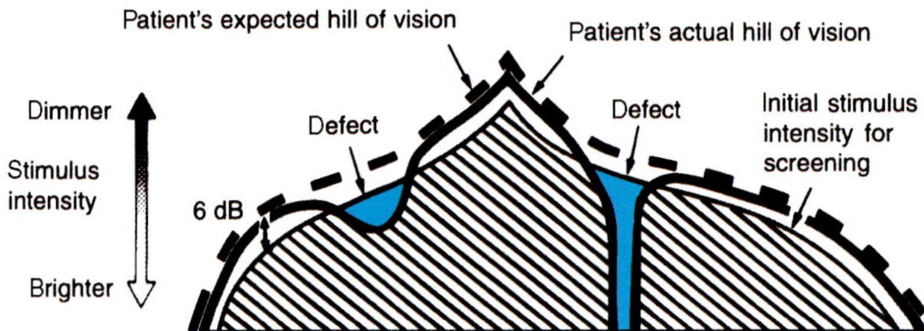

Figure 3-23 Threshold-related screening strategy records tested points as seen or not seen. Screening is done at an intensity 6 dB brighter than the expected threshold, and points missed twice at that level are recorded as defects. *(Reproduced with permission from* The Field Analyzer Primer. *San Leandro, CA: Allergan Humphrey; 1989.)*

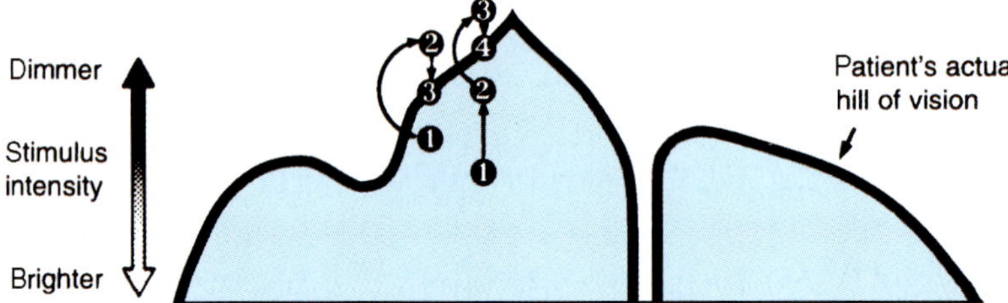

Figure 3-24 Full-threshold strategy determines retinal sensitivity at each tested point by altering the stimulus intensity in 4-dB steps until the threshold is crossed. It then recrosses the threshold, moving in 2-dB steps, in order to check and refine the accuracy of the measurement. *(Reproduced with permission from* The Field Analyzer Primer. *San Leandro, CA: Allergan Humphrey; 1989.)*

brightness to determine if a defect is relative or absolute. This type of test is designed to screen for moderate to severe defects and is only appropriate for screening; it cannot be used to follow patients.

2. *Threshold-related strategy:* The threshold is determined at a few points, and a presumed hill of vision is extrapolated from these points. Then a stimulus 6 dB brighter is presented, and the results are recorded as either seen or not seen. This type of test will detect moderate to severe defects, but it may miss mild defects (see Figs 3-23 and 3-24).
3. *Threshold:* Threshold testing is the current standard for automated perimetry in glaucoma management. As described earlier, threshold may be determined by a variety of bracketing and statistical strategies. Several points are tested twice to determine a patient's variability, and occasional tests are done to monitor fixation and to assess the frequency of a given individual's false-positive and false-negative responses.
4. *Efficient Threshold Strategies:* Full-threshold testing algorithms suffer from patient fatigue, high variability, and generally poor patient acceptance. Although shorter threshold-testing algorithms, such as FASTPAC, have been developed, the variability of the results of these shorter tests remains a concern that tempers confidence in their results. In an attempt to achieve shorter threshold testing with good

accuracy and reproducibility, the *Swedish interactive thresholding algorithm (SITA)* was developed. Unlike the discrete intervals used to step toward threshold employed by staircase strategies, SITA employs a logical "best guess," or forecasting, approach to threshold estimation. Briefly, the "best guess" intensity of SITA's initial stimulus presentation at each test location corresponds to the intensity associated with the highest probability of being seen by an age-matched individual. Depending on the patient's response to this first stimulus, the intensity of each subsequent presentation is modified. This iterative procedure is repeated until the likely threshold measurement error is reduced to below a predetermined level, with at least 1 reversal occurring at every test location. SITA also uses neighborhood comparisons to optimize the "best guess" procedure: if adjacent test locations show lower or higher sensitivity than expected, the initial stimulus intensity is altered. SITA monitors the timing of patient responses in order to interactively pace the test. Similar to the SITA test strategy for the HFA, the *tendency-oriented perimeter (TOP)* algorithm was developed for the Octopus perimeter as an alternative to the lengthy staircase threshold procedures. The intent of both of these strategies was to provide a faster, more efficient test procedure that maintained the same degree of accuracy and reliability as the staircase procedures.

Comparisons between SITA testing algorithms and older thresholding algorithms have suggested that the SITA Standard yields visual field results comparable to, although not exactly the same as, full-threshold testing. Both SITA (Standard and Fast) strategies yield marginally higher values for differential light sensitivity compared with other algorithms. Average test time with SITA Standard is approximately 50% the full-thresholding strategy time, and SITA Fast results in an additional reduction of approximately 30% compared with SITA Standard. The significantly reduced test time with SITA Standard appears to be achieved without significant sacrifice of accuracy or increase in variability or noise levels within the test. SITA Fast should be reserved for patients with glaucomatous visual field loss who are unable to perform SITA Standard because of mental or physical limitations.

Screening tests

These tests may or may not be threshold-related, and they cover varying areas of the visual field. Suprathreshold tests are not recommended for glaucoma suspects because they do not provide a good reference for future comparison, but they are appropriate for screening people not suspected of having glaucoma. On a full-field screening test, such as the Octopus 07 or Humphrey full-field 120-point test, a field should be considered abnormal if more than 10 points are missed or if 2 or more adjacent points are missed. A threshold field should be performed on such patients unless a cause other than glaucoma is apparent on examination.

Threshold tests

The most common programs for glaucoma testing are the central 24° and 30° programs, such as the Octopus 32 and G1 and the Humphrey 24-2 and 30-2 (Fig 3-25). These programs test the central field using a 6° grid. They test points 3° above and 3° below the horizontal midline and facilitate diagnosis of defects that respect this line. For patients

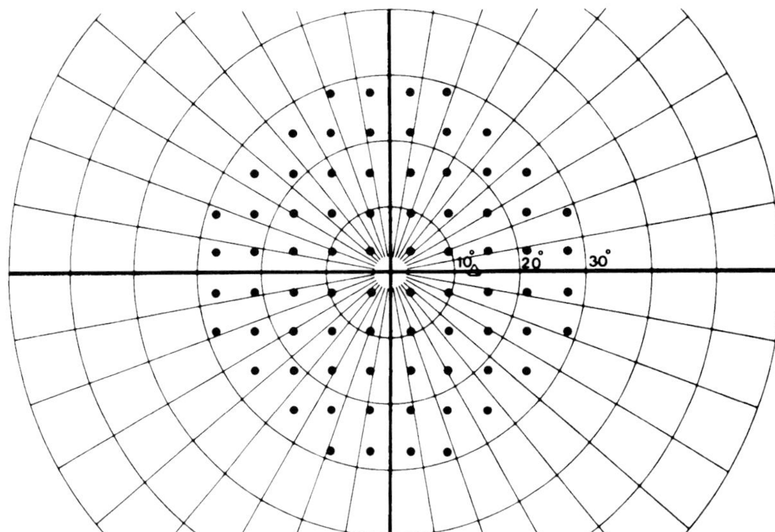

Figure 3-25 Central 30-2 threshold test pattern, right eye. *(Reproduced with permission from* The Field Analyzer Primer. *San Leandro, CA: Allergan Humphrey; 1989.)*

with advanced visual field loss that threatens fixation, serial 10-2 or C8 visual fields should be used. These visual fields concentrate on the central 8°–10° of the visual field and test points every 1°–2°, which enables the physician to follow many more test points within the central island and improve the detection of progression.

Although a 30°–60° program is available on most static threshold perimeters, it is rarely performed. The abandonment of peripheral testing, which has accompanied the shift from manual to automated perimetry, is the subject of ongoing discussion, but no trend to move beyond the central program has emerged after more than 2 decades of static threshold perimetry.

Interpretation of a Single Field

Quality

The first aspect of the field to be evaluated is its quality. The percentage of fixation losses, the false positives and false negatives, and the fluctuations of doubly determined points are assessed. Damaged areas of the field demonstrate more variability than normal areas. Glaucomatous damage may cause an increase in false-negative responses unrelated to patient reliability. In general, the average fluctuation between 2 determinations should be less than 2 dB in a normal field, less than 3 dB in a field with early damage, and less than 4 dB in a field with moderate damage. Patient reliability can be evaluated by looking at the least damaged areas in a badly damaged visual field.

Normality or abnormality

Next to be assessed is normality or abnormality. When tested under photopic conditions, the normal visual field demonstrates the greatest sensitivity centrally, with sensitivity falling steadily toward the periphery. A cluster of 2 or more points depressed ≥5 dB compared with surrounding points is suspicious. A single point depressed >10 dB is very unusual but is of less value on a single visual field than a cluster, because cluster points confirm one another. Corresponding points above and below the horizontal midline should not vary markedly; normally the superior field is depressed 1–2 dB compared with the inferior field.

To aid the clinician in interpreting the numerical data generated by threshold tests, field indices have been developed by perimeter manufacturers. In addition to the mean difference from normal and the test–retest variability, other measures of the irregularity of the visual field include Humphrey pattern standard deviation and Octopus loss variance indices. These indices highlight localized depressions in the field. When corrected for short-term fluctuation, the indices are termed *corrected pattern standard deviation* and *corrected loss variance.*

These corrected indices help to distinguish between generalized field depression and localized loss. An abnormal pattern deviation has greater diagnostic specificity than a generalized loss of sensitivity. An abnormally high pattern standard deviation indicates that some points of the visual field are depressed relative to other points in the field after correction for the patient's moment-to-moment variability. Such a finding is suggestive of focal damage such as that occurring with glaucoma (and many other conditions). Although a normal pattern standard deviation in an eye with an abnormal visual field indicates a generalized depression of the hill of vision such as that occurring with media opacity, such generalized loss may also occur with diffuse glaucomatous damage.

The Humphrey STATPAC 2 program performs an additional calculation on a single field to determine the likelihood that a field shows glaucomatous damage. This test is designed only for glaucoma and involves comparison of corresponding points above and below the horizontal midline (Fig 3-26). This hemifield analysis is at least as accurate as other methods for the classification of single visual fields.

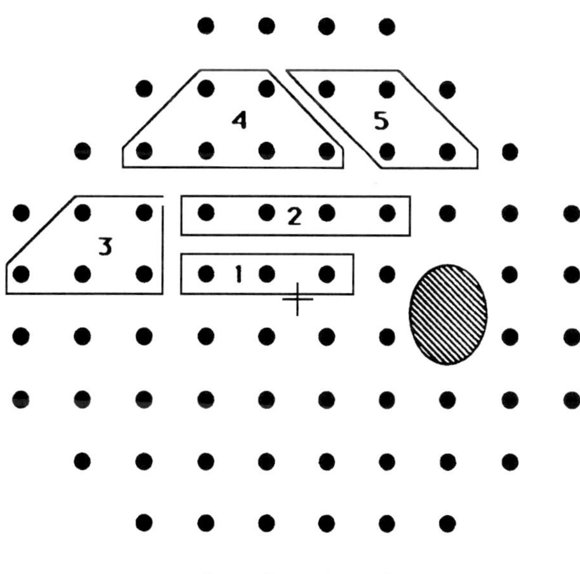

Figure 3-26 Superior field zones used in the glaucoma hemifield test. *(Reproduced with permission from* The STATPAC User's Guide. *San Leandro, CA: Allergan Humphrey; 1989.)*

Comparison of various perimetric techniques

With the introduction of new perimetric techniques into the clinical arena, clinicians may be asked to derive important clinical information from several perimetric printouts. The association between glaucoma and short-wavelength (blue) color vision deficits has been known for some time. Sensitivity to blue stimuli is believed to be mediated by a small subpopulation of morphologically distinct ganglion cells, the small bistratified ganglion cells, that typically have large receptive fields, little receptive field overlap, and relatively large axon diameters. If early ganglion cell loss in open-angle glaucoma preferentially affects either sparsely represented cell groups or those with larger axons, either scenario may produce reduced short-wavelength (blue) sensitivity. Using special stimuli and background illumination conditions, it is possible to isolate and test the sensitivity of short-wavelength mechanisms throughout the visual field with *short-wavelength automated perimetry (SWAP).* SWAP is available on the HFA II (700 series) and the Octopus 1–2–3. Data are analyzed using a STATPAC procedure and are presented using the same layout as for standard automated perimetry. SWAP is suitable for identifying individuals likely to develop SAP field loss. Repeatable field loss on SWAP should be carefully monitored. Analyses of local loss such as glaucoma hemisphere test (GHT) and pattern threshold deviations are the best statistical tools to identify glaucomatous SWAP deficits and separate them from artifacts resulting from media opacities.

The *frequency-doubling technology (FDT)* perimeter was developed to measure contrast detection thresholds for frequency-doubled test targets. The high temporal frequency and low spatial frequency attributes of the stimulus that causes frequency doubling means that the stimulus is an M-cell task. Whether it is because of the isolation of specific cell populations, which are susceptible to early damage in glaucoma, or because of the reduced redundancy allowing earlier identification of defects, visual function tests that employ frequency-doubled stimuli may be useful for detection of early defects. The greater sensitivity of both SWAP and FDT for detection of early glaucomatous damage are illustrated in Figure 3-27. Standard perimetric results reveal a small, localized region of reduced sensitivity nasally, whereas both SWAP and FDT show more extensive amounts of visual field damage.

Artifacts

Identification of artifacts is the next step in evaluating the visual field. The following are common artifacts seen on automated perimetry:

- *lens rim:* If the patient's corrective lens is decentered or set too far from the eye, the lens rim may project into the central 30° (Fig 3-28).
- *incorrect corrective lens:* If an incorrect corrective lens is used, the resulting field will be generally depressed. In practice, such an error is rarely noted, but it probably accounts for the occasional inexplicably depressed field that improves on follow-up testing. This appears to be less of a problem with FDT perimetry.
- *cloverleaf field:* If a patient stops paying attention and ceases to respond partway through a visual field, a distinctive field pattern may develop, depending on the test logic of a given perimeter. Figure 3-29 shows a cloverleaf field, the result of the test logic of the Humphrey 30-2 perimeter, which begins testing with the points circled and works outward. This pattern may also be seen if a patient is malingering.

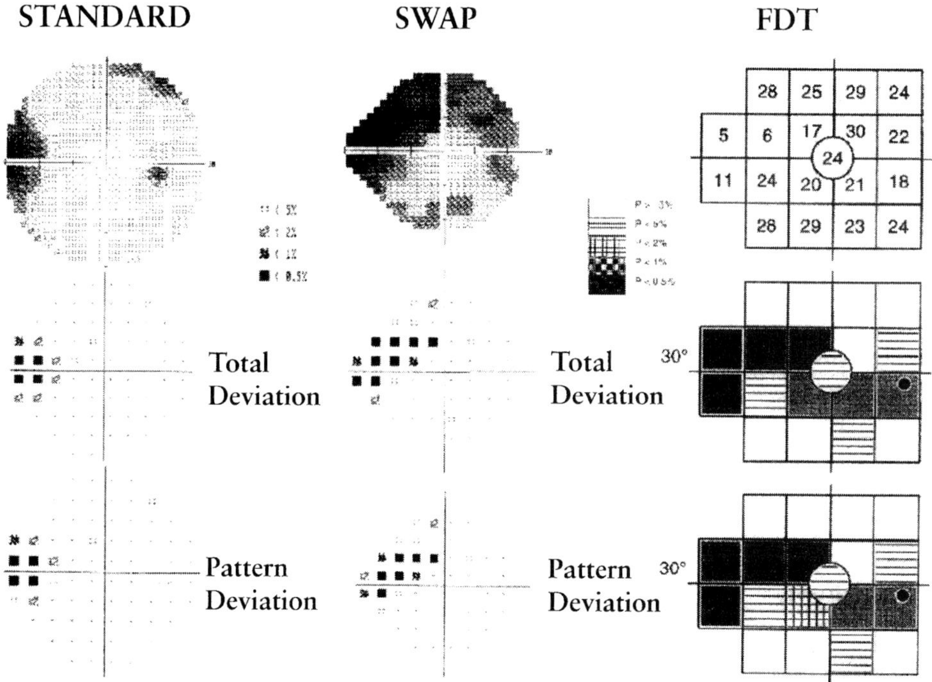

Figure 3-27 Comparison of standard automated perimetry (SAP), short-wavelength automated perimetry (SWAP), and frequency-doubling technology (FDT) in the right eye of a patient with early glaucomatous optic neuropathy. Note the more extensive superior arcuate scotoma and nasal loss detected by SWAP and FDT perimetry testing. These tests frequently detect visual field loss earlier than SAP. *(Reproduced with permission from Johnson CA, Spry PGD. Automated perimetry.* Focal Points: Clinical Modules for Ophthalmologists. *San Francisco; American Academy of Ophthalmology; 2002, module 10.)*

- *high false-positive rate:* When a patient responds at a time when no test stimulus is being presented, a false-positive response is recorded. False-positive rates greater than 33% suggest an unreliable test that can mask or minimize an actual scotoma. A high false-positive response rate can, in extreme cases, result in a field with impossibly high threshold values (Fig 3-30). A high false-positive and a high fixation-loss rate will also occur if the instrument records fixation losses by presenting stimuli in the blind spot. Careful instruction of the patient may sometimes resolve this artifact.
- *high false-negative rate:* When a patient fails to respond to a stimulus presented in a location where a dimmer stimulus was previously seen, a false-negative response is recorded. False-negative rates greater than 33% suggest test unreliability. A high false-negative rate should alert the clinician to the likelihood that the patient's actual visual field might not be as depressed as suggested by the test result. However, it should also be noted that patients with significant visual field loss, including scotomata with steep edges, can demonstrate high false-negative rates that do not indicate unreliability. This effect appears to arise from presentation of stimuli at the edges of deep scotomata, where short-term threshold fluctuation can be quite variable.

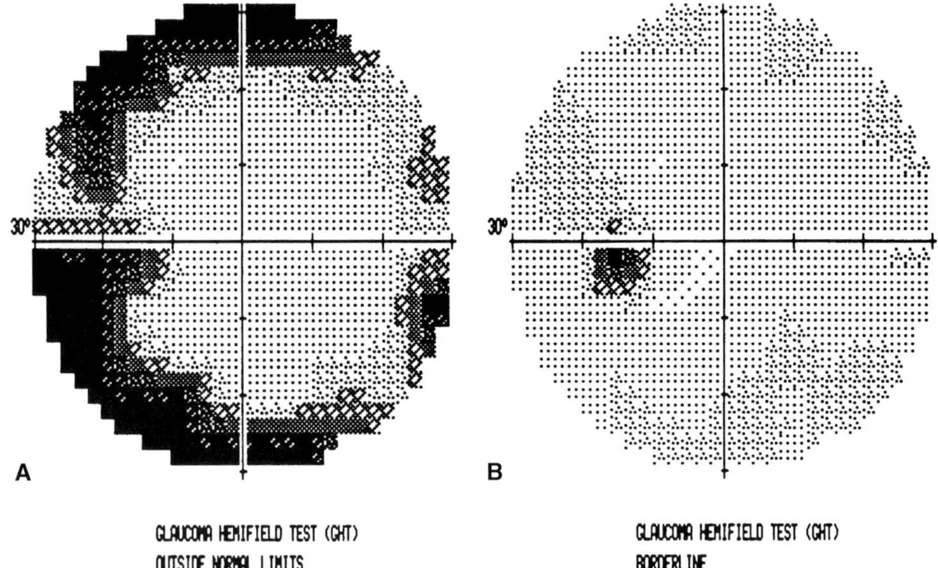

Figure 3-28 Lens rim artifact. The two visual fields shown were obtained 9 days apart. The field on the left, **A,** shows a typical lens rim artifact, whereas the corrective lens was positioned appropriately for the field on the right, **B** (Humphrey 30-2 program).

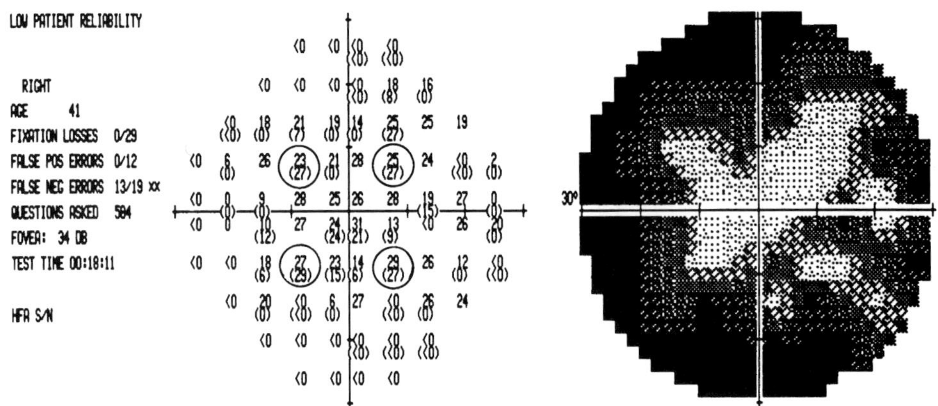

Figure 3-29 Cloverleaf field. The Humphrey visual field perimeter test is designed so that four circled points are checked initially and the testing in each quadrant proceeds outward from these points. If the patient ceases to respond after only a few points have been tested, the result is some variation of the cloverleaf field shown at right (Humphrey 30-2 program).

Interpretation of a Series of Fields

Interpretation of serial visual fields should meet 2 goals:

1. separating real change from ordinary variation
2. using the information from the field testing to determine the likelihood that a change is related to glaucomatous progression

DATE 10-02-86

LOW PATIENT RELIABILITY

LEFT
AGE 52
FIXATION LOSSES 24/33 xx
FALSE POS ERRORS 9/23 xx
FALSE NEG ERRORS 8/21 xx
QUESTIONS ASKED 689
FOVEA: 33 DB ::
TEST TIME 00:22:31

HFA S/N

30°

GLAUCOMA HEMIFIELD TEST (GHT)
ABNORMALLY HIGH SENSITIVITY

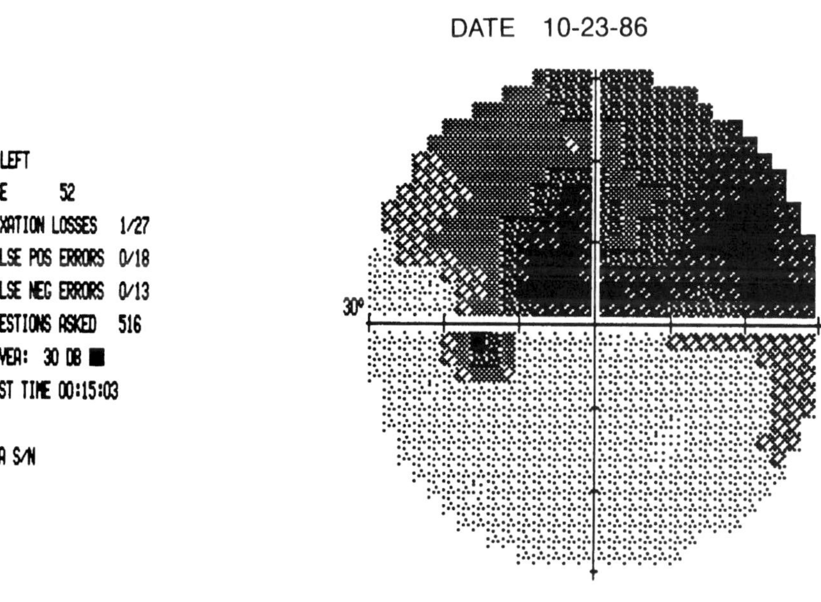

GLAUCOMA HEMIFIELD TEST (GHT)
OUTSIDE NORMAL LIMITS

Figure 3-30 High false-positive rate. The top visual field contains characteristic "white scotomata," which represent areas of impossibly high retinal sensitivity. Upon return visit 3 weeks later, the patient was carefully instructed to respond only when she saw the light, resulting in the bottom visual field, which shows good reliability and demonstrates the patient's dense superior visual field loss (Humphrey 30-2 program).

A number of methods can be employed to analyze a series of visual fields for glaucomatous change. Point-by-point analysis by hand, in the absence of a statistical program package, is extremely cumbersome. The mountain of data present in a series of visual fields cannot be effectively analyzed by hand. Fortunately, statistical programs are available from the major instrument manufacturers (for example, the Humphrey STATPAC 2 or Octopus Delta programs); these are valuable aids in point-by-point series analysis. The application of each of these packages is described clearly in the owner's manual that comes with the program.

Calculation and comparison of visual field indices is another method that can be useful in visual field series analysis. Examination of visual field indices can reveal global trends that may be missed using point-by-point analysis. Raw perimetric data can also be transferred to independent software programs for change analysis. Even when computed statistical methods are employed, however, separation of true pathologic progression from normal test-to-test variability remains a difficult challenge. Moreover, the examiner interpreting a series of visual fields must keep in mind that test variability is increased as part of the pathophysiology of glaucoma.

Whatever method the clinician uses, the fundamental requirement for adequate interpretation over time is a good *baseline* visual field. Often the patient experiences a learning effect, and the second visual field may show substantial improvement over the first (Fig 3-31). At least 2 visual fields should be obtained as early in a patient's course as possible. If they are quite different, a third test should be performed. Subsequent visual fields should be compared to these baseline fields. Any follow-up visual field that appears to be quite different should be repeated for confirmation of the suspected change from baseline.

Progression

No hard-and-fast rules define what determines visual field progression, but the following are reasonable guidelines:

- Deepening of an existing scotoma is suggested by the reproducible depression of a point in an existing scotoma by ≥7 dB.
- Enlargement of an existing scotoma is suggested by the reproducible depression of a point adjacent to an existing scotoma by ≥9 dB.
- Development of a new scotoma is suggested by the reproducible depression of a previously normal point in the visual field by ≥11 dB, or of 2 adjacent, previously normal points by ≥5 dB.

Cases such as that shown in Figure 3-32 are easy to recognize. A general decrease in sensitivity may be secondary to glaucoma or may be related to media opacity, and clinical correlation is required, which is often difficult. Two causes of general decline in sensitivity that may confuse interpretation are variable miosis (often related to use of eyedrops) and cataract (Fig 3-33). To help avoid the problem of variable pupil size, the pupil size should be recorded at each examination and should remain constant from field to field if at all possible.

Suspected new defects or progression of existing defects should be reproduced on subsequent visual fields to determine their validity. Definitions of progression have varied

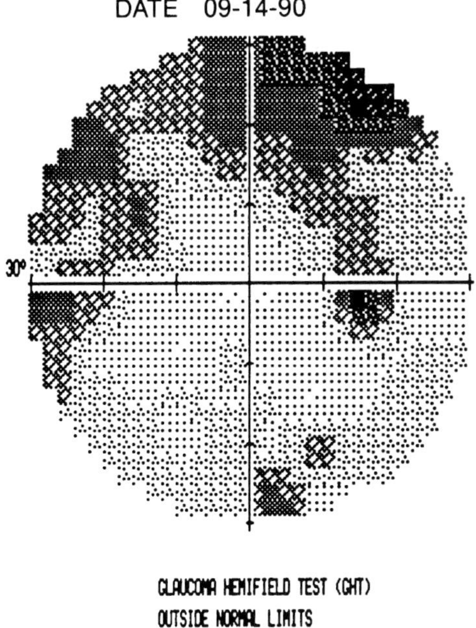

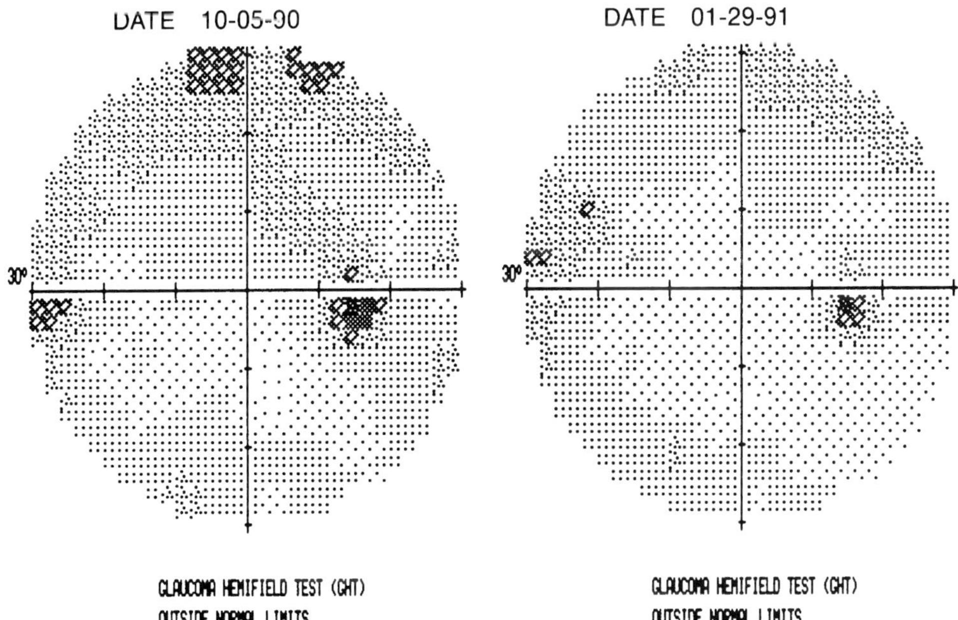

Figure 3-31 Learning effect. These 3 visual fields were obtained within the first 3½ months of diagnosis in a patient with very early, clinically stable, glaucoma. They illustrate the learning effect between the first and second visual field. The third field is similar to the second field, and the second and third visual fields provided a baseline for subsequent follow-up of the patient (Humphrey 30-2 program).

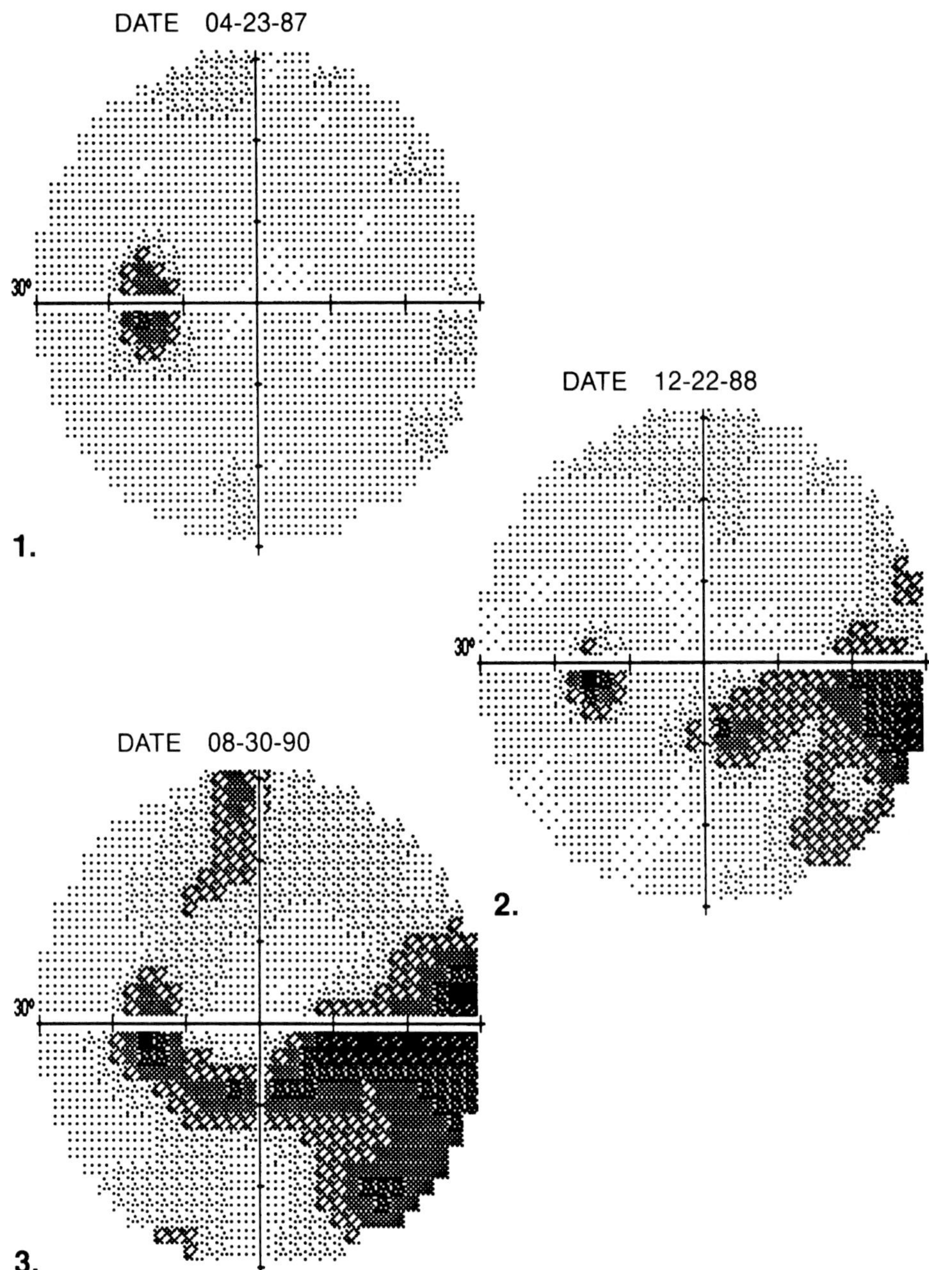

Figure 3-32 Progression of glaucomatous damage. The three fields shown illustrate the development and advancement of a visual field defect. Between the first and second visual fields, the patient developed a significant inferior nasal step. The third visual field illustrates the extension of this defect to the blind spot, as well as the development of superior visual field loss (Humphrey 30-2 program).

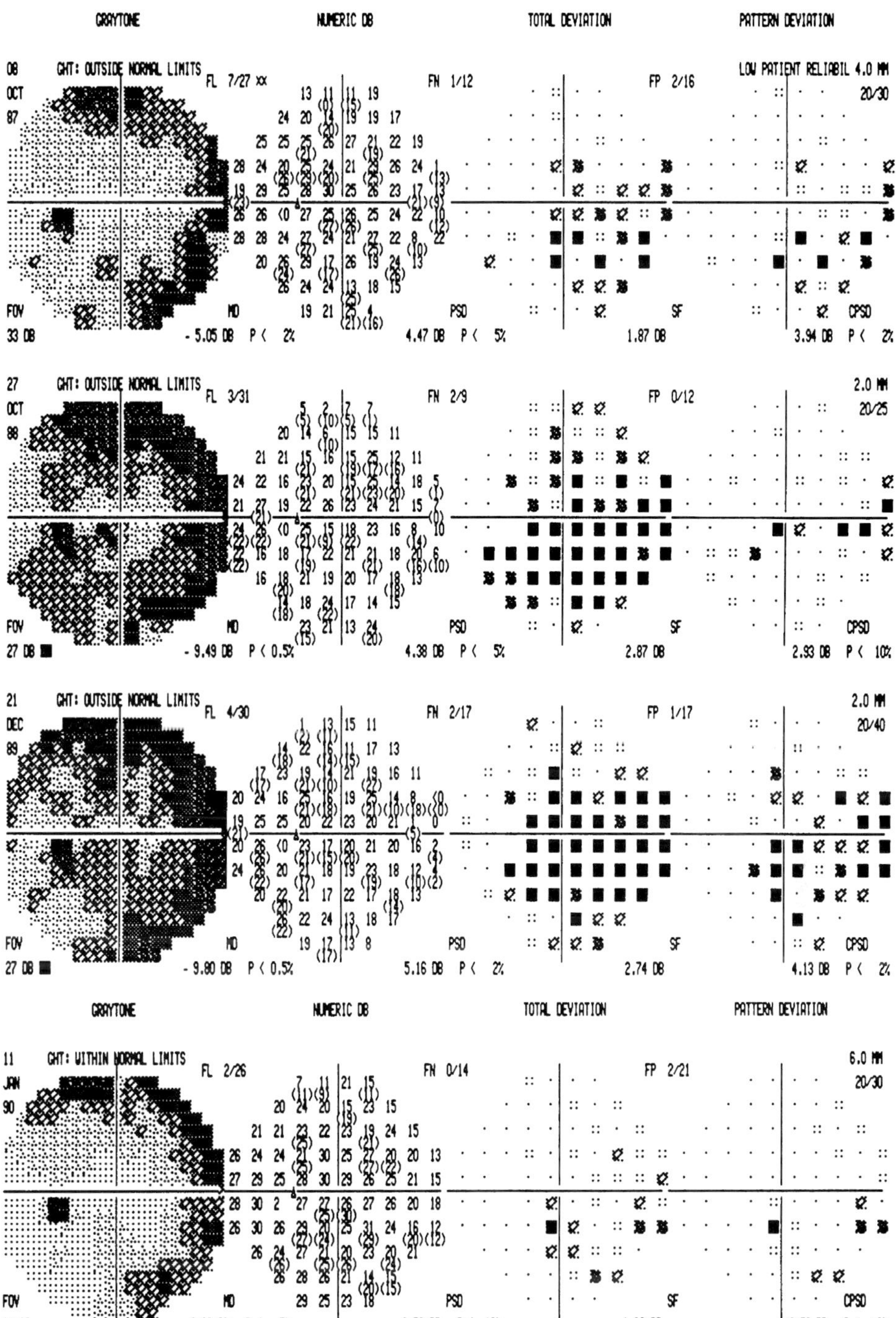

Figure 3-33 Pupil size. The first field in this series was obtained before the patient began pilocarpine therapy. The second and third fields were obtained with a miotic pupil. Before the fourth field was obtained, the patient's pupil was dilated (Humphrey 30-2 program).

in the numerous clinical trials; these definitions will continued to be refined with additional years of experience and further improvements in computer software.

Correlation with optic disc

It is important to correlate changes in the visual field with the optic disc. If such correlation is lacking, other causes of visual loss should be considered, such as ischemic optic neuropathy, demyelinating or other neurologic disease, pituitary tumor, and so on. This consideration is especially important in the following situations:

- The patient's optic disc seems less cupped than would be expected for the degree of field loss.
- The pallor of the disc is more impressive than the cupping.
- The progression of the visual field loss seems excessive.
- The pattern of visual field loss is uncharacteristic for glaucoma—for example, it respects the vertical midline.
- The location of the cupping or thinning of the neural rim does not corrrespond to proper location of the visual field defect.

Anderson DR, Patella VM. *Automated Static Perimetry.* 2nd ed. St Louis: Mosby; 1999.

Drake MV. A primer on automated perimetry. *Focal Points: Clinical Modules for Ophthalmologists.* San Francisco: American Academy of Ophthalmology; 1993, module 8.

Drance SM, Anderson DR, eds. *Automatic Perimetry in Glaucoma: A Practical Guide.* Orlando, FL: Grune & Stratton; 1985.

Harrington DO, Drake MV. *The Visual Fields: A Textbook and Atlas of Clinical Perimetry.* 6th ed. St Louis: Mosby; 1989.

Lieberman MF. Glaucoma and automated perimetry. *Focal Points: Clinical Modules for Ophthalmologists.* San Francisco: American Academy of Ophthalmology; 1993, module 9.

Spry PGD, Johnson CA: Advances in automated perimetry. *Focal Points: Clinical Modules for Ophthalmologists.* San Francisco: American Academy of Ophthalmology; 2002, module 10.

Walsh TJ, ed. *Visual Fields: Examination and Interpretation.* 2nd ed. Ophthalmology Monograph 3. San Francisco: American Academy of Ophthalmology; 1996.

Manual Perimetry

The 2 goals of perimetry—to identify abnormalities and to define and record visual function for comparison over time—are most commonly pursued in manual perimetry using *the Armaly-Drance screening technique.* This screening technique for the detection of early glaucomatous visual field loss was originally developed for the Goldmann perimeter but has been adapted for a number of instruments. It combines a kinetic examination of the peripheral isopters with a suprathreshold static examination of the central field (Fig 3-34).

With this technique, the kinetic perimeter—usually the Goldmann I-2e—is used to determine the stimulus that is just suprathreshold for the central 25°. The central isopter is then plotted kinetically with this stimulus to detect nasal, temporal, or vertical steps, with special attention to the 15° straddling the horizontal and vertical meridians. The blind spot is mapped with the same stimulus moving from the center of the blind spot

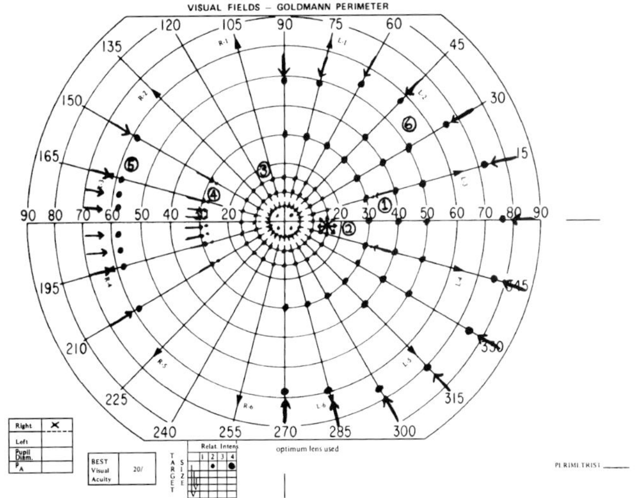

Figure 3-34 Armaly-Drance screening technique on Goldmann perimeter.

outward in 8 directions. The same stimulus is then used in static presentations to search for paracentral and arcuate defects. A more intense stimulus, often the equivalent of a Goldmann I-4e, is used to search for both nasal step and temporal sector defects to prepare a kinetic plot of the peripheral isopter.

A different perimetric technique must be used for quantifying defects and for following patients with established glaucomatous damage. This form of perimetry quantifies visual field defects by size, shape, and depth and determines whether the disease is progressing or not. If the examiner is using a kinetic technique, targets of different size and brightness must be employed. The technique of quantifying defects with kinetic perimetry is well described in standard texts. An example of a quantified defect is shown in Figure 3-35.

Progression of glaucomatous field loss generally occurs in areas damaged previously. Scotomata become larger and deeper, and new scotomata appear in the same hemifield. Arcuate scotomata extend to the peripheral boundaries on the nasal side and break through to the periphery. The ophthalmologist who quantifies defects with precision can use this pattern of progression to determine a patient's ongoing stability or progression.

Because high-quality manual threshold perimetry requires a well-trained and conscientious perimetrist, and even the best perimetrist varies from day to day, automated field testing has become increasingly widespread. Computerized static perimetry has shown itself to be at least as good as the best-quality manual perimetry in the detection and quantification of glaucomatous defects. However, manual perimetry remains helpful in documenting defects outside the central 30° and in monitoring endstage visual field loss.

Anderson DR. *Perimetry With and Without Automation.* 2nd ed. St Louis: Mosby; 1987.

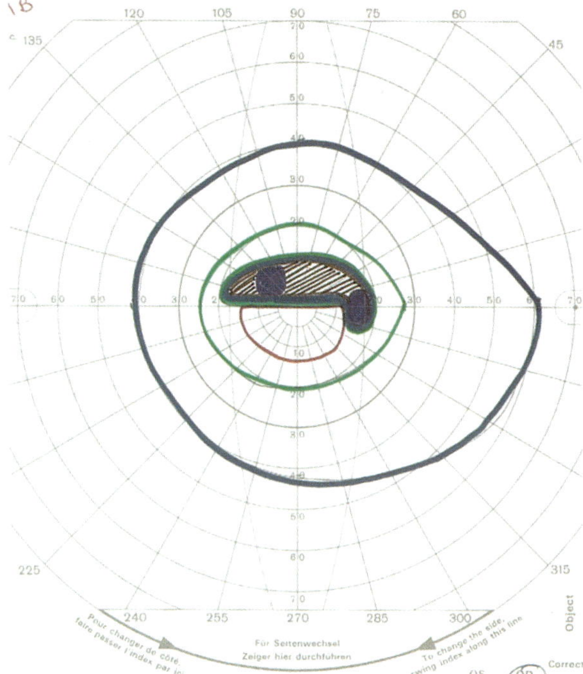

Figure 3-35 Split fixation (Goldmann perimeter).

Other Tests

Several other tests may be helpful in selected patients. Many of these tests are described elsewhere in the BCSC series, and the reader is advised to consult the *Master Index* for the following:

- fluorescein angiography
- corneal pachymetry
- measurement of episcleral venous pressure
- carotid noninvasive vascular studies
- ocular blood-flow measurements
- ultrasonography

Although it is not currently widely available, ultrasound biomicroscopy (UBM) provides valuable information about several types of glaucoma. The test employs shorter-wavelength sound waves than does conventional ocular ultrasound, limiting the penetration but increasing the resolution tenfold. The test allows detailed examination of the anterior segment, the posterior chamber, and the ciliary body (Fig 3-36).

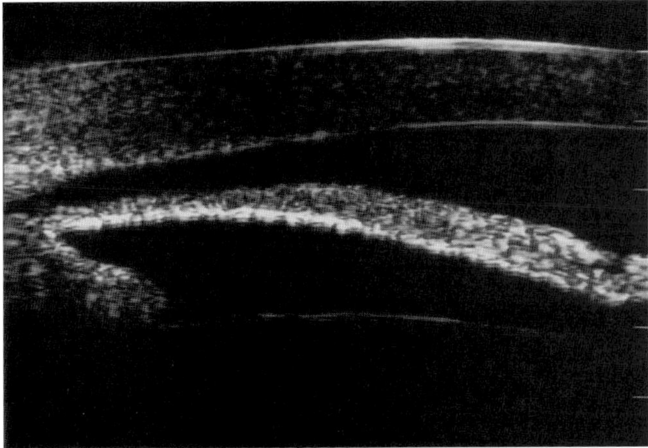

Figure 3-36 Pupillary block as shown by ultrasound biomicroscopy. Note the elevation above the lens of the peripheral iris on the left compared with the central iris on the right. *(Photograph courtesy of Charles J. Pavlin, MD.)*

CHAPTER 4

Open-Angle Glaucoma

Primary Open-Angle Glaucoma

Primary open-angle glaucoma (POAG) is characterized as a chronic, slowly progressive, optic neuropathy with characteristic patterns of optic nerve damage and visual field loss. POAG lacks the identifiable contributing factors of the secondary open-angle glaucomas, such as pigment dispersion in pigmentary glaucoma or the exfoliative material seen in exfoliation syndrome. IOP is an important risk factor for POAG; other factors, such as race, central corneal thickness (CCT), age, and family history, also contribute to the risk of developing this disease. Reduced perfusion to the optic nerve, abnormalities of axonal or ganglion cell metabolism, and disorders of the extracellular matrix of the lamina cribrosa may be contributory factors. Unfortunately, the puzzle of the interplay of the multiple causes of POAG remains unsolved.

Clinical Features

POAG is usually insidious in onset, slowly progressive, and painless. Although usually bilateral, it can be quite asymmetric. Because central visual acuity is relatively unaffected until late in the disease, visual loss may be significant before symptoms are noted. POAG is diagnosed by assessing a combination of findings, including IOP levels, optic disc appearance, and visual field loss, as described in Chapter 3.

Intraocular pressure

Large, population-based epidemiologic studies have revealed a mean IOP of approximately 16 mm Hg, with a standard deviation of approximately 3 mm Hg. This led to the definition of "normal" IOP as 2 standard deviations above and below the mean IOP, or approximately 10–22 mm Hg.

Although IOP greater than 22 mm Hg has in the past been defined as "abnormal," this definition has a number of shortcomings. First, it is now known that IOP in the general population is not represented by a Gaussian distribution but is skewed toward higher pressures (see Fig 2-3). IOPs of 22 mm Hg and above would thus not necessarily represent abnormality from a statistical standpoint. More importantly, IOP distribution curves in glaucomatous and nonglaucomatous eyes show a great deal of overlap. An IOP screening value of 21 or 22 mm Hg thus has no real clinical significance. Several studies have indicated that as many as 30%–50% of individuals in the general population who have glaucomatous optic neuropathy and/or visual field loss have initial screening IOPs below 22 mm Hg. Furthermore, because of diurnal fluctuation, elevations of IOP may occur only intermittently in some glaucomatous eyes, with as many as one third of the measurements being normal.

The IOP in an untreated glaucoma patient may vary rapidly, by 15 mm Hg or more, over a 24-hour period. Most patients without glaucoma show a diurnal range of 5 mm Hg or less; glaucoma patients have been reported to have average diurnal fluctuations in IOP of 4.8–11.3 mm Hg. Patterns of diurnal fluctuation have been broken into several types depending on time of peak pressure: morning (the most common, with highest pressure in the first hours after wakening), day, night, or flat (meaning little diurnal variation). Most individuals manifest similar patterns from day to day; however, 10%–20% of patients are "erratic," manifesting different patterns of diurnal IOP fluctuation over time.

Zeimer RC. Circadian variations in intraocular pressure. In: Ritch R, Shields MB, Krupin T. *The Glaucomas.* 2nd ed. St. Louis: Mosby; 1996: ch 21, 429–445.

Corneal thickness affects the measurement of IOP. Thicker corneas resist the indentation inherent to nearly all methods of IOP measurement, including applanation, air-puff, Tonopen, and pneumotonometry. Average corneal thickness is approximately 534 μm (optical measurement) or 544 μm (ultrasound measurement) in normal eyes; it has been found to be thicker in groups of patients with ocular hypertension and thinner in patients with normal-tension glaucoma. The exact effect corneal thickness has on IOP is not known, but IOP has been estimated to increase at 2–7 mm Hg per 100 μm of increased corneal thickness. Corneal thickness may be measured (pachymetry) by optical and ultrasonic methods. Corneal curvature may also play a role in the measurement of IOP, as more sharply curved (steeper) corneas resist indentation more.

Bhan A, Browning AC, Shah S, et al. Effect of corneal thickness on intraocular pressure measurements with the pneumotonometer, Goldmann applanation tonometer, and Tono-Pen. *Invest Ophthalmol Vis Sci.* 2002;43:1389–1392.

Brandt JD, Beiser JA, Kass MA, et al. Central corneal thickness in the Ocular Hypertension Treatment Study (OHTS). *Ophthalmology.* 2001;108:1779–1788.

Doughty MJ, Zaman ML. Human corneal thickness and its impact on intraocular pressure measures: a review and meta-analysis approach. *Surv Ophthalmol.* 2000;44:367–408.

Herndon LW, Choudhri SA, Cox T, et al. Central corneal thickness in normal, glaucomatous, and ocular hypertensive eyes. *Arch Ophthalmol.* 1997;115:1137–1141.

Optic disc appearance and visual field loss

Although elevated IOP is still considered a key risk factor for glaucoma, it is no longer considered essential to its diagnosis. Optic nerve head appearance and visual field defects have assumed predominant roles in the diagnosis of POAG, although treatment at this time remains aimed at lowering the IOP. Table 4-1 and Clinical Trials 4-1 through 4-4 summarize recent clinical trials to evaluate control of IOP and POAG.

Careful periodic evaluation of the optic disc and visual field is vital in the follow-up of glaucoma patients. Stereophotographic documentation or computerized imaging of

Table 4-1 Controlled Clinical Trials with Published Results

Name/Date of Published Results	Study Design	Recruitment (No. of Patients)	Follow-Up Duration (Years)	Finding
Scottish Glaucoma Trial/ 1989	Newly diagnosed POAG: medicine vs trabeculectomy	99	3–5	Trabeculectomy lowered IOP more than medicine; medicine group lost more visual function than trabeculectomy group.
Moorfields Primary Treatment Trial/1994	Newly diagnosed POAG: medicine vs laser trabeculoplasty vs trabeculectomy	168	5+	Trabeculectomy lowered IOP the most; laser trabeculoplasty and medicine groups lost more visual function than trabeculectomy group.
Glaucoma Laser Trial (GLT)/1990	Newly diagnosed POAG: medicine vs laser trabeculoplasty	271	2.5–5.5	Initial laser trabeculoplasty is at least as effective as initial treatment with topical timolol maleate to reduce IOP and preserve vision.
Glaucoma Laser Trial Follow-up Study/1995	Participants in the GLT	203	6–9	Initial laser trabeculoplasty is at least as effective as initial treatment with topical timolol maleate to reduce IOP and preserve vision.
Fluorouracil Filtering Surgery Study/1989, 1996	Patients at high risk for surgical failure: results of trabeculectomy with or without 5-fluorouracil	213	5+	Substantial improvements in IOP reduction with adjunctive 5-fluorouracil.
Collaborative Normal Tension Glaucoma Study/1998	POAG in eyes with normal IOP: rate of progression, effect of IOP reduction on progression rate	200	5+	Lowering IOP 30% reduced progression from 35% to 12%.
Advanced Glaucoma Intervention Study (AGIS) 1998	POAG after medical treatment failure with no previous surgery: laser trabeculoplasty vs trabeculectomy	591 (789 eyes)	4–7	After 5 years, white patients had less progression (field and acuity loss) if treated with trabeculectomy first (although acuity loss was greater earlier with trabeculectomy). Black patients had less progression if treated with ALT first.
Collaborative Initial Glaucoma Treatment Study (CIGTS)/2001	Newly diagnosed POAG: medicine vs trabeculectomy	607	5	After 5 years, the outcomes were very similar between the 2 groups; surgical group had slightly more ocular symptoms and slightly worse visual acuity early in the study. IOP goals for both groups were more aggressive and the overall rate of progression was low.
Ocular Hypertension Treatment Study (OHTS)/2002	Ocular hypertensive patients: medication vs observation	1636	5	Greater age, cup–disc ratio, IOP, PSD, and reduced central corneal thickness were associated with greater risk of glaucoma development; IOP reduction reduced the development of glaucoma from 9.5% to 4.4%.
Early Manifest Glaucoma Trial (EMGT)/2002	Newly diagnosed POAG: betaxolol and ALT vs observation	255	4	The treated group experienced less, and later, progression than the observation group (30% vs 49%).

(Modified from Preferred Practice Patterns Committee, Glaucoma Panel. *Primary Open-Angle Glaucoma.* San Francisco: American Academy of Ophthalmology; 2000.)

the disc enhances the clinician's ability to detect subtle changes over time. Pertinent clinical signs of glaucoma affecting the optic disc include the following:

- asymmetry of the neuroretinal rim area or cupping
- focal thinning or notching of the neuroretinal rim
- optic disc hemorrhage
- any acquired change in the disc rim appearance or the surrounding retinal nerve fiber layer

Visual field loss should correlate with the appearance of the optic disc. Significant discrepancies in the pattern of field loss and optic nerve damage warrant additional investigation, as noted in Chapter 3.

Gonioscopy should be performed in all patients evaluated for glaucoma and repeated periodically in patients with open-angle glaucoma to detect possible progressive angle closure caused by miotic therapy or age-related lens changes, especially in patients with hyperopia. Repeated gonioscopy is also indicated when the chamber becomes shallow, when strong miotics are prescribed, after laser trabeculoplasty or iridectomy, and when IOP rises.

Jonas JB, Budde WM, Panda-Jonas S. Ophthalmoscopic evaluation of the optic nerve head. *Surv Ophthalmol.* 1999;43:293–320.

Preferred Practice Patterns Committee, Glaucoma Panel. *Primary Open-Angle Glaucoma.* San Francisco: American Academy of Ophthalmology; 2003.

Risk factors for POAG other than IOP

Age is an important risk factor for the presence of POAG. The Baltimore Eye Survey found that the prevalence of glaucoma increases dramatically with age, particularly among blacks, exceeding 11% in those 80 years of age or older (Table 4-2). In the Collaborative Initial Glaucoma Treatment Study (CIGTS), visual field defects were 7 times more likely to develop in patients 60 years of age or older than in those under 40 years of age. Although increased IOP with age has been observed in many populations and may account for part of the relationship between age and glaucoma, studies in Japan have shown a relationship between glaucoma and age even with no increase in IOP in the population. Thus, age appears to be an independent risk factor for the development of glaucoma. The Ocular Hypertension Treatment Study (OHTS) found an increased risk of open-angle glaucoma with age (per decade), of 43% in the univariate analysis and 22% in the multivariate analysis.

Race is another important risk factor for POAG (see Table 4-2). The prevalence of POAG is 4 to 5 times greater in African Americans than in others. Blindness from glaucoma is 4 to 8 times more common in African Americans than in white Americans in the United States. Glaucoma is more likely to be diagnosed at a younger age and likely to be at a more advanced stage at time of diagnosis in black vs white patients. In the OHTS, black patients were more likely to develop glaucoma than whites in a univariate analysis (59%), but this relationship was not present after corneal thickness and baseline vertical cup–disc ratio were factored into the multivariate analysis (blacks had thinner corneas and larger baseline vertical cup–disc ratios on average).

Clinical Trial 4-1

Ocular Hypertension Treatment Study Essentials

Purpose: To evaluate the safety and efficacy of topical ocular hypotensive medications in preventing or delaying the onset of visual field loss and/or optic nerve damage in subjects with ocular hypertension

Participants: 1637 patients with ocular hypertension recruited between 1994 and 1996

Study Design: Multicenter randomized, controlled clinical trial comparing observation to medical therapy for ocular hypertension

Results: Topical ocular hypotensive medication was effective in delaying or preventing the onset of POAG: a 22.5% decrease in IOP in the treatment group (vs 4.0% in controls) was associated with a reduction of the development of POAG from 9.5% in controls to 4.4% in treated patients at 60 months' follow-up. Topical medications were generally well tolerated.

Increased risk of the onset of POAG was associated with increased age (10 years: 22% increase in relative risk), vertical and horizontal cup–disc ratio (0.1 increase: 32% and 27% increases in relative risk, respectively), pattern standard deviation (0.2 dB increase: 22% increase in relative risk), and IOP at baseline (1 mm Hg increase: 10% increase in relative risk). Central corneal thickness (CCT) was found to be a powerful predictor for the development of POAG (relative risk of POAG increased 81% for every 40 μm thinner).

OHTS subjects had thicker corneas than the general population. African-American subjects had thinner corneas than white subjects in the study. The effect of CCT may influence the accuracy of applanation tonometry in the diagnosis, screening, and management of patients with glaucoma and ocular hypertension.

Repeat testing failed to confirm visual field abnormalities in 604 (85.9%) of 703 reliable but abnormal visual fields.

Family history is also a risk factor for glaucoma. The Baltimore Eye Survey found that the relative risk of having POAG is increased approximately 3.7-fold for individuals having a sibling with POAG. A Finnish twin cohort study showed a 10.2% inheritance for chronic open-angle glaucoma.

Wilson MR, Martone JF. Epidemiology of chronic open-angle glaucoma. In: Ritch R, Shields MB, Krupin T. *The Glaucomas.* 2nd ed. St. Louis: Mosby; 1996: ch 35, 753–768.

Associated Disorders

The following conditions are also associated, although not as strongly, with glaucoma. Some of these conditions are discussed in greater detail elsewhere in the BCSC series. See also Section 1, *Update on General Medicine* (diabetes and cardiovascular disease), and Section 12, *Retina and Vitreous* (diabetes and retinal vein occlusion).

Clinical Trial 4-2

Early Manifest Glaucoma Trial Essentials

Purpose: To compare immediate lowering of intraocular pressure with observation on the progression of newly detected open-angle glaucoma

Participants: Newly diagnosed patients 50 to 80 years of age with early glaucomatous visual field defects were mainly identified from a population-based screening of more than 44,000 residents of Malmö and Helsingborg, Sweden. Exclusion criteria were advanced visual field loss; mean IOP greater than 30 mm Hg or any IOP greater than 35 mm Hg; visual acuity less than 0.5 (20/40). 255 patients were randomized between 1993 and 1997.

Study Design: Multicenter randomized, controlled clinical trial comparing observation to betaxolol and laser trabeculoplasty for open-angle glaucoma.

Results: After 6 years, 53% of patients progressed. In multivariate analyses, progression risk was halved by treatment (HR = 0.50; 95% CI, 0.35–0.71). Predictive baseline factors were higher IOP, exfoliation, and having both eyes eligible, worse mean deviation, and older age. Progression risk decreased by about 10% with each millimeter of mercury of IOP reduction from baseline to the first follow-up visit. The percentage of patient follow-up visits with disc hemorrhages was also related to progression (HR = 1.02 per percent higher; 95% CI, 1.01–1.03).

Myopia

An association has been reported between POAG and myopia. It is possible that individuals with myopia may be at increased risk for the development of glaucoma. Another possible explanation is that the association between myopia and POAG is influenced by selection bias, because people who have refractive errors are more likely to seek eye care and thus have a higher probability than individuals with emmetropia of having glaucoma detected early. An association between myopia and the development of glaucoma was not observed in OHTS.

The concurrence of POAG and myopia may complicate both diagnosis and management. Disc evaluation is particularly complicated in the presence of myopic fundus changes, such as tilting of the disc and posterior staphylomas, which may make an assessment of cupping difficult. Myopia-related retinal changes can cause visual field abnormalities apart from any glaucomatous process. High refractive error may also make it difficult to perform accurate perimetric measurement and to interpret visual field abnormalities. In addition, the magnification of the disc associated with the myopic refractive error interferes with optic disc evaluation.

Wong TY, Klein BE, Klein R, et al. Refractive errors, intraocular pressure, and glaucoma in a white population. *Ophthalmology.* 2003;110:211–217.

Diabetes mellitus

Studies have reported a higher prevalence of both elevated mean IOP and POAG among persons with diabetes. In addition, glaucoma patients have been reported to have a higher

Clinical Trial 4-3

Collaborative Initial Glaucoma Treatment Study (CIGTS) Essentials

Purpose: To determine whether patients with newly diagnosed open-angle glaucoma are better treated by initial treatment with medications or by immediate filtration surgery

Participants: 607 patients with open-angle glaucoma (primary, pigmentary, or pseudoexfoliative) recruited between 1993 and 1997.

Study Design: Multicenter randomized, controlled clinical trial comparing initial medical to initial surgical therapy for open-angle glaucoma

Results: Initial medical and initial surgical therapy resulted in similar visual field outcomes after up to 5 years of follow-up. Early visual acuity loss was greater in the surgery group, but the differences between groups converged over time.

The quality of life (QOL) impact reported by the 2 treatment groups was very similar. The most persistent QOL finding was the increased impact of local eye symptoms reported by the surgical group compared with the medical group.

The overall rate of progression was lower than in many clinical trials, potentially the result of more aggressive IOP goals. Over the course of follow-up, IOP in the medical therapy group averaged 17–18 mm Hg, whereas that in the surgery group averaged 14–15 mm Hg. The rate of cataract removal was greater in the surgically treated group.

prevalence of abnormal glucose metabolism. Some authorities believe that the small-vessel involvement in diabetes may cause the optic nerve to become more susceptible to pressure-related damage. Whether diabetes is an independent risk factor for the development of POAG remains controversial. Diabetes was not associated with an increased risk of progression to glaucoma in OHTS.

Cardiovascular disease

Positive associations between blood pressure and IOP and between blood pressure and POAG have been reported. The hypothesis that systemic hypertension, with its possible microcirculatory effects on the optic nerve, may increase susceptibility to glaucoma is biologically plausible. However, evidence that cardiovascular disease is a risk factor for glaucoma is weak. The possible role of arteriosclerotic and ischemic vascular disease is also unclear, but these factors may be important in the development of some cases of glaucoma, particularly those with IOP in the normal range. Evidence is accumulating that suggests vascular autoregulatory abnormalities in individuals with glaucoma, and ongoing research into the pathophysiology of glaucoma may expand on these findings in the future. Systemic hypotension may also predispose the optic nerve to damage through reduced perfusion.

Clinical Trial 4-4

Advanced Glaucoma Intervention Study (AGIS) Essentials

Purpose: To compare the clinical outcomes of 2 treatment sequences: argon laser trabeculoplasty–trabeculectomy–trabeculectomy (ATT) and trabeculectomy–argon laser trabeculoplasty–trabeculectomy (TAT)

Participants: 789 eyes of 591 patients with medically uncontrolled open-angle glaucoma recruited from 1988 to 1992

Study Design: Multicenter randomized, controlled clinical trial comparing 2 treatment sequences (ATT and TAT) for patients with open-angle glaucoma uncontrolled by medical therapy

Results

AGIS 4: Black patients had less combined visual acuity and visual field loss if treated with the ATT sequence. White patients had less combined visual acuity and visual field loss at 7 years if treated with the TAT sequence. In the first years of follow-up in the white patients, the TAT group had greater visual acuity loss than the ATT group, but by 7 years the groups' acuities were equivalent.

AGIS 5: Encapsulated blebs were more common in male patients and in patients with prior ALT. By 1 year postop and with the resumption of medical therapy, eyes with encapsulated blebs had similar IOP control to others.

AGIS 7: Lower IOP was associated with less visual field loss. Eyes with average IOP of 14 mm Hg or less over the first 18 months, or eyes with IOP of 18 mm Hg or less at all visits throughout the study had significantly less visual field loss.

AGIS 8: Approximately half of the study patients developed cataract in the first 5 years of follow-up. Trabeculectomy increases the relative risk of cataract formation by 78%.

AGIS 9: Trabeculectomy retards the progression of glaucoma more effectively in white than in black patients. ALT was slightly more effective in blacks than in whites.

AGIS 11: ALT failure is associated with younger age and higher IOP. Trabeculectomy failure was associated with younger age, higher IOP, diabetes, and postoperative complications such as particularly elevated IOP and marked inflammation.

Retinal vein occlusion

Patients with central retinal vein occlusion (CRVO) may present with elevated IOP or glaucoma. This relationship may be obscured by the temporary hypotony that often follows the vein occlusion. In susceptible individuals, eyes with elevated IOP are at risk of developing CRVO. Thus, elevated IOP in the fellow eye of an eye affected with retinal vein occlusion must be kept as low as reasonably possible.

Table 4-2 Prevalence of Definite Primary Open-Angle Glaucoma by Age and Race

Age (Years)	No. Screened	No. of Cases	Observed Rate/100 (95% CI)*	Adjusted Rate/100 (95% CI)
White Americans				
40–49	543	1	0.18 (0.02–1.03)	0.92 (0–2.72)
50–59	618	2	0.32 (0.03–1.17)	0.41 (0–0.98)
60–69	915	7	0.77 (0.31–1.57)	0.88 (0.14–1.62)
70–79	631	18	2.85 (1.70–4.50)	2.89 (1.44–4.34)
≥80	206	4	1.94 (0.49–4.95)	2.16 (0. 05–4.26)
Total	2913	32	1.10 (0.75–1.55)	1.29 (0.80–1.78)
African Americans				
40–49	632	6	0.95 (0.35–2.07)	1.23 (0.23–2.24)
50–59	699	25	3.58 (2.32–5.26)	4.05 (2.47–5.63)
60–69	614	31	5.05 (3.42–7.17)	5.51 (3.57–7.46)
70–79	349	27	7.74 (4.94–10.54)	9.15 (5.83–12.48)
≥80	101	11	10.89 (4.81–16.97)	11.26 (4.52–18.00)
Total	2395	100	4.18 (3.38–4.98)	4.74 (3.81–5.67)

* CI = confidence interval.

(Modified from Tielsch JM, Sommer A, Katz J, et al. Racial variations in the prevalence of primary open-angle glaucoma. The Baltimore Eye Survey. *JAMA*. 1991;266:369–374.)

Prognosis

Most patients with POAG will retain useful vision for their entire lives. The incidence of blindness has been variously reported and has been estimated at 27% and 9% (unilateral vs bilateral) at 20 years following diagnosis (Hattenhauer et al.) and at a prevalence of bilateral blindness of 8% in blacks and 4% in whites (Quigley and Vitale). The age and severity at diagnosis are clearly important prognostic factors.

Hattenhauer MG, Johnson DH, Ing HH, et al. The probability of blindness from open-angle glaucoma. *Ophthalmology.* 1998;105:2099–2104.

Quigley HA, Vitale S. Models of open-angle glaucoma prevalence and incidence in the United States. *Invest Ophthalmol Vis Sci.* 1997;38:83–91.

Treatment with medications, lasers, and surgeries to lower IOP has been shown to significantly slow or possibly halt the progression of the disease. Many clinical trails have confirmed the efficacy of IOP reduction and compared various treatments at various points in the clinical course (see Table 4-1 and Clinical Trials 4-1 through 4-4). In the Early Manifest Glaucoma Treatment Study (EMGTS), a 25% reduction in IOP reduced progression from 49% to 30% of patients at 4 years' follow-up. The CIGTS showed relatively equivalent outcomes between initial surgery and initial medications for glaucoma treatment after 5 years, with significant visual progression in only 10%–13% of participants. In the Advanced Glaucoma Intervention Study (AGIS), the group of patients in whom IOP was always less than 18 mm Hg did not show progressive visual field loss; patients with average IOP of 14 mm Hg or less over the first 18 months fared better than those with average IOP greater than 17.5 mm Hg (AGIS 7). The results of AGIS also suggest that African American patients do better if treated with argon laser trabeculoplasty (ALT) before trabeculectomy after failing medical therapy (AGIS 4). For Caucasians, the data suggest that after 5 years, the trabeculectomy-first patients had less combined visual field or visual acuity loss than the ALT group, although the ALT group still had better visual acuity (with worse visual field loss) (AGIS 4).

Comparison of treatment outcomes within race: seven-year results. Advanced Glaucoma Intervention Study (AGIS): 4. *Ophthalmology.* 1998;105:1146–1164.

Preferred Practice Patterns Committee, Glaucoma Panel. *Primary Open-Angle Glaucoma.* San Francisco: American Academy of Ophthalmology; 2003.

The relationship between control of intraocular pressure and visual field deterioration. Advanced Glaucoma Intervention Study (AGIS): 7. The AGIS Investigators. *Am J Ophthalmol.* 2000;130:429–440.

Wilson MR, Brandt JD. Update on glaucoma clinical trials. *Focal Points: Clinical Modules for Ophthalmologists.* San Francisco: American Academy of Ophthalmology; 2003, module 9.

Open-Angle Glaucoma Without Elevated IOP (Normal-tension Glaucoma)

Considerable controversy remains about whether normal-tension glaucoma represents a distinct disease entity or is simply POAG with IOP within the average range. Because IOP is a continuous variable with no firm dividing line between normal and abnormal, many authorities believe the terms *low-tension glaucoma* and *normal-tension glaucoma* should be abandoned. This debate is likely to persist. Whatever the outcome, the concept of normal-tension glaucoma has undeniably had a strong influence on the classification and understanding of glaucoma.

Clinical Features

As previously emphasized, elevated IOP is an important risk factor in the development of glaucoma, but it is not the only risk factor. In normal-tension glaucoma, other risk factors, most of which are currently unknown, may play a more important role. Many authorities have hypothesized that local vascular factors may have a significant part in the development of this disorder. Studies have suggested that patients with normal-tension glaucoma show a higher prevalence of vasospastic disorders such as migraine headache and Raynaud phenomenon, ischemic vascular diseases, autoimmune diseases, and coagulopathies compared with patients who have high-tension glaucoma. However, these findings have not been consistent. Vascular autoregulatory defects have also been described in studies of eyes with normal-tension glaucoma.

The condition is characteristically progressive, often despite the lowering of IOP. The association between IOP and normal-tension glaucoma has long been controversial. Studies have indicated that in glaucomatous eyes with normal but asymmetric IOP, the worse damage usually occurs in the eye with the higher IOP. The Collaborative Normal-Tension Glaucoma Study (CNTGS) found that reducing IOP by greater than 30% reduced the rate of visual field progression from 35% to 12%, confirming a clear role of IOP in this disease. However, because some patients did progress despite the reduction in IOP, other factors may be operative as well. In addition, progression of the visual field loss, when it did occur, tended to be slow. It should be noted that the protective effect of IOP reduction was only evident after adjusting for the effect of cataracts, which were more frequent in the treated group.

Cartwright MJ, Anderson DR. Correlation of asymmetric damage with asymmetric intraocular pressure in normal-tension glaucoma (low-tension glaucoma). *Arch Ophthalmol.* 1988; 106:898–900.

Comparison of glaucomatous progression between untreated patients with normal-tension glaucoma and patients with therapeutically reduced intraocular pressures. Collaborative Normal-Tension Glaucoma Study Group. *Am J Ophthalmol.* 1998;126:487–497.

Another area of considerable debate concerns patterns of optic disc damage and visual field loss in normal-tension glaucoma compared with POAG. In eyes matched for total visual field loss, the neuroretinal rim has been reported to be thinner, especially inferiorly and inferotemporally, in those with normal-tension glaucoma. Varied patterns of peripapillary atrophy may also be characteristic for normal-tension glaucoma. Some authorities have separated normal-tension glaucoma into 2 groups based on disc appearance:

- a *senile sclerotic group* with shallow, pale sloping of the neuroretinal rim (primarily in older patients with vascular disease)
- a *focal ischemic group* with deep, focal, polar notching in the neuroretinal rim

The visual field defects in normal-tension glaucoma tend to be more focal, deeper, and closer to fixation, especially early in the course of the disease, compared with those commonly seen in POAG. A dense paracentral scotoma encroaching on fixation is not an unusual finding as the initial defect. Although many reports have described these differences between the presentation of normal-tension glaucoma and POAG, others have failed to confirm them.

Differential Diagnosis

Normal-tension glaucoma can be mimicked by many conditions, as summarized in Table 4-3. Several of these conditions can cause arcuate-type visual field defects; some may be progressive. Great care must be taken to distinguish normal-tension glaucoma from these other etiologies, as appropriate treatment may vary greatly. Diurnal IOP measurement is useful to determine peak IOP, which aids in determining target IOP.

Elevated IOP can be obscured in patients taking systemic medication, particularly systemic beta blockers, and by artifactually low tonometric readings caused, for example, by reduced scleral rigidity and corneal thickness. Assessment of central corneal thickness (CCT) is recommended in patients suspected of having normal-tension glaucoma, as a thin central cornea may lead to artifactually low IOP readings. In studies to date, the average CCT has ranged between 510 and 520 μm in patients with normal-tension glaucoma vs 540 μm in unaffected patients. Corneal thickness is therefore especially of interest in patients who have undergone refractive surgery. Many patients with myopia may have anomalous discs or myopic field changes, further complicating the diagnosis of glaucoma. Other conditions to consider in the differential diagnosis include normalized IOP in an

Table 4-3 Differential Diagnosis of Normal-Tension Glaucoma

Undetected high-tension glaucoma
- Primary open-angle glaucoma with diurnal IOP variation
- Intermittent IOP elevation
  - Angle-closure glaucoma
  - Glaucomatocyclitic crisis
- Previously elevated IOP
  - Old secondary glaucoma (eg, corticosteroid-induced glaucoma, uveitic glaucoma, pigmentary glaucoma)
  - Normalized IOP in an eye with previously elevated IOP
- Use of medication that may cause IOP lowering (systemic beta blocker)
- Tonometric error (reduced corneal thickness, low scleral rigidity)

Nonglaucomatous optic nerve disease
- Congenital anomalies (coloboma, optic nerve pits)
- Compressive lesions of optic nerve and chiasm
- Shock optic neuropathy
- Anterior ischemic optic neuropathy
- Retinal disorders (ie, retinal detachment, retinoschisis, vascular occlusions, chorioretinitis, syphilis)
- Optic nerve drusen

eye with previously elevated IOP, intermittent angle-closure glaucoma, and previous corticosteroid-induced or other secondary glaucoma.

Diagnostic Evaluation

It is difficult to know how often glaucomatous damage occurs with IOP in the normal range. Population-based epidemiologic studies have suggested that as many as 30%–50% of glaucomatous eyes may have IOP below 21 mm Hg on a single reading. Repeated testing would undoubtedly have detected elevated IOP in many of these eyes. The prevalence of normal-tension glaucoma appears to vary among different populations. Studies have suggested that among Japanese patients, a particularly high proportion of open-angle glaucoma occurs with IOP in the normal range. Among clinic-based patients, a diagnosis of normal-tension glaucoma is influenced by how thoroughly other possible causes of optic neuropathy are considered and eliminated.

Before making a diagnosis of normal-tension glaucoma, the clinician should measure the patient's IOP by applanation tonometry at various times during the day. Gonioscopy should be performed to rule out angle closure, angle recession, or evidence of previous intraocular inflammation. Careful stereoscopic disc evaluation is essential to rule out other congenital or acquired disc anomalies, such as optic nerve coloboma, drusen, and physiologically enlarged cups. The clinician must also consider the patient's medical history, particularly any record of cardiovascular disease and low blood pressure caused by hemorrhage, myocardial infarction, or shock. Field loss consistent with glaucoma has been noted after a decrease in blood pressure following a hypotensive crisis. However, damage secondary to such a specific precipitating event tends to be stable and does not progress once the underlying problem has been corrected. Similarly, a prior episode of prolonged, elevated IOP, such as that related to the use of topical steroids in susceptible individuals, may create optic nerve damage that later mimics normal-tension glaucoma but is not progressive. Most cases of normal-tension glaucoma are not caused by a sudden precipitating event.

Sometimes a diagnosis cannot be established on the basis of a single or even multiple ophthalmic examinations, particularly if findings are atypical, such as unilateral disease, decreased central vision, or visual field loss not consistent with the optic disc appearance. In such cases, medical and neurologic evaluation should be considered, including tests for anemia, heart disease, syphilis, and temporal arteritis or other causes of systemic vasculitis. Auscultation and palpation of the carotid arteries should be performed, and noninvasive tests of carotid circulation may be helpful. Increasing attention is being focused on assessment of ocular blood flow, but techniques for these measurements are generally still investigational. Evaluation of the optic nerve in the chiasmal region with computed tomography (CT) or magnetic resonance imaging (MRI) may be warranted in some cases to rule out compressive lesions, especially if the visual field loss is at all suggestive of congruous, bitemporal, or other neurologic defects (see also BCSC Section 5, *Neuro-Ophthalmology*).

Greenfield DS, Siatkowski RM, Glaser JS, et al. The cupped disc. Who needs neuroimaging? *Ophthalmology.* 1998;105:1866–1874.

Prognosis and Therapy

Therapy for normal-tension glaucoma can be difficult and controversial. It is generally initiated for normal-tension glaucoma unless the optic neuropathy is determined to be stable. The results of the Collaborative Normal-Tension Glaucoma Study support aggressive reduction in IOP by greater than 30% in an attempt to reduce progressive visual field loss. The criteria for initiating therapy in this study were visual field loss threatening fixation, disc hemorrhage, and documented visual field or optic nerve progression. This study demonstrated that disease in some patients (65%) did not progress over the length of the study despite the lack of treatment, whereas in others (12%) it did progress despite aggressive reduction in IOP, demonstrating the extremely variable clinical course. The potential role of neuroprotective agents is experimental and remains under investigation (see Chapter 7). In vivo and animal studies are promising; clinical trials of these agents in humans are currently ongoing. The goal of therapy should be to achieve an IOP as low as possible without inducing complications, using the knowledge currently available.

Systemic medications such as calcium channel blockers are advocated by some authorities because of the possible beneficial effects of increasing capillary perfusion of the optic nerve head. The efficacy of this treatment, however, has not been conclusively demonstrated. If systemic treatment with calcium channel blockers is undertaken, it should be coordinated with the patient's primary care physician because of possible side effects. Systemic hypotension, a possible complication of this therapy, may adversely affect ocular blood flow.

As with POAG, medical therapy is the most common initial approach in treating normal-tension glaucoma. As with all glaucomas, it is useful for the ophthalmologist to change or add medications to one eye at a time so the contralateral eye can be used as a control to assess therapeutic response. If medications are inadequate in controlling the disease, laser trabeculoplasty can be effective in reducing IOP. Glaucoma filtering surgery may be indicated in an attempt to obtain the lowest IOP. An antifibrotic agent, 5-fluorouracil or mitomycin C, may be used to improve the success rate of filtering surgery and to reduce the postoperative and long-term IOP in these patients with low target IOPs (see Chapter 8).

Bhandari A, Crabb DP, Poinoosawmy D, et al. Effect of surgery on visual field progression in normal-tension glaucoma. *Ophthalmology.* 1997;104:1131–1137.

Comparison of glaucomatous progression between untreated patients with normal-tension glaucoma and patients with therapeutically reduced intraocular pressures. Collaborative Normal-Tension Glaucoma Study Group. *Am J Ophthalmol.* 1998;126:487–497.

The effectiveness of intraocular pressure reduction in the treatment of normal-tension glaucoma. Collaborative Normal-Tension Glaucoma Study Group. *Am J Ophthalmol.* 1998;126: 498–505.

Mikelberg FS. Normal tension glaucoma. *Focal Points: Clinical Modules for Ophthalmologists.* San Francisco: American Academy of Ophthalmology; 2000, module 12.

The Glaucoma Suspect

A glaucoma suspect is defined as an adult who has one of the following findings in at least 1 eye:

- an optic nerve or nerve fiber layer defect suggestive of glaucoma (enlarged cup–disc ratio, asymmetric cup-disc ratio, notching or narrowing of the neural rim, a disc hemorrhage, or diffuse or local abnormality in the nerve fiber layer)
- a visual field abnormality consistent with glaucoma
- an elevated IOP consistently greater than 22 mm Hg

Usually, if 2 or more of these findings are present, the diagnosis of POAG is supported, especially in the presence of other risk factors, such as age >50, family history of glaucoma, and African descent. Diagnosis of a glaucoma suspect is also dependent on a normal open angle on gonioscopy.

A frequent finding warranting this diagnosis is elevated IOP in the absence of identifiable optic nerve damage or visual field loss, a condition often termed *ocular hypertension.* Estimates of the prevalence of ocular hypertension vary considerably; some authorities believe it may be as high as 8 times that of definite POAG. Analysis of studies that have followed individuals with elevated IOP for variable time periods indicates that the higher the baseline IOP, the greater the risk of developing glaucoma. However, it is important to note that even among individuals with elevated IOP, the majority never develop glaucoma.

Differentiating between diagnoses of ocular hypertension versus early POAG is often difficult. The ophthalmologist must look carefully for signs of early damage to the optic nerve, such as focal notching, asymmetry of cupping, splinter disc hemorrhage, nerve fiber layer dropout, or subtle visual field defects. The increasing use of short-wavelength and frequency-doubling automated perimetry may improve our ability to recognize early glaucomatous visual field loss in these patients (see Chapter 3). If these signs of optic nerve damage are present, the diagnosis of early POAG should be considered and treatment initiated. However, in uncertain cases, the ophthalmologist should not hesitate to closely monitor patients without therapy to confirm either initial findings or progressive change in order to better establish the diagnosis prior to initiating therapy.

No clear consensus exists on whether elevated IOP should be treated in the absence of signs of early damage. Some clinicians select and treat those individuals thought to be at greatest risk for developing glaucoma after assessing all risk factors.

The Ocular Hypertension Treatment Study (OHTS) identified elevated IOP, reduced central corneal thickness (CCT), and increased cup–disc ratio as important risk factors for the development of glaucoma in patients with ocular hypertension. The OHTS included patients with IOP between 24 and 32 mm Hg and randomized patients to observation or to the reduction of IOP by topical medications (Fig 4-1). In OHTS, 4.4% of patients treated (with topical antiglaucoma medications to reduce IOP 20%) progressed to glaucoma over 5 years, based on the development of optic nerve or visual field damage. More than twice as many of the untreated observation group, 9.5%, progressed. Thus, topical medications were definitively shown to reduce the risk of glaucoma in patients with ocular hypertension; however, most untreated patients did not get worse over a

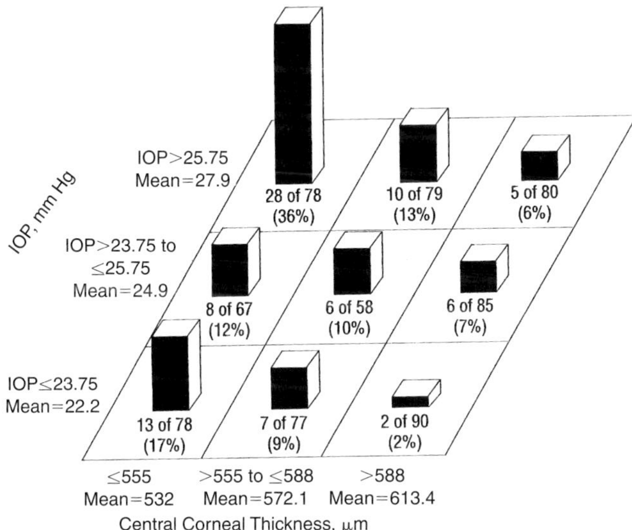

Figure 4-1 The percentage of participants in the observation group who developed POAG (median follow-up, 72 months) grouped by baseline intraocular pressure (IOP) of ≤23.75 mm Hg, >23.75 mm Hg to ≤25.75 mm Hg, and >25.75 mm Hg and by central corneal thickness measurements of ≤555 μm, >555 μm to ≤588 μm, and >588 μm. These percentages are not adjusted for length of follow-up. The means are not identical to those given in the text, which includes all participants in the Ocular Hypertension Treatment Study rather than just the observation group. *(From Wilson RM, Brandt JD, Update on glaucoma clinical trials.* Focal Points: Clinical Modules for Ophthalmologists. *San Francisco: American Academy of Ophthalmology; 2003, module 9. Reprinted with permission from Gordon MO, Beiser JA, Brandt JD, et al. The Ocular Hypertension Treatment Study: baseline factors that predict the onset of primary open-angle glaucoma.* Arch Ophthalmol. *2002;120:718:Fig 1. Copyrighted 2002, American Medical Association.)*

5-year period. Each millimeter of elevated baseline IOP increased the risk of glaucomatous change by about 10%. For each 0.1 increment in vertical cup–disc ratio, the risk was increased by 30%.

CCT has been recognized to affect the IOP measurement, probably because a thicker cornea resists indentation by applanation, resulting in a higher measured IOP. However, the increase in risk of progression to glaucoma was not fully explained in OHTS by the anticipated artifactual change in measured IOP from differences in CCT. In this study, every 40 μm of reduced corneal thickness increased the risk of glaucomatous change by 70%. Thus, in this population of patients with baseline IOP of 24–32 mm Hg, CCT is very important in assessing the risk of developing glaucoma.

Other potential risk factors such as myopia, diabetes mellitus, family history, migraine, and high or low blood pressure were not confirmed in this study to be significant risk factors in the univariate or multivariate analysis. As mentioned previously, African-American origin was found to increase the risk of developing glaucoma in the univariate but not in the multivariate analysis, apparently as a result of the thinner average corneal thickness and greater baseline vertical cup–disc ratio in this population.

All available data must be weighed in assessing the patient's risk for developing glaucoma and deciding whether to treat elevated IOP. The following risk factors should be considered:

- level of IOP
- CCT (corneal pachymetry)
- cup–disc ratio
- family history of glaucoma
- race
- age
- associated disease states (diabetes mellitus, systemic hypertension, and cardiovascular disease)

Based on the findings of the examination and the results of the OHTS study, an assessment of the patient's risk of developing glaucoma can be derived. The clinician and the patient can together decide if this risk warrants the inconvenience, cost, and potential side effects of therapy. Care must be taken that the risks of therapy do not exceed the risks of the disease. Additional factors that may affect the decision to start ocular antihypertensive therapy include the desires of the patient, compliance, availability for follow-up visits, reliability of visual fields, and ability to examine the optic disc.

Gordon MO, Beiser JA, Brandt JD, et al. The Ocular Hypertension Treatment Study: baseline factors that predict the onset of primary open-angle glaucoma. *Arch Ophthalmol.* 2002; 120:714–720.

Kass MA, Heuer DK, Higginbotham EJ, et al. The Ocular Hypertension Treatment Study: a randomized trial determines that topical ocular hypotensive medication delays or prevents the onset of primary open-angle glaucoma. *Arch Ophthalmol.* 2002;120:701–713.

Preferred Practice Patterns Committee, Glaucoma Panel. *Primary Open-Angle Glaucoma Suspect.* San Francisco: American Academy of Ophthalmology; 2002.

Wilson MR, Brandt JD. Update on glaucoma clinical trials. *Focal Points: Clinical Modules for Ophthalmologists.* American Academy of Ophthalmology; 2003, module 9.

Secondary Open-Angle Glaucoma

Exfoliation Syndrome (Pseudoexfoliation)

Exfoliation syndrome is characterized by the deposition of a distinctive fibrillar material in the anterior segment of the eye. Histologically, this material has been found in and on the lens epithelium and capsule, pupillary margin, ciliary epithelium, iris pigment epithelium, iris stroma, iris blood vessels, and subconjunctival tissue. Although the origin of this material is not known precisely, it probably arises from multiple sources as part of a generalized basement membrane disorder. Histochemically, the material resembles amyloid.

Deposits occur in a targetlike pattern on the anterior lens capsule and are best seen after pupil dilation. A central area and a peripheral zone of deposition are usually separated by an intermediate clear area, where iris movement presumably rubs the material from the lens (Fig 4-2). The material is often visible on the iris at the edge of the pupil. Deposits also occur on the zonular fibers of the lens, ciliary processes, inferior anterior chamber angle, and corneal endothelium (Fig 4-3). In aphakic individuals, these deposits may be seen on the anterior hyaloid as well.

The chamber angle is often characterized by a trabecular meshwork that is heavily pigmented with dark, almost black, pigment, usually in a variegated fashion. An inferior pigmented deposition, scalloped in nature, is often present anterior to Schwalbe's line. This pigmented line is often referred to as Sampaolesi's line (Fig 4-4). The chamber angle

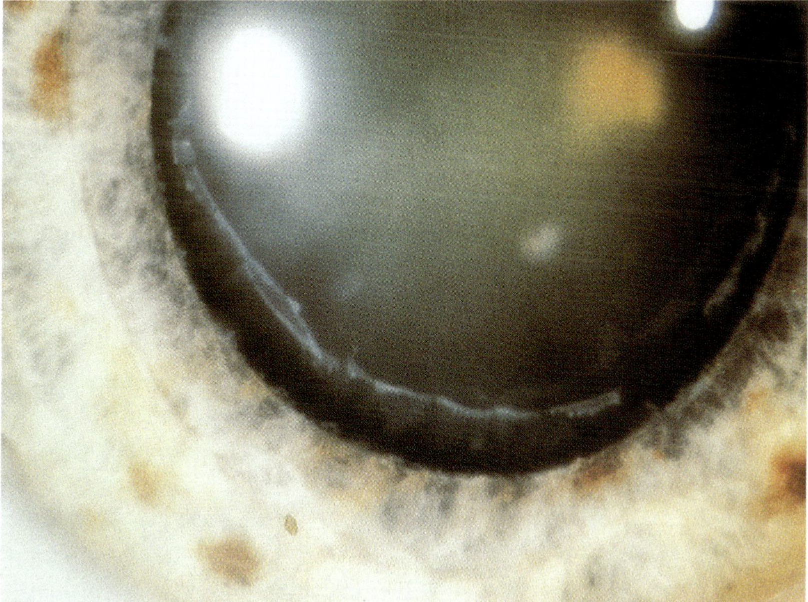

Figure 4-2 Evidence of exfoliative material deposited on the anterior lens capsule. Exfoliative material may also be deposited on other structures within the anterior segment, including the iris, ciliary processes, peripheral retina, and the conjunctiva.

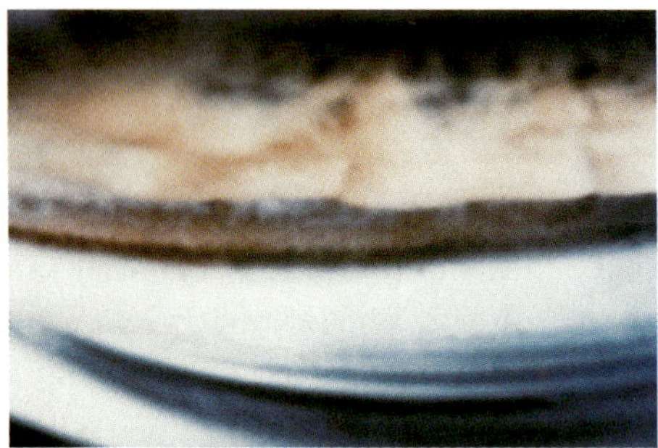

Figure 4-3 Exfoliative debris collecting on iris processes in inferior anterior chamber angle. *(Photograph courtesy of Steven T. Simmons, MD.)*

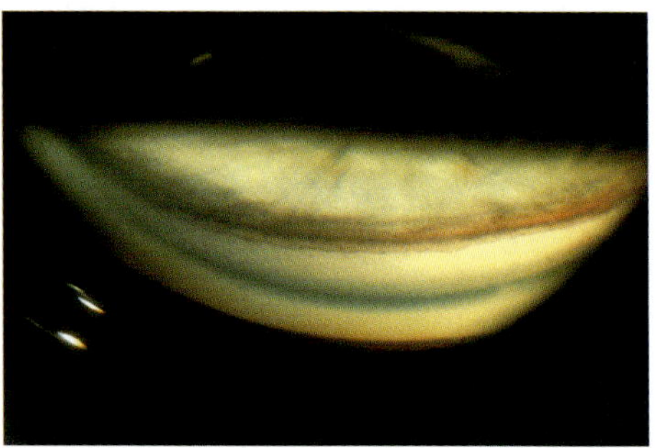

Figure 4-4 Sampaolesi's line in the inferior anterior chamber angle of a patient who has exfoliation syndrome. *(Photograph courtesy of L. J. Katz, MD.)*

is often narrow, presumably as a result of anterior movement of the lens-iris diaphragm related to zonular weakness.

In addition to the typical deposits and pigmentation, other anterior segment abnormalities are also noted. Fine pigment deposits often appear on the iris surface, and peripupillary atrophy with transillumination of the pupillary margin is common. A more scattered, diffuse depigmentation may also occur, with transillumination defects over the entire sphincter region. The pupil often dilates poorly. Phacodonesis and iridodonesis are not uncommon; they are related to zonular weakness, which may predispose affected eyes to zonular dehiscence; vitreous loss; and other complications, including lens dislocation, during cataract surgery (see also BCSC Section 11, *Lens and Cataract*). Iris angiography has demonstrated abnormalities of the iris vessels with fluorescein leakage.

Exfoliation syndrome may be monocular or binocular with varying degrees of asymmetry. Often the disorder is clinically apparent in only 1 eye, although the uninvolved fellow eye often develops the syndrome at a later time. Exfoliation syndrome is associated with open-angle glaucoma in all populations, but the prevalence varies considerably. In Scandinavian countries, exfoliation syndrome accounts for more than 50% of cases of open-angle glaucoma. The odds of the exfoliation syndrome leading to glaucoma vary widely, and range up to 40% over a 10-year period. This syndrome is strongly age-related: it is rarely seen under the age of 50 and occurs most commonly in individuals over the age of 70.

The open-angle glaucoma associated with exfoliation syndrome is thought to be caused by the fibrillar material obstructing flow through, and causing damage to, the trabecular meshwork. Exfoliation glaucoma differs from POAG in often presenting monocularly and showing greater pigmentation of the trabecular meshwork. Furthermore, the IOP is often higher, with greater diurnal fluctuations than in POAG, and the overall prognosis is worse. Laser trabeculoplasty can be very effective, but the response may not last as long as with POAG. Lens extraction does not alleviate the condition. Trabeculectomy results are similar to those with POAG, but there may be an increase in postoperative inflammation. In fact, increased ocular inflammation can be seen following all ocular surgery in patients with this condition.

Ritch R. Perspective on exfoliation syndrome. *J Glaucoma.* 2001;10 (Suppl 1):S33–S35.
Ritch R. Exfoliation syndrome. In: Ritch R, Shields MB, Krupin T, eds. *The Glaucomas.* 2nd ed. St. Louis: Mosby; 1996: ch 47, 993–1022.

Pigmentary Glaucoma

The *pigment dispersion syndrome* consists of pigment deposition on the corneal endothelium in a vertical spindle pattern (Krukenberg spindle), in the trabecular meshwork, and on the lens periphery (Fig 4-5), and, typically, midperipheral iris transillumination defects. The spindle pattern on the posterior cornea is caused by the aqueous convection currents and subsequent phagocytosis of pigment by the corneal endothelium. The presence of Krukenberg spindles is not absolutely necessary to make the diagnosis of pigment dispersion syndrome, and it may occur in other diseases such as exfoliation syndrome. Characteristic spokelike loss of the iris pigment epithelium occurs that is manifested as transillumination defects in the iris midperiphery (Fig 4-6). The peripheral iris transillumination defects appear in front of the lens zonular fibers, suggesting that mechanical contact between the zonular fibers and the iris causes the iris pigment release.

Gonioscopy reveals a homogeneous, densely pigmented trabecular meshwork with a speckled ring of pigment at or anterior to Schwalbe's line (Fig 4-7). The midperipheral iris is often concave in appearance, bowing posterior toward the zonular fibers. When dilated, pigment deposits can be seen on the zonular fibers and both the anterior and posterior lens capsule near the equator of the lens (Zentmayer's line; Fig 4-8).

This syndrome does not universally lead to glaucoma. An individual with pigment dispersion syndrome may never develop elevated IOP, and various studies have suggested that the risk of an affected individual developing glaucoma is approximately 25%–50%. Pigmentary glaucoma occurs most commonly in white males with myopia between the ages of 20 and 50 years. Affected females tend to be older than affected males.

Pigmentary glaucoma is characterized by wide fluctuations in IOP, which can exceed 50 mm Hg in untreated eyes. High IOP often occurs when pigment is released into the aqueous humor, such as following exercise or pupillary dilation. Symptoms may include halos, intermittent visual blurring, and ocular pain.

Posterior bowing of the iris with "reverse pupillary block" configuration is noted in many eyes that have pigmentary glaucoma. This iris configuration may result in greater

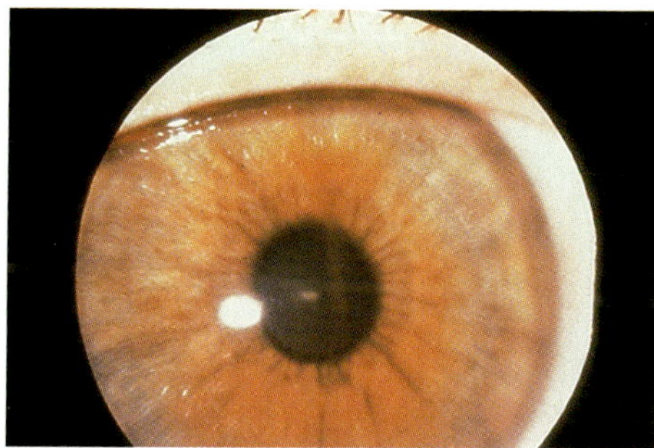

Figure 4-5 Krukenberg spindle. *(Photograph courtesy of L. J. Katz, MD.)*

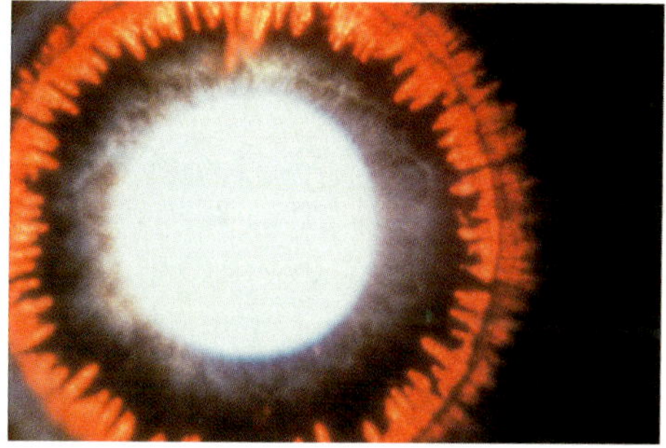

Figure 4-6 Classic spokelike iris transillumination defects seen in pigmentary dispersion syndrome. *(Photograph courtesy of L. J. Katz, MD.)*

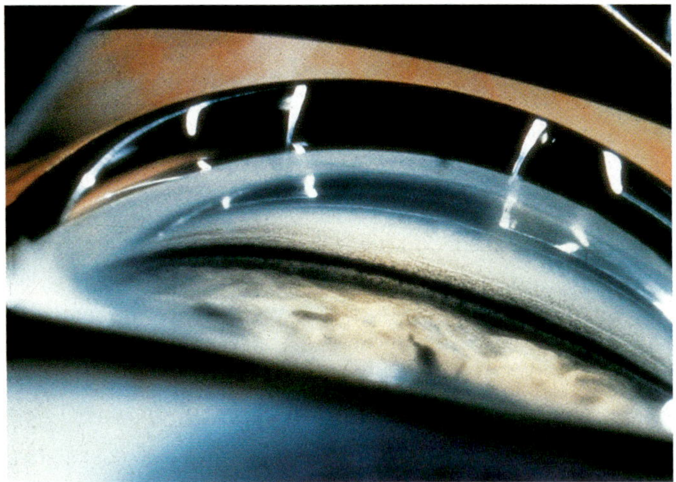

Figure 4-7 Characteristic heavy, uniform pigmentation of the trabecular meshwork seen in the pigment dispersion syndrome and pigmentary glaucoma. *(Photograph courtesy of M. Roy Wilson, MD.)*

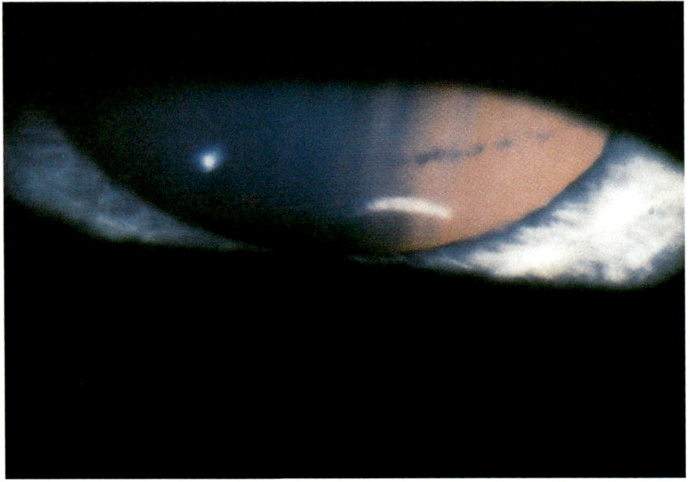

Figure 4-8 In pigmentary dispersion syndrome, pigment deposits can be seen on the anterior and posterior lens capsule and on the lens zonules with gonioscopy in dilated eye. *(Photograph courtesy of Steven T. Simmons, MD.)*

contact of the zonular fibers with the posterior iris surface, with a subsequent increase of pigment release. Laser iridectomy has been proposed as a means of minimizing posterior bowing of the iris (Fig 4-9). However, its effectiveness in treating pigmentary glaucoma has not been established.

Gandolfi SA, Vecchi M. Effect of a YAG laser iridotomy on intraocular pressure in pigment dispersion syndrome. *Ophthalmology.* 1996;103:1693–1695.

With age, the signs and symptoms of pigment dispersion may decrease in some individuals, possibly as a result of normal growth of the lens and an increase in physio-

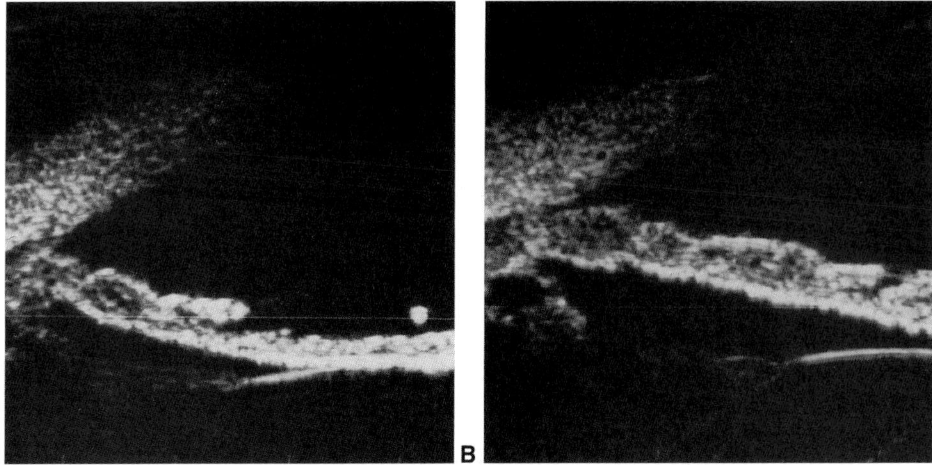

Figure 4-9 **A,** Ultrasound biomicroscopy image of concave iris configuration in pigmentary glaucoma, pre–laser treatment. **B,** Same eye, post–laser treatment. *(Photographs courtesy of Charles J. Pavlin, MD.)*

logic pupillary block, moving the iris forward, away from contact with the zonular fibers. Loss of accommodation may also be a factor. As pigment dispersion is reduced, the deposited pigment may fade from the trabecular meshwork, anterior iris surface, and corneal endothelium. Transillumination defects may also gradually disappear.

Medical treatment is often successful in reducing IOP. Patients respond reasonably well to laser trabeculoplasty, although the effect may be short-lived. The heavy trabecular pigmentation allows increased absorption of laser energy, in turn allowing lower energy levels for trabeculoplasty. Spikes in IOP may be seen more frequently with higher energy settings in pigment dispersion syndrome following laser trabeculoplasty. Filtering surgery is usually successful; however, extra care is warranted, as young patients with myopia may be at increased risk for hypotony maculopathy.

Liebmann JM. Pigmentary glaucoma: new insights. *Focal Points: Clinical Modules for Ophthalmologists.* San Francisco: American Academy of Ophthalmology; 1998, module 2.

Yang JW, Sakiyalak D, Krupin T. Pigmentary glaucoma. *J Glaucoma.* 2001;10 (Suppl 1): S30–S32.

Lens-Induced Glaucoma

The lens may cause both open-angle and angle-closure glaucomas, and these are summarized in Table 4-4. The open-angle, lens-induced glaucomas are divided into 3 clinical entities:

- phacolytic glaucoma
- lens particle glaucoma
- phacoanaphylaxis

See also BCSC Section 9, *Intraocular Inflammation and Uveitis,* and Section 11, *Lens and Cataract.*

Phacolytic glaucoma

Phacolytic glaucoma is an inflammatory glaucoma caused by the leakage of lens protein through the capsule of a mature or hypermature cataract (Fig 4-10). As the lens ages, its protein composition becomes altered, with an increased concentration of high-molecular-weight lens protein. In a mature or hypermature cataract, these proteins are released through microscopic openings in the lens capsule. The proteins precipitate a secondary glaucoma as these lens proteins, phagocytizing macrophages, and other inflammatory debris obstruct the trabecular meshwork.

The clinical picture usually involves an elderly patient with a history of poor vision who has sudden onset of pain, conjunctival hyperemia, and worsening vision. Examination reveals a markedly elevated IOP, microcystic corneal edema, prominent cell and flare reaction without keratic precipitates (KP), and an open anterior chamber angle (Fig 4-11). The lack of KP helps distinguish phacolytic glaucoma from phacoanaphylaxis. Cellular debris may be seen layering in the anterior chamber angle, and a hypopyon may be present. Large white particles (clumps of lens protein) may also be seen in the anterior chamber. A mature, hypermature, or morgagnian cataract is present, often with wrinkling of the anterior lens capsule representing loss of volume and the release of lens material (see Fig 4-10). Although medications to control the IOP should be used immediately, definitive therapy requires cataract extraction.

Lens particle glaucoma

Lens particle glaucoma occurs when lens cortex obstructs the trabecular meshwork following cataract extraction, capsulotomy, or ocular trauma. The extent of the glaucoma depends on the quantity of lens material released, the degree of inflammation, the ability of the trabecular meshwork to clear the lens material, and the functional status of the ciliary body, which is often altered following surgery or trauma.

Table 4-4 Lens-Induced Glaucomas

Open-angle	**Angle-closure** (see Chapter 5)
Phacolytic glaucoma	Phacomorphic
Lens particle glaucoma	Ectopia lentis
Phacoanaphylaxis	

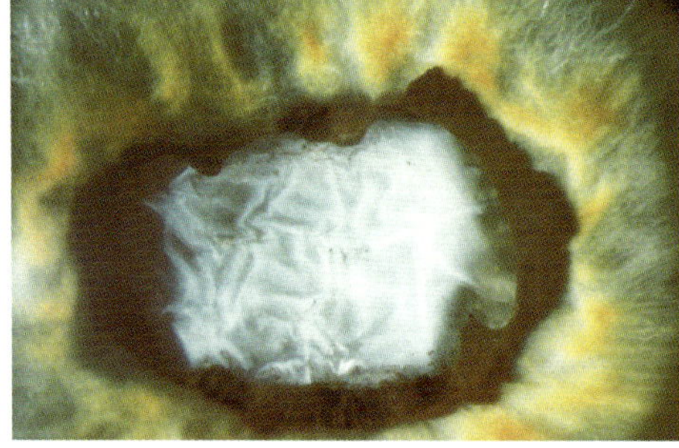

Figure 4-10 Characteristic appearance of hypermature cataract with loss of cortical volume and wrinkling of the anterior lens capsule. Extensive posterior synechiae are present, confirming the presence of previous inflammation. *(Photograph courtesy of Steven T. Simmons, MD.)*

Lens particle glaucoma usually occurs within weeks of the initial surgery or trauma, but it may occur months or years later (Figs 4-12, 4-13). Clinical findings include free cortical material in the anterior chamber, elevated IOP, moderate anterior chamber reaction, microcystic corneal edema, and, with time, the development of posterior and peripheral anterior synechiae.

If possible, medical therapy should be initiated to control the IOP while the residual lens material resorbs. Appropriate therapy includes medications to decrease aqueous formation, mydriatics to inhibit posterior synechiae formation, and topical corticosteroids to reduce inflammation. If the glaucoma cannot be controlled, surgical removal of the lens material is necessary.

Phacoanaphylaxis

Phacoanaphylaxis is a rare entity in which patients become sensitized to their own lens protein following surgery or penetrating trauma, resulting in a granulomatous inflammation. The clinical picture is quite variable, but most patients present with a moderate anterior chamber reaction with KP on both the corneal endothelium and the anterior

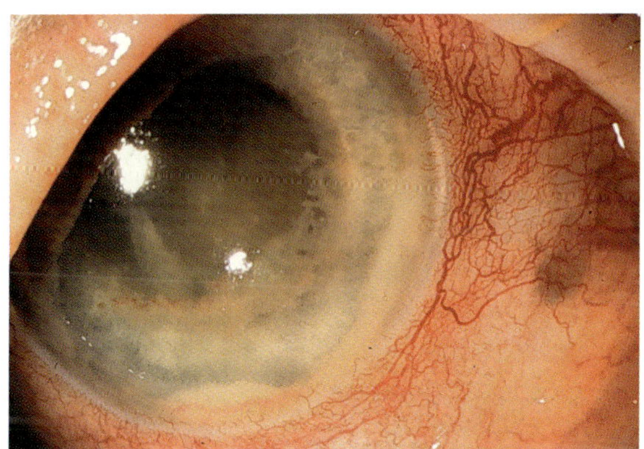

Figure 4-11 Phacolytic glaucoma. Conjunctival hyperemia, microcystic corneal edema, mature cataract, and prominent anterior chamber reaction is the typical presentation of phacolytic glaucoma, as demonstrated in this photograph. Note lens protein deposits on endothelium and layering in the angle, creating a pseudohypopyon. *(Courtesy of George A. Cioffi, MD.)*

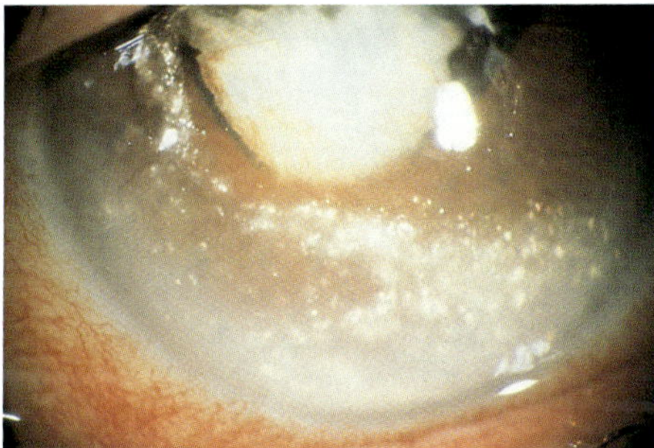

Figure 4-12 Lens particle glaucoma. Cortical lens material obstructs the trabecular meshwork following traumatic disruption of the anterior lens capsule. *(Photograph courtesy of Steven T. Simmons, MD.)*

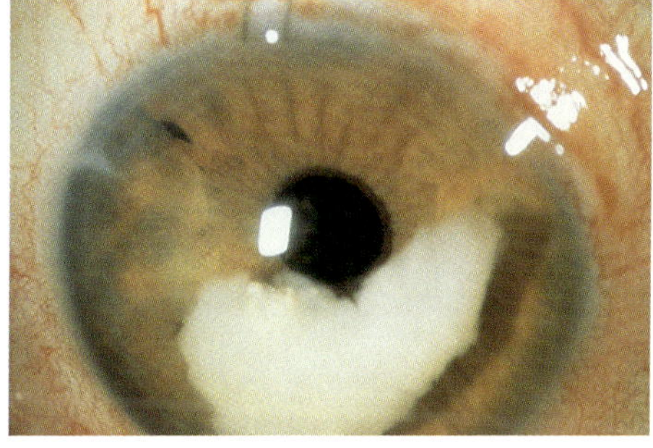

Figure 4-13 Lens particle glaucoma. Despite the large amount of lens cortex remaining in the anterior chamber following cataract surgery, this eye is relatively quiet and the IOP remained normal. *(Photograph courtesy of the Wills Eye Hospital slide collection, 1986.)*

lens surface. In addition, a low-grade vitritis, synechial formation, and residual lens material in the anterior chamber may be found. Glaucoma, although it may occur, is not common in eyes with phacoanaphylaxis. Phacoanaphylaxis is treated medically with corticosteroids and aqueous suppressants to reduce inflammation and IOP. If medical treatment is unsuccessful, residual lens material should be removed.

Intraocular Tumors

A variety of tumors can cause unilateral chronic glaucoma. Many of the tumors described in this section are discussed in greater detail in BCSC Section 4, *Ophthalmic Pathology and Intraocular Tumors.* The glaucoma can result from several different mechanisms, depending on the size, type, and location of the tumor:

- direct tumor invasion of the anterior chamber angle
- angle closure by rotation of the ciliary body or by anterior displacement of the lens–iris diaphragm (see Chapter 5)
- intraocular hemorrhage
- neovascularization of the angle
- deposition of tumor cells, inflammatory cells, and cellular debris within the trabecular meshwork

Choroidal melanomas and other choroidal and retinal tumors tend to cause secondary angle-closure glaucoma as the result of a forward shift in the lens–iris diaphragm and closure of the anterior chamber angle. Inflammation caused by necrotic tumors may cause posterior synechiae, which can exacerbate this angle closure through a pupillary-block mechanism. Choroidal melanomas, medulloepitheliomas, and retinoblastomas can also cause anterior segment neovascularization, which can result in angle closure.

The most common cause of glaucoma in primary or metastatic tumors of the ciliary body is direct angle invasion. This glaucoma can be exacerbated by anterior segment hemorrhage and inflammation, which further obstruct outflow. Necrotic tumor and tumor-filled macrophages may cause obstruction of the trabecular meshwork and result in a secondary open-angle glaucoma. Tumors causing glaucoma in adults include uveal melanoma, metastatic carcinoma, lymphomas, and leukemia. Glaucoma in children is associated with retinoblastoma, juvenile xanthogranuloma, and medulloepithelioma.

Shields CL, Materin MA, Shields JA, et al. Factors associated with elevated intraocular pressure in eyes with iris melanoma. *Br J Ophthalmol.* 2001;85:666–669.

Ocular Inflammation and Secondary Open-Angle Glaucoma

Inflammatory glaucoma is a secondary glaucoma that often combines components of open-angle and angle-closure disease. In uveitis, elevated IOP occurs when the trabecular dysfunction exceeds the ciliary body hyposecretion seen with acute inflammation. Often the ocular inflammation is nonspecific. When the inflammation is accompanied by increased IOP, the physician's dilemma is whether the cause of the increased IOP is the active inflammation and insufficient anti-inflammatory therapy, chronic structural damage related to the underlying inflammation, or corticosteroid therapy.

Open-angle inflammatory glaucoma is caused by a variety of mechanisms:

- edema of the trabecular meshwork
- trabecular meshwork endothelial cell dysfunction
- blockage of the trabecular meshwork by fibrin and inflammatory cells
- prostaglandin-mediated breakdown of the blood–aqueous barrier
- steroid-induced reduction in aqueous outflow through the trabecular meshwork

Most cases of anterior uveitis are idiopathic, but uveitides commonly associated with open-angle inflammatory glaucoma include herpes zoster iridocyclitis, herpes simplex keratouveitis, toxoplasmosis, rheumatoid arthritis, and pars planitis. See also BCSC Section 9, *Intraocular Inflammation and Uveitis.*

The presence of KP and a miotic pupil suggests iritis as the cause of IOP elevation. Gonioscopic evaluation may reveal subtle trabecular meshwork precipitates. Sometimes, peripheral anterior synechiae (PAS) or posterior synechiae with iris bombé may develop, resulting in angle closure. The treatment of inflammatory glaucoma is complicated by the fact that corticosteroid therapy may increase IOP, either by reducing inflammation and improving aqueous production or by decreasing outflow. Miotic agents should be avoided in patients with iritis, because they may aggravate the inflammation and cause posterior synechiae. In these entities, inadequately controlled inflammation with elevated IOP is often mistaken for steroid-induced glaucoma. In the face of active inflammation, elevated IOP should be presumed to be inflammation-related rather than steroid-induced.

Glaucomatocyclitic crisis (Posner-Schlossman syndrome)

Glaucomatocyclitic crisis, an uncommon form of open-angle inflammatory glaucoma, is characterized by recurrent bouts of markedly increased IOP and low-grade anterior chamber inflammation. First described by Posner and Schlossman in 1948, the condition affects middle-aged patients and usually presents with unilateral blurred vision and mild eye pain. The iritis is mild with few KP that are small, discrete, and round in nature and usually resolve spontaneously within a few weeks. KP may be seen on the trabecular meshwork on gonioscopy, suggesting a "trabeculitis." The IOP is usually markedly elevated, in the 40–50 mm Hg range, and corneal edema may be present. In between bouts, the IOP usually returns to normal, but, with increasing numbers of attacks, a chronic secondary glaucoma may develop, resulting in visual loss. The etiology of the disease remains unknown, but a prostaglandin-mediated mechanism has been proposed. There is no evidence that chronic suppressive therapy with topical nonsteroidal anti-inflammatory agents or mild steroids is effective in preventing attacks. Recurrent attacks of acute angle-closure glaucoma have been mistaken for this condition.

Fuchs heterochromic iridocyclitis

Fuchs heterochromic iridocyclitis, a relatively rare, chronic form of iridocyclitis, is characterized by iris heterochromia with loss of iris pigment in the affected eye; low-grade anterior chamber reaction with small, stellate KP; posterior subcapsular cataracts; and secondary open-angle glaucoma. The condition is insidious and unilateral, affecting the hypochromic eye, and presents equally in middle-aged men and women. The secondary open-angle glaucoma occurs in approximately 15% of the cases. Gonioscopy reveals multiple fine vessels that cross the trabecular meshwork (Fig 4-14). These vessels, unlike those in iris neovascularization, do not appear to be associated with a fibrous membrane and usually do not lead to PAS and secondary angle closure, although in rare cases the neovascularization may be progressive. These vessels are fragile and may cause an anterior chamber hemorrhage, either spontaneously or with trauma, including cataract or glaucoma surgery (Fig 4-15).

The glaucoma does not correspond to the degree of inflammation and may be difficult to control. Corticosteroids are generally not effective in treating this condition. Medical therapy starts with aqueous suppressants, which are often effective in controlling IOP.

Elevated Episcleral Venous Pressure

Episcleral venous pressure is an important factor in the regulation of IOP. Normal episcleral venous pressure is 8–10 mm Hg, but it can be raised by a variety of clinical entities that either obstruct venous outflow or involve arteriovenous malformations. A partial list of entities that increase episcleral venous pressure is presented in Table 4-5.

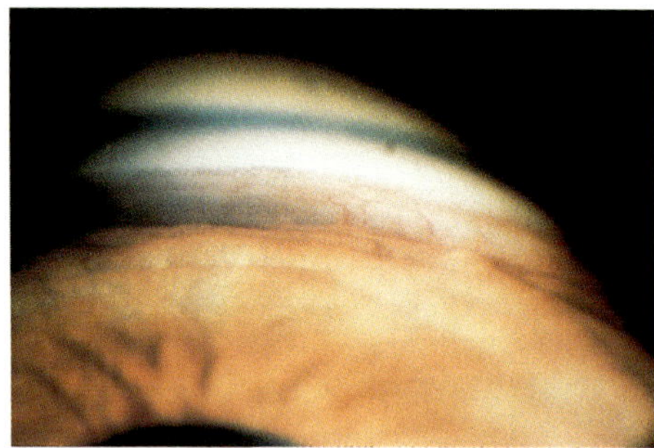

Figure 4-14 Fuchs heterochromic iridocyclitis. Fine vessels are seen crossing the trabecular meshwork. This neovascularization is not accompanied by a fibrovascular membrane and does not result in peripheral anterior synechiae formation and secondary angle closure. *(Photograph courtesy of Steven T. Simmons, MD.)*

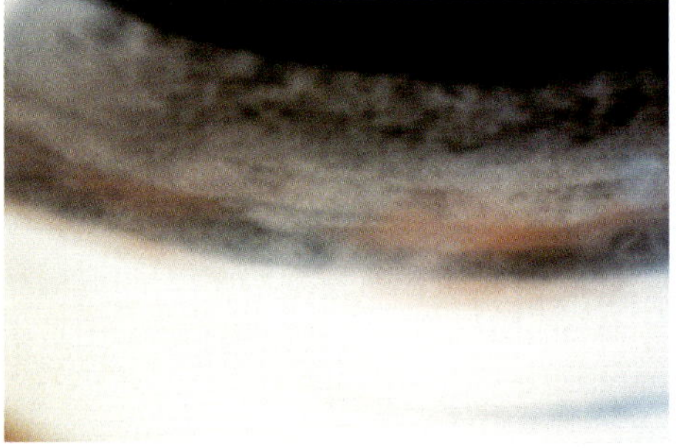

Figure 4-15 The atypical vessels seen in the anterior chamber angle of patients with Fuchs heterochromic iridocyclitis are fragile and can result in a filiform hemorrhage. This hemorrhage often occurs spontaneously or with minimal trauma, as demonstrated in this photograph. *(Photograph courtesy of Steven T. Simmons, MD.)*

Table 4-5 Causes of Increased Episcleral Pressure

Causes
Arteriovenous malformations
Arteriovenous fistula (carotid–dural)
Orbital varix
Sturge-Weber syndrome
Venous obstruction
Retrobulbar tumor
Thyroid ophthalmopathy
Superior vena cava syndrome

Patients may note a chronic red eye without discomfort or allergic symptoms. Occasionally, a distant history of significant head trauma may suggest the cause of a carotid-cavernous or dural sinus fistula. However, most cases are idiopathic, often without angiographic abnormalities, and may be familial. Clinically, patients with increased episcleral venous pressure present with tortuous, dilated episcleral veins (Fig 4-16). These vascular changes may be unilateral or bilateral depending on the location of the vascular anomaly. The anterior segment appears normal in most of these patients, except for elevated IOP and the gonioscopic finding of blood in Schlemm's canal. Rarely, signs of ocular ischemia or venous stasis may be present. Sudden, severe carotid-cavernous fistulas may be accompanied by proptosis and other orbital or neurologic signs. These cases may require neurosurgical intervention.

Medications that reduce aqueous humor formation are more effective than drugs that increase aqueous outflow. Laser trabeculoplasty is not effective unless there are secondary changes in the outflow channels. Glaucoma filtering surgery may be complicated by a ciliochoroidal effusion or a suprachoroidal hemorrhage.

Accidental and Surgical Trauma

Nonpenetrating, or blunt, trauma to the eye causes a variety of anterior segment injuries:

- hyphema
- angle recession (cleavage)
- iridodialysis
- iris sphincter tear
- cyclodialysis
- lens subluxation

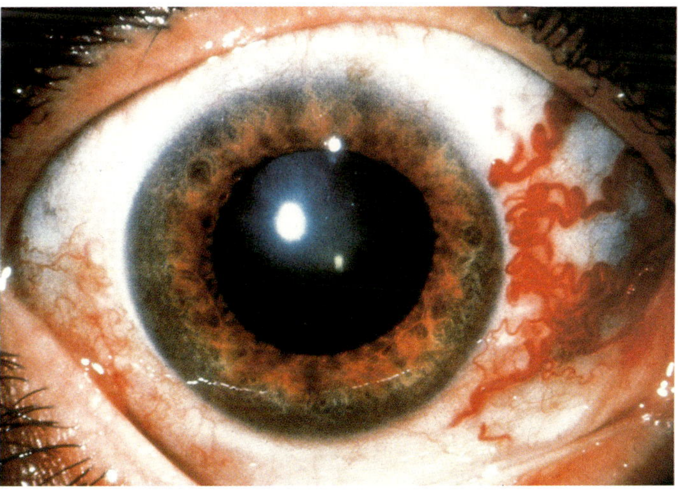

Figure 4-16 Elevated episcleral pressure. Prominent episcleral vessels are seen in a patient with Sturge-Weber syndrome. Patients with increased episcleral pressure present with tortuous, dilated episcleral vessels. *(Photograph courtesy of Steven T. Simmons, MD.)*

A combination of posttraumatic inflammation, presence of blood and red blood cells, and direct injury to the trabecular meshwork often results in elevated IOP initially after trauma. This elevation tends to be short in duration but may be protracted, with the risk of corneal blood staining (Fig 4-17) and glaucomatous optic nerve damage.

Open-angle glaucoma is one of the long-term sequelae of *siderosis* or *chalcosis* from a retained intraocular metallic foreign body in penetrating or perforating injuries. Chemical injuries, particularly alkali, may cause acute secondary glaucoma as a result of inflammation, shrinkage of scleral collagen, release of chemical mediators such as prostaglandins, direct damage to the chamber angle, or compromise of the anterior uveal circulation. Trabecular damage or inflammation may cause glaucoma to develop months or years after a chemical injury.

Hyphema

Glaucoma may result from hyphema through several mechanisms (Fig 4-18). Increased IOP is more common following recurrent hemorrhage or rebleeding following a traumatic hyphema. The reported frequency of rebleeding following hyphema varies considerably in the literature, with an average incidence of 5%–10%. Rebleeding usually occurs within 3–7 days after the initial hyphema and may be related to normal clot retraction and lysis. In most cases, the size of the hyphema associated with rebleeding is greater than the primary hyphema. In general, the larger the hyphema, the higher the incidence of increased IOP, although small hemorrhages may also be associated with marked elevation of IOP, especially in the already compromised angle. Increased IOP is a result of obstruction of the trabecular meshwork with red blood cells, inflammatory cells, debris, and fibrin, and direct injury to the trabecular meshwork from the blunt trauma.

Individuals with sickle cell hemoglobinopathies have an increased incidence of elevated IOP following hyphema. Normal red blood cells generally pass through the trabecular meshwork without difficulty. However, in the sickle cell hemoglobinopathies

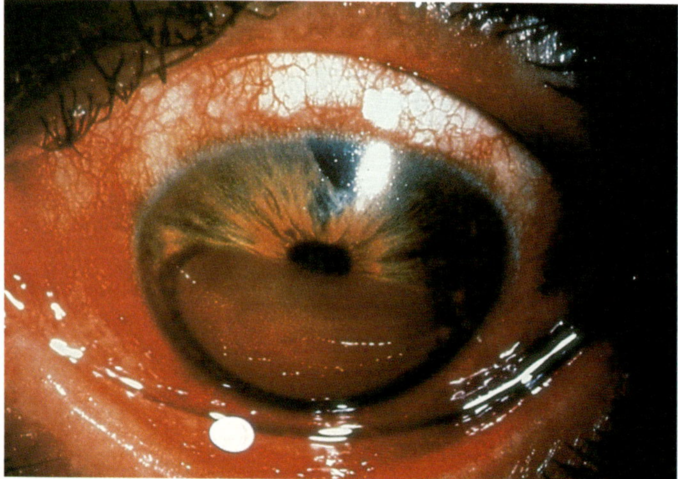

Figure 4-17 Corneal blood staining following trauma. *(Photograph courtesy of Steven T. Simmons, MD.)*

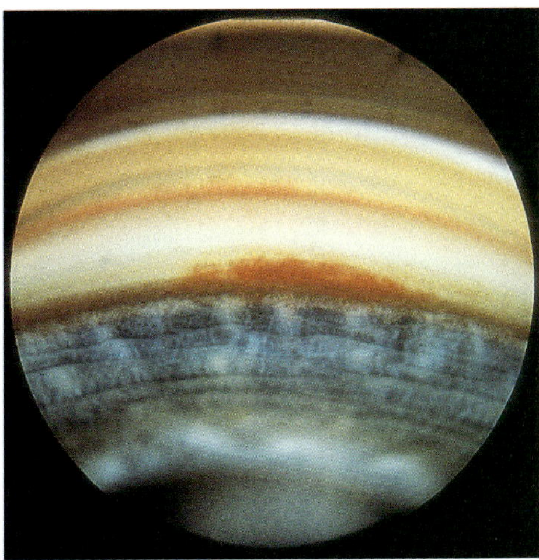

Figure 4-18 A small hyphema seen gonioscopically in the inferior chamber angle with layering of blood on the trabecular meshwork. *(Photograph courtesy of Steven T. Simmons, MD.)*

(including sickle trait), the red blood cells tend to sickle in the anterior chamber due to the acidity of the stagnant aqueous humor. These more rigid cells have great difficulty passing out of the eye through the trabecular meshwork. Even small amounts of blood in the anterior chamber may therefore result in marked elevations of IOP. In addition, the optic nerves of patients with sickle cell disease are much more sensitive to elevated IOP and are prone to ischemic injuries, such as anterior ischemic optic neuropathy and central retinal artery occlusion, as a result of compromised microvascular perfusion.

In general, an uncomplicated hyphema should be managed conservatively, with an eye shield, limited activity, and head elevation. Topical and systemic corticosteroids may reduce associated inflammation, although their effect on rebleeding is debatable. If significant ciliary spasm or photophobia occurs, cycloplegic agents may be helpful, but they have no proven benefit in terms of rebleeding. Systemic administration of aminocaproic acid has been shown to reduce rebleeding in some studies. However, this has not been confirmed in all studies, and systemic side effects, such as hypotension, syncope, abdominal pain, and nausea can be significant and limit the use of aminocaproic acid. Patching and bed rest are also advocated by some authors, although these precautions are of unproven value.

If the IOP is elevated, aqueous suppressants and hyperosmotic agents are recommended. It has been suggested that patients with sickle cell hemoglobinopathies should avoid carbonic anhydrase inhibitors, as they may increase the sickling tendency in the anterior chamber by increasing aqueous levels of ascorbic acid; however, this relationship has not been firmly established. Physicians should be aware of the potential of systemic carbonic anhydrase inhibitors and hyperosmotic agents to induce sickle crises in susceptible individuals who are significantly dehydrated. Sickling may be enhanced by both drugs, as they may each exacerbate dehydration, and carbonic anhydrase inhibitors may additionally promote acidosis. Adrenergic agonists with significant $alpha_1$ agonist effects (apraclonidine, dipivefrin, epinephrine) should also be avoided in sickle cell disease because of concerns regarding anterior segment vasoconstriction. Parasympathomimetic agents should be avoided in all patients with hyphemas.

Clinicians should have a lower threshold for surgical intervention in sickle cell patients given the increased risk of complications from elevated IOP. The potential of inducing amblyopia if the hyphema or corneal staining significantly obstructs vision may justify early surgical intervention in very young children. If surgery for increased IOP becomes necessary, an anterior chamber irrigation or washout procedure is commonly performed first. If a total hyphema is present, pupillary block may occur, and an iridectomy is helpful at time of washout. If the IOP remains uncontrolled, a trabeculectomy may be required. Some surgeons prefer to perform a trabeculectomy as the initial surgical procedure with the anterior chamber washout in order to obtain immediate IOP control and relief of any pupillary block.

Hemolytic and ghost cell glaucoma

Hemolytic and/or ghost cell glaucoma may develop after vitreous hemorrhage. In *hemolytic glaucoma,* hemoglobin-laden macrophages block the trabecular outflow channels. Red-tinged cells are seen floating in the anterior chamber, and a reddish brown discoloration of the trabecular meshwork is often present.

Ghost cell glaucoma is a transient secondary open-angle glaucoma caused by degenerated red blood cells (ghost cells) blocking the trabecular meshwork. Ghost cells are red blood cells that have lost their intracellular hemoglobin and appear as small, khaki-colored cells that are less pliable than normal red blood cells (Fig 4-19). This loss of pliability results in obstruction of the trabecular meshwork and secondary glaucoma. The cells develop within 1–3 months following a vitreous hemorrhage. They gain access to

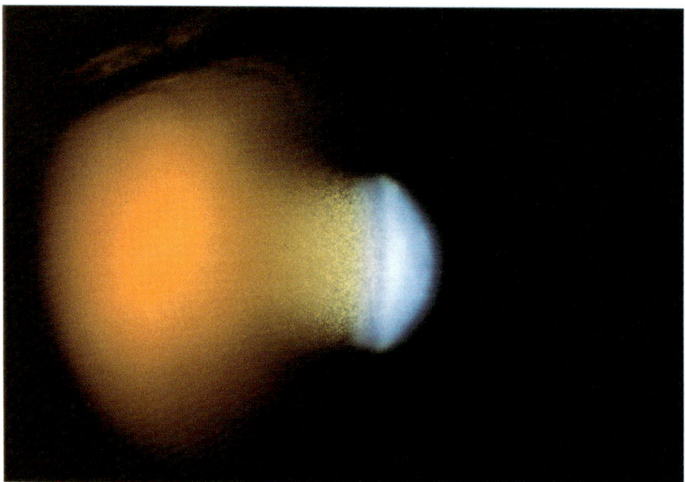

Figure 4-19 Ghost cell glaucoma: the classic appearance of ghost cells in the anterior chamber. These khaki-colored cells are small and can become layered, as is seen in a hyphema and hypopyon. As a result of their loss of pliability, they remain longer in the anterior chamber, causing obstruction of the trabecular meshwork and secondary glaucoma. *(Photograph courtesy of Ron Gross, MD.)*

the anterior chamber through a disrupted hyaloid face, which can occur from previous surgery (pars plana vitrectomy, cataract extraction, or capsulotomy), trauma, or spontaneous disruption.

Clinically, patients present with increased IOP and history of vitreous hemorrhage resulting from trauma, surgery, or preexisting retinal disease. The IOP may be markedly elevated, causing corneal edema. The anterior chamber is filled with small, circulating, tan-colored cells (see Fig 4-19). The cellular reaction appears out of proportion to the aqueous flare, and the conjunctiva tends not to be inflamed unless the IOP is markedly elevated. Gonioscopically, the angle appears normal except for the layering of ghost cells over the trabecular meshwork inferiorly. The vitreous has the appearance of old hemorrhage, with characteristic khaki coloration and clumps of extracellular pigmentation from degenerated hemoglobin.

Both hemolytic and ghost cell glaucoma generally resolve once the hemorrhage has cleared. Medical therapy with aqueous suppressants is the preferred initial approach. If medical therapy fails to control marked elevations of IOP, some patients may require irrigation of the anterior chamber, pars plana vitrectomy, and/or a trabeculectomy to control the condition.

Traumatic, or angle-recession, glaucoma

An angle recession, or cleavage, is a tear in the ciliary body that splits between the longitudinal and circular muscle fibers. Angle recessions are often associated with injury to the trabecular meshwork as well. Angle recession glaucoma is a chronic, unilateral secondary open-angle glaucoma that usually occurs months to years following ocular trauma. It resembles primary open-angle glaucoma in presentation and clinical course but can usually be distinguished by its classic gonioscopic findings (Figs 4-20, 4-21):

- broad angle recess
- absent or torn iris processes
- white glistening scleral spur

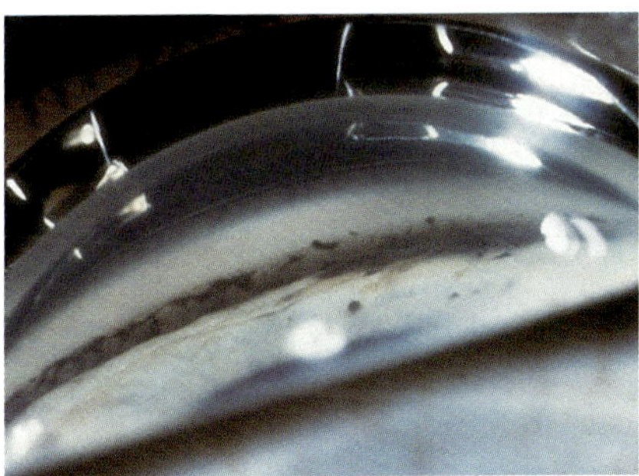

Figure 4-20 An angle recession occurs when the ciliary body is torn between the longitudinal and circular fibers of the ciliary body. There is a deepened angle recess as a result of atrophy of the circular fibers. *(Photograph courtesy of Joseph Krug, MD.)*

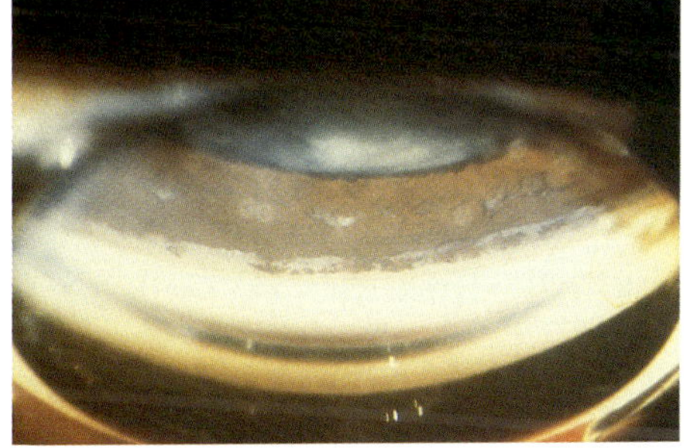

Figure 4-21 Typical angle appearance of an angle recession. Torn iris processes; a whitened, increasingly visible scleral spur; and a localized depression of the trabecular meshwork are seen. *(Photograph courtesy of Steven T. Simmons, MD.)*

- depression in the overlying trabecular meshwork
- localized PAS at the border of the recession

The degree of angle involvement and underlying patient predisposition play an important role in determining whether a secondary glaucoma will develop. A significant proportion (up to 50%) of fellow eyes may develop increased IOP, suggesting that perhaps many eyes with angle-recession glaucoma may have been predisposed to open-angle glaucoma.

Angle-recession glaucoma should be considered in patients presenting with unilateral elevations in IOP. History may reveal the contributing incident; however, often this has been forgotten. Careful examination may show findings consistent with previous trauma, such as corneal scars, tears in the pupil margin, changes in the angle as above, focal anterior subcapsular cataracts, and a loose or subluxated lens.

A greater extent of angle recession is associated with a greater the risk of glaucoma. Even with substantial angle recession, this risk is not high, but all eyes with angle recession must be followed because it is not possible to predict which eyes will develop glaucoma. Although the risk of developing glaucoma decreases appreciably after several years, the risk is still present even 25 years or more following injury, and these eyes should continue to be examined annually.

The treatment of angle-recession glaucoma is often best accomplished with aqueous suppressants, hypotensive lipids, and alpha$_2$-adrenergic agonists. Miotics may be useful, but paradoxical responses with increased IOP may occur. Laser trabeculoplasty has a limited role and a reduced chance of success.

Surgical trauma

Operative procedures such as cataract extraction, filtering surgery, or corneal transplantation may be followed by an increase in IOP. Similarly, laser surgery—including trabeculoplasty, iridectomy, and posterior capsulotomy—may be complicated by posttreatment IOP elevation. Although the IOP may rise as high as 50 mm Hg or more, these elevations are usually transient, lasting from a few hours to a few days. The exact mechanism is not always known, but pigment release, presence of inflammatory cells and debris, mechanical deformation of the trabecular meshwork, and angle closure may all be implicated.

In addition, agents used as adjuncts to intraocular surgery may cause secondary IOP elevations. For example, the injection of viscoelastic substances such as sodium hyaluronate into the anterior chamber may result in a transient and possibly severe postoperative increase in IOP. Dispersive viscoelastics (sodium hyaluronate), especially in higher-molecular-weight forms, may be more likely to cause IOP increases than retentive viscoelastic agents (chondroitin sulfate).

Such postoperative pressure elevation can cause considerable damage to the optic nerve of a susceptible individual even in a short time. Eyes with preexisting glaucoma are at particular risk for further damage. Elevated IOP may increase the risk of retinal and optic nerve ischemia. It is thus important to measure IOP soon after surgery or laser treatment. If a substantial rise in IOP does occur, therapy may be required. Usually, use of beta-adrenergic antagonists, alpha$_2$-adrenergic agonists, or carbonic anhydrase inhibitors is adequate. However, hyperosmotic agents are sometimes necessary. See Chapter 7, Medical Management of Glaucoma, for discussion of these agents.

The implantation of an intraocular lens (IOL) can lead to a variety of secondary glaucomas:

- uveitis-hyphema-glaucoma (UGH) syndrome (Fig 4-22)
- secondary pigmentary glaucoma (Fig 4-23)
- pseudophakic pupillary block (see Chapter 5)

Uveitis-hyphema-glaucoma (UGH) syndrome is a form of secondary inflammatory glaucoma caused by chronic irritation that is usually the result of a malpositioned or rotating anterior chamber IOL (see Fig 4-22). Characterized by chronic inflammation, secondary iris neovascularization, and recurrent hyphemas, this condition often results in an intractable form of secondary glaucoma following the chafing of the iris by the IOL or erosion of the lens haptics through the iris or ciliary body. This condition may also occur following implantation of a posterior chamber or suture-fixated IOL. Gonioscopy and ultrasound biomicroscopy (UBM) may be helpful in revealing the IOL's exact relation to the iris and ciliary body. Persistent or recurrent cases occasionally require lens repositioning or lens exchange, which can be technically challenging, as many of these eyes may have synechiae and/or an open posterior capsule. This syndrome may be mimicked in patients with neovascularization of the internal lip of a corneoscleral wound. These patients may have recurrent spontaneous hypemas, which can lead to elevated IOP. Argon laser ablation of the vessels may successfully resolve these cases.

Jarstad JS, Hardwig PW. Intraocular hemorrhage from wound neovascularization years after anterior segment surgery (Swan syndrome). *Can J Ophthalmol.* 1987;22:271–275.

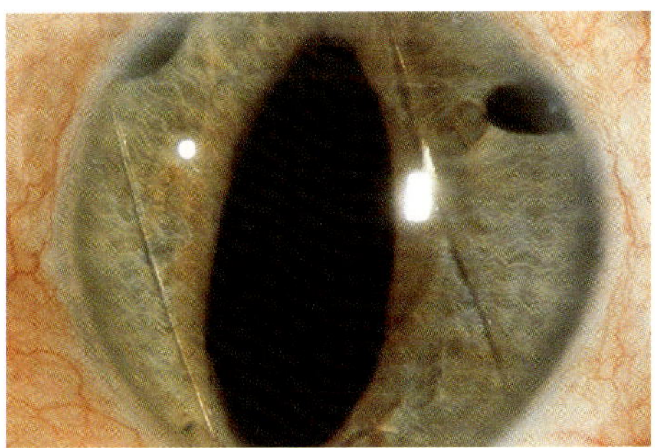

Figure 4-22 Uveitis-glaucoma-hyphema (UGH) syndrome is a form of secondary inflammatory glaucoma caused by chronic inflammation from a malpositioned anterior chamber IOL. The early rigid anterior chamber IOLs, such as this one, were more susceptible to this entity than the more modern lenses used today. *(Photograph courtesy of L. J. Katz, MD.)*

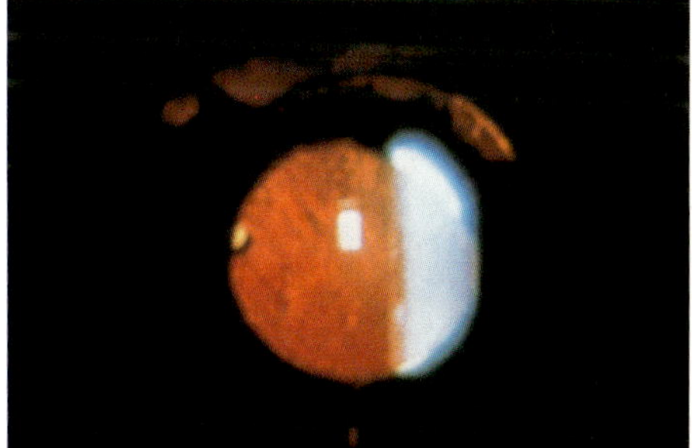

Figure 4-23 Secondary pigmentary glaucoma. Superior iris transillumination is seen in this photograph caused by the underlying optic and haptic of the posterior chamber IOL. The release of iris pigmentation can lead to trabecular meshwork dysfunction and secondary glaucoma. *(Photograph courtesy of Wills Eye Hospital slide collection, 1986.)*

Schwartz's syndrome (Schwartz-Matsuo syndrome)

Rhegmatogenous retinal detachments typically lower IOP, presumably as a result of increased outflow by active pumping of fluid through the exposed retinal pigment epithelium. Schwartz first described elevated IOP in association with a rhegmatogenous retinal detachment, and Matsuo later demonstrated photoreceptor outer segments in the aqueous humor in a group of similar patients. The postulated mechanism of IOP elevation is that a chronic rhegmatogenous retinal detachment leads to the liberation of photoreceptor outer segments, which, migrating through the retinal tear, reach the anterior chamber and impede aqueous outflow through the trabecular meshwork. The photoreceptor segments may be mistaken for an anterior chamber inflammatory reaction or pigment. The IOP tends to normalize after successful retinal reattachment.

Glaucoma and penetrating keratoplasty

Secondary glaucoma is a common complication of penetrating keratoplasty, and it occurs with increased frequency in the aphakic/pseudophakic patient and with repeat grafts. The different mechanisms of the glaucoma are outlined in Table 4-6. Wound distortion of the trabecular meshwork and a progressive angle closure are the most common causes of long-standing glaucoma, and attempts to minimize these secondary glaucomas with oversized donor grafts, peripheral iridectomies, and surgical repair of the iris sphincter have been only partially successful. BCSC Section 8, *External Disease and Cornea,* discusses penetrating keratoplasty in detail.

Drugs and Glaucoma

Corticosteroid-induced glaucoma is an open-angle glaucoma caused by prolonged use of topical, periocular, inhaled, or systemic corticosteroids. It mimics POAG in its presentation and clinical course. Approximately one third of all patients demonstrate some responsiveness to corticosteroids, but only a small percentage will have a clinically significant elevation in IOP. The type and potency of the agent, the means and frequency of its administration, and the susceptibility of the patient all affect the duration of time before the IOP rises and the extent of this rise. A high percentage of patients with POAG demonstrate this response to topical corticosteroids. Systemic administration of corticosteroids may also raise IOP in some individuals, although less frequently than topical administration. The elevated IOP is a result of an increased resistance to aqueous outflow in the trabecular meshwork.

Table 4-6 Mechanism of Secondary Glaucoma Following Penetrating Keratoplasty

Open Angle	Closed Angle
Inflammatory	Chronic PAS/angle closure
Corticosteroid induced	Pupillary block
Viscoelastic	
Wound distortion of trabecular meshwork	Fibrous/epithelial ingrowth
Fibrous/epithelial ingrowth	Inflammatory

Corticosteroid-induced glaucoma may develop at any time during long-term corticosteroid administration. IOP thus needs to be monitored regularly in patients receiving corticosteroid treatment. Some corticosteroid preparations such as fluorometholone (FML), rimexolone (Vexol), medrysone (HMS), or loteprednol (Lotemax) are less likely to raise IOP than are prednisolone or dexamethasone. However, even weaker corticosteroids or lower concentrations of stronger drugs can raise IOP in susceptible individuals.

A corticosteroid-induced rise in pressure may cause glaucomatous optic nerve damage in some patients. This condition can mimic POAG in patients of any age.

The cause of the elevation in IOP is not always related to the use of a corticosteroid and may be instead related to underlying ocular disease such as anterior uveitis. Following discontinuation of the corticosteroid, the IOP usually decreases with a time course similar to or slightly longer than the onset of elevation. However, unmasked POAG or secondary open-angle inflammatory glaucoma may remain.

Patients with excessive levels of endogenous corticosteroids (eg, Cushing syndrome) can also develop increased IOP. Generally, IOP returns to normal when the corticosteroid-producing tumor or hyperplastic tissue is excised.

Cycloplegic drugs can increase IOP in individuals with open angles. Routine dilation for ophthalmoscopy may increase IOP; those at greater risk include patients with POAG, exfoliation syndrome, or pigment dispersion syndrome, and those on miotic therapy.

Epstein DL, Allingham RR, Schuman JS, eds. *Chandler and Grant's Glaucoma.* 4th ed. Baltimore: Williams & Wilkins; 1997.

Shields MB. *Textbook of Glaucoma.* 4th ed. Philadelphia: Williams & Wilkins; 2000.

CHAPTER 5

Angle-Closure Glaucoma

Introduction

Of the nearly 67 million patients with glaucoma worldwide, it has been estimated that one half are affected by angle-closure glaucoma. Primary angle-closure glaucoma (PACG) has been called the most common form of glaucoma in the world, and the leading cause of bilateral blindness. Occurring less often in the West, it is the predominant form of glaucoma in East Asia. PACG is responsible for 91% of the bilateral blindness in China and affects over 1.5 million Chinese.

The modern history of PACG goes back almost 150 years. In 1856, von Graefe performed an iridectomy on a staphylomatous eye and demonstrated the first cure for acute "inflammatory glaucoma." However, the pathophysiology of primary angle closure and how the iridectomy brought about this cure remained in question for another century. In 1873, Leber wrote that aqueous was secreted from the ciliary processes, traveled through the pupil, and entered into the anterior chamber. He felt that the forward movement of the iris could lead to elevated IOP and angle-closure glaucoma. In the later part of the 19th century, Weber and later Priestly Smith hypothesized that angle closure occurred as a result of swelling of the ciliary processes, which pushed the iris forward over the trabecular meshwork. In 1920, Edward Curran proposed the mechanism of pupillary block and the importance of an iridectomy in breaking this impeded aqueous flow. His initial observations and theories on PACG were finally accepted in 1951, following papers and presentations by Joseph Haas, Harold Scheie, and Paul Chandler, confirming the principle of "relative pupillary block." Advances in gonioscopy prior to 1940, by Barkan, Trantus, Koeppe, Salzmann, and Troncoso further helped define and distinguish the angle-closure glaucomas. The development of the Goldmann lens in 1938 allowed more universal use of gonioscopy, further advancing our knowledge and understanding of the anterior chamber angle.

The angle-closure glaucomas include a large and diversified group of diseases, which are unified by the presence of peripheral anterior synechiae and/or iridotrabecular apposition. Their presentation can be acute, with profound symptoms, or chronic, with asymptomatic visual loss. The physician must identify the anatomic changes that have occurred and the underlying pathophysiology that has precipitated these changes in order to initiate the appropriate therapy for each type of angle-closure glaucoma. Early diagnosis and treatment in most forms of angle-closure glaucoma can be invaluable, if not curative, and so understanding and identifying the various forms of pathophysiology is essential if proper treatment is to be initiated. Also, screening patients at greatest risk for angle closure can be beneficial in reducing the number of patients developing these diseases and reduce the risk of blindness.

Any discussion of angle-closure glaucoma is constrained by the lack of uniform terminology in describing the various disease entities, especially primary angle closure. Traditionally, the angle-closure glaucomas are broken down into 2 main categories: primary and secondary angle closure. Each category is further divided by the symptomatology, etiology, and duration of each of the diseases. Often, each entity ends in glaucoma, even though in some cases glaucomatous visual field loss or glaucomatous optic neuropathy has not occurred. Recent trends have been to separate the various diseases depending on whether glaucomatous optic nerve damage is or is not present. This trend is seen especially with primary angle closure, where researchers have attempted to make its terminology more similar to that used with primary open-angle disease.

In primary angle closure, there is no underlying pathology; there is only an anatomic predisposition. In secondary angle closure, an underlying pathologic cause, such as an intumescent lens, iris neovascularization, corneal endothelial migration, or epithelial downgrowth, initiates the angle closure.

Foster PJ, Johnson GJ. Glaucoma in China: how big is the problem? *Br J Ophthalmol.* 2001;85:1277–1282.

Kim YY, Jung HR. Clarifying the nomenclature for primary angle-closure glaucoma. *Surv Ophthalmol.* 1997;42:125–136.

Lowe RF. A history of primary angle closure glaucoma. *Surv Ophthalmol.* 1995;40:163–170.

Pathogenesis and Pathophysiology of Angle Closure

Angle closure is defined by the apposition of the peripheral iris to the trabecular meshwork and the resulting reduced drainage of aqueous humor through the anterior chamber angle. In considering the underlying pathogenesis of angle closure, it is important to assess the relative and absolute size and position of each of the anterior segment structures and the pressure gradients between the posterior and anterior chambers. Conceptually, the mechanism of angle closure falls into 2 categories (Table 5-1):

- mechanisms that push the iris forward from behind
- mechanisms that pull the iris forward into contact with the trabecular meshwork

Pupillary Block

Pupillary block is the most frequent cause of angle closure and is the underlying cause of most cases of primary angle closure. The flow of aqueous from the posterior chamber through the pupil is impeded, and this obstruction creates a pressure gradient between the posterior and anterior chambers, causing the peripheral iris to bow forward against the trabecular meshwork (Fig 5-1). Absolute pupillary block occurs when there is no movement of aqueous through the pupil as a result of 360° of posterior synechiae (secluded pupil). These posterior synechiae can form between the iris and the crystalline lens, an intraocular lens, capsular remnants, and/or the vitreous face. Relative pupillary block occurs when there is restricted movement of aqueous through the pupil because

Table 5-1 Underlying Mechanisms of Angle Closure

Iris pushed forward from behind, into the angle:
- relative pupillary block
- absolute pupillary block
- aqueous misdirection-malignant glaucoma
- ciliary body swelling, inflammation, or cysts
- anteriorly located ciliary processes (plateau iris configuration/syndrome)
- choroidal swelling, serous or hemorrhagic choroidal detachments or effusions
- posterior segment tumors or space-occupying lesions (silicone oil, gas bubble)
- contracting retrolental tissue (retinopathy of prematurity)
- anteriorly displaced lens
- encircling retinal bands/buckles

Iris pulled forward into contact with the angle:
- contraction of inflammatory membrane or fibrovascular tissue
- migration of corneal endothelium [iridocorneal endothelial (ICE) syndrome]
- fibrous ingrowth
- epithelial downgrowth
- iris incarceration in traumatic wound or surgical incision

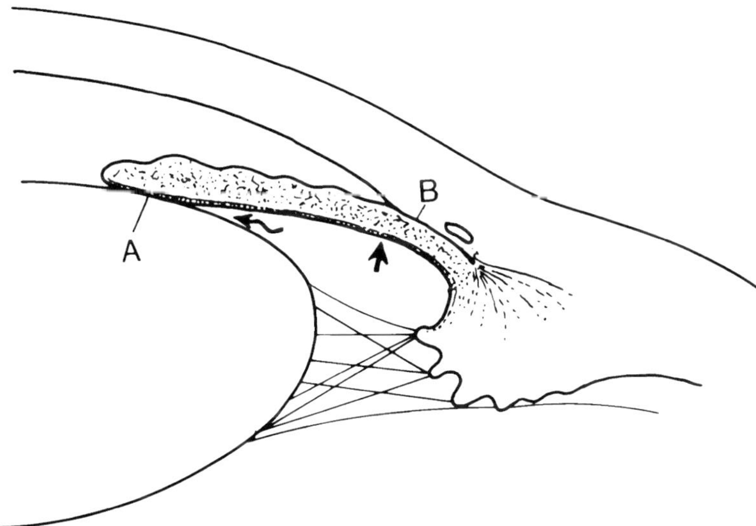

Figure 5-1 Pupillary-block glaucoma. A functional block between the lens and iris **(A)** leads to increased pressure in the posterior chamber *(arrows)* with forward shift of the peripheral iris and closure of the anterior chamber angle **(B)**. *(Reproduced with permission from Shields MB.* Textbook of Glaucoma. *3rd ed. Baltimore: Williams & Wilkins; 1992.)*

of iris contact with the lens, intraocular lens, capsular remnants, anterior hyaloid, or vitreous space-occupying substance (air, silicone oil). Relative and absolute pupillary block are broken by an unobstructed peripheral iridectomy.

Angle Closure Without Pupillary Block

Angle closure may occur without pupillary block. Iridotrabecular apposition, or synechiae, can result from the iris and/or lens being pushed, rotated, or pulled forward for a variety of reasons, as outlined in Table 5-1. Each of these underlying mechanisms can usually be identified by a comprehensive examination, including gonioscopy. Many patients may present with multiple underlying causes for their angle closure.

Lens-Induced Angle-Closure Glaucoma

Intumescent or dislocated lenses (complete zonular dehiscence) may increase pupillary block and cause angle closure. Angle closure from an unusually large or intumescant lens is often referred to as *phacomorphic glaucoma.* With lens subluxation (partial zonular dehiscence), as in Marfan syndrome or hemocystinuria, pupillary block from the lens or vitreous may occur. Lens block (Mobile lens syndrome) is a recently coined phrase that highlights an underlying mechanism of primary angle closure, in which the lens has a tendency to rotate forward, especially in the prone position, aggravating the relative pupillary block and angle closure.

Iris-Induced Angle Closure

Iris-induced angle closure occurs when the peripheral iris is the cause of the iridotrabecular apposition. This can occur with an anterior iris insertion into the scleral spur; a thick peripheral iris, which on dilatation "rolls" into the trabecular meshwork; and/or anteriorly displaced ciliary processes, which rotate the peripheral iris forward (plateau iris). In addition, the angle closure seen in aniridia, where the rudimentary iris leaflets, lacking support, rotate into the angle and cause secondary angle closure, is an example of iris-induced angle closure.

Primary Angle Closure

Primary angle closure is a complex disease entity that is the leading cause of glaucoma worldwide. Relative pupillary block is felt to be the underlying cause of over 90% of cases of primary angle closure, although recently plateau iris and lens block (anterior lens movement) have been implicated as causes or partial causes of chronic primary angle closure, especially seen in East Asia.

Risk Factors for Developing Primary Angle Closure

Race

The prevalence of PACG in patients over the age of 40 varies greatly depending on race: 0.1%–0.6 % in whites, 0.1%–0.2% in Africans, 2.1–5.0% in Inuits, 0.4%–1.4% in East Asians, 0.3% in Japanese, and 2.3% in a mixed ethnic group in South Africa. Some of these differences can be explained by the difference in the biometric parameters (anterior chamber depth, axial length) of the different white and Inuit populations, whereas the increased incidence in the Chinese and East Asian populations cannot be explained by biometric parameters alone. In addition, some races present more commonly with acute forms (whites), whereas Africans and Asians present more frequently with asymptomatic chronic disease.

Bonomi L, Marchini G, Marraffa M, et al. Epidemiology of angle-closure glaucoma: prevalence, clinical types, and association with peripheral anterior chamber depth in the Egna-Neumarket Glaucoma Study. *Ophthalmology.* 2000;107:998–1003.

Congdon N, Wang F, Tielsch JM. Issues in the epidemiology and population-based screening of primary angle-closure glaucoma. *Surv. Ophthalmol.* 1992;36:411–423.

Dandona L, Dandona R, Mandal P, et al. Angle-closure glaucoma in an urban population in southern India: the Andhra Pradesh Eye Disease Study. *Ophthalmology.* 2000;107: 1710–1716.

Erie JC, Hodge DO, Gray DT. The incidence of primary angle-closure glaucoma in Olmstead County, Minnesota. *Arch Ophthalmol.* 1997;115:177–181.

Foster PJ, Oen FT, Machin D, et al. The prevalence of glaucoma in Chinese residents of Singapore: a cross-sectional population survey of the Tanjong Pagar district. *Arch Ophthalmol.* 2000;118:1105–1111.

Rotchford AP, Johnson GJ. Glaucoma in Zulus: a population-based cross-sectional survey in a rural district in South Africa. *Arch Ophthalmol.* 2002;120:471–478.

Ocular biometrics

Patients who develop primary angle closure have small, "crowded" anterior segments and short axial lengths. The most important factors predisposing to angle closure are a shallow anterior chamber, a thick lens and increased anterior curvature of the lens, a short axial length, and small corneal diameter and radius of curvature. An anterior chamber depth of less than 2.5 mm predisposes patients to primary angle closure, whereas most patients with primary angle closure have an anterior chamber depth less than 2.1 mm.

Congdon NG, Youlin Q, Quigley H, et al. Biometry and primary angle-closure glaucoma among Chinese, white, and black populations. *Ophthalmology.* 1997;104:1489–1495.

Devereux JG, Foster PJ, Baasanhu J, et al. Anterior chamber depth measurement as a screening tool for primary angle closure glaucoma in an East Asian population. *Arch Ophthalmol.* 2000;118:257–263.

Marchini G, Pagliarusco A, Toscano A, et al. Ultrasound biomicroscopic and conventional ultrasonographic study of ocular dimensions in primary angle-closure glaucoma. *Ophthalmology.* 1998;105:2091–2098.

Age

Primary angle closure is rare in patients under the age of 40; its prevalence increases with each decade after 40. This increased incidence with age has been explained by the increasing thickness of the lens, its forward movement with age, and the resultant increase in iridolenticular contact.

Gender

Primary angle closure occurs 2 to 4 times more commonly in woman than in men, irrespective of race. In studies assessing ocular biometry, women tend to have smaller anterior segments and axial lengths than do men. This difference, however, is not large enough to explain this sexual predilection.

Family history

The incidence of primary angle closure is increased in first-degree relatives. In whites, the prevalence of primary angle closure in first-degree relatives has been reported to be between 1% and 12%, whereas in a Chinese population survey, the risk was 6 times greater in patients with any family history. In Inuits, the relative risk in patients with a family history is increased 3.5 times compared to the general Inuit population.

Refraction

Primary angle closure occurs more commonly in patients with hyperopia irrespective of race. Increasing rates of myopia, especially in Asia, may eventually influence the prevalence of this disease.

Acute Primary Angle Closure

Acute primary angle closure (PAC) occurs when IOP rises rapidly as a result of relatively sudden blockage of the trabecular meshwork by the iris. It is typically manifested by ocular pain, headache, blurred vision, rainbow-colored halos around lights, nausea, and vomiting. The rise in IOP to relatively high levels causes corneal epithelial edema, which is responsible for the visual symptoms. Signs of acute angle closure include

- high IOP
- middilated, sluggish, and often irregular pupil
- corneal epithelial edema
- congested episcleral and conjunctival blood vessels
- shallow anterior chamber
- a mild amount of aqueous flare and cells

The optic nerve may be swollen during an acute attack.

Definitive diagnosis depends on the gonioscopic verification of angle closure. Gonioscopy should be possible in almost all cases of acute angle closure, although medical treatment of elevated IOP and clearing of corneal edema with topical glycerin may be necessary to enable visualization of the chamber angle. Dynamic (compression/indentation) gonioscopy may help the physician determine if the iris–trabecular meshwork blockage is reversible (appositional closure) or irreversible (synechial closure), and it may be therapeutic in breaking the attack of acute angle closure. Gonioscopy of the fellow eye in a patient with PAC usually reveals a narrow, occludable angle.

During an acute attack, IOP may be high enough to cause glaucomatous optic nerve damage, ischemic nerve damage, and/or retinal vascular occlusion. Peripheral anterior synechiae (PAS) can form rapidly, and IOP-induced ischemia may produce sector atrophy of the iris. Such atrophy releases pigment and causes pigmentary dusting of the iris surface and corneal endothelium. Iris ischemia, specifically of the iris sphincter muscle, may cause the pupil to become permanently fixed and dilated. *Glaukomflecken,* characteristic small anterior subcapsular lens opacities, may also develop as a result of ischemia. These findings are helpful in detecting previous episodes of acute angle-closure glaucoma.

The definitive treatment for acute angle closure is an iridectomy, laser or surgical; this is discussed in detail in Chapter 8. Mild attacks may be broken by cholinergic agents (pilocarpine 1%–2%), which induce miosis that pulls the peripheral iris away from the trabecular meshwork. Stronger miotics should be avoided, as they may increase the vascular congestion of the iris or rotate the lens–iris diaphragm more anteriorly, increasing the pupillary block. However, when the IOP is quite elevated (eg, above 40–50 mm Hg), the pupillary sphincter may be ischemic and unresponsive to miotic agents alone. In this case, the patient should be treated with some combination of a topical beta-adrenergic antagonist; $alpha_2$-adrenergic agonists; an oral, topical, or intravenous carbonic anhydrase inhibitor; and, when necessary, a hyperosmotic agent. This treatment is used to reduce IOP to the point where the miotic agent will constrict the pupil and open the angle. Globe compression and compression gonioscopy have also been described to treat acute angle-closure glaucoma. Nonselective adrenergic agonists or medications with significant $alpha_1$-adrenergic activity (apraclonidine) should be avoided to prevent further pupillary dilation and iris ischemia.

The fellow eye, which shares the anatomic predisposition for increased pupillary block, is at high risk for developing acute angle closure. In addition, the pain and emotional upset resulting from the involvement of the first eye may increase sympathetic flow to the fellow eye and produce pupillary dilation. It is recommended that a peripheral iridectomy be performed in the other eye if a similar angle configuration is present. If it is not, specific secondary angle-closure glaucomas must be strongly considered in the differential diagnosis. In general, PAC is a bilateral disease, and its occurrence in a patient whose fellow eye has a deep chamber angle raises the possibility of a secondary cause, such as a posterior segment mass or ICE syndrome.

An untreated fellow eye has a 40%–80% chance of developing an acute attack of angle closure over the next 5–10 years. Long-term pilocarpine administration is not effective in preventing acute attacks in many cases. Thus, prophylactic iridectomy should be performed in the contralateral eye unless the angle clearly appears to be nonoccludable.

Laser iridectomy is the treatment of choice for primary angle closure secondary to pupillary block. Surgical iridectomy is indicated when laser iridectomy cannot be accomplished. Once an iridectomy has been performed, pupillary block is relieved and the iris is no longer pushed forward into contact with the trabecular meshwork, as the pressure gradient between the posterior and anterior chambers approaches zero. If a laser iridectomy cannot be performed, the acute attack may be broken by flattening the peripheral iris with a laser iridoplasty or by relieving the pupillary block with a laser pupilloplasty.

Once the attack is broken and the cornea is of adequate clarity, a peripheral iridectomy should be performed. Following resolution of the acute attack, it is important to reevaluate the angle by gonioscopy to assess the degree of residual synechial angle closure and to confirm the reopening of at least part of the angle.

The IOP may remain low for weeks following acute angle closure because of ciliary body ischemia and poor aqueous production; it is a poor indicator of angle function or anatomy. Repeat or serial gonioscopy is therefore essential in following the patient for the development of chronic angle closure.

Seah SK, Foster PJ, Chew PT, et al. Incidence of acute angle closure glaucoma in Singapore: an island-wide survey. *Arch Ophthalmol.* 1997;115:1436–1440.

Subacute or Intermittent Angle Closure

Subacute (intermittent or prodromal) angle closure is a condition characterized by episodes of blurred vision, halos, and mild pain caused by elevated IOP. These symptoms resolve spontaneously, especially during sleep-induced miosis, and IOP is usually normal between the episodes, which occur periodically over days or weeks. These episodes may be confused with headaches or migraines. The correct diagnosis can be made only with a high index of suspicion and gonioscopy. The typical history and the gonioscopic appearance of a narrow chamber angle with or without PAS help establish the diagnosis. Laser iridectomy is the treatment of choice in subacute angle closure. This condition can progress to chronic angle closure or to an acute attack that does not resolve spontaneously.

Chronic Angle Closure

Chronic angle closure may develop either after acute angle closure in which synechial closure persists or when the chamber angle closes gradually and IOP rises slowly as enough angle is compromised. The later form of chronic angle closure, in which there is gradual asymptomatic angle closure, is the most common. This disease tends to be diagnosed in its later stages and is a major cause of blindness in Asia. In discussing the mechanism of chronic primary angle closure, the term *creeping angle closure* is often used. Creeping angle closure defines the slow formation of PAS, which advance forward circumferentially, moving the iris insertion gradually forward onto the trabecular meshwork. The cause of the phenomenon is uncertain, but evidence suggests that multiple mechanisms are involved, including pupillary block, iris thickness and position, and plateau iris configuration.

In chronic angle-closure glaucoma, permanent PAS are present, as determined by indentation gonioscopy. The clinical course resembles that of open-angle glaucoma in its lack of symptoms, modest elevation of IOP, progressive cupping of the optic nerve head, and characteristic glaucomatous loss of visual field. The diagnosis of chronic angle-closure glaucoma is frequently overlooked, and it is commonly confused with chronic open-angle glaucoma. Gonioscopic examination of all glaucoma patients is important to enable the ophthalmologist to make the correct diagnosis.

Even if miotics and other agents lower IOP, an iridectomy is necessary to relieve the pupillary block component and reduce the potential for further permanent synechial angle closure. Without an iridectomy, the closure of the angle usually progresses and makes the glaucoma more difficult to control. Even with a patent peripheral iridectomy, progressive angle closure can occur, and repeated periodic gonioscopy is imperative. An iridectomy with or without chronic use of ocular hypotensive medication will control the disease for most chronic angle-closure glaucoma patients. Others may require subsequent filtering surgery or goniosynechialysis.

No clinical test can reliably determine whether an iridectomy alone will control the disease for an individual patient. However, because laser iridectomy is a relatively low-risk procedure compared to other surgical procedures, it should be performed prior to a more invasive or risky operative procedure. Individuals with extensive PAS and elevated IOP following acute angle closure may be helped by argon laser gonioplasty or goniosynechialysis.

Alsagoff Z, Aung T, Ang LP, et al. Long-term clinical course of primary angle-closure glaucoma in an Asian population. *Ophthalmology.* 2000;107:2300–2304.

Ritch R, Lowe RF. Angle closure glaucoma: mechanisms and epidemiology. In: Ritch R, Shields MB, Krupin T, eds. *The Glaucomas.* 2nd ed. St Louis: Mosby; 1996: ch 37, 801–819.

Ritch R, Lowe RF. Angle closure glaucoma: clinical types. In: Ritch R, Shields MB, Krupin T, eds. *The Glaucomas.* 2nd ed. St Louis: Mosby; 1996: ch 38, 821–840.

The Occludable, or Narrow, Anterior Chamber Angle

Only a small percentage of patients with shallow anterior chambers develop angle-closure glaucoma. Many clinicians have attempted to predict which asymptomatic patients with normal IOP will develop angle closure by performing a variety of provocative tests. These tests are designed to precipitate a limited form of angle closure, which can then be detected by gonioscopy and IOP measurement. The methods commonly used include pharmacologic pupillary dilation and prone-darkroom testing. An IOP increase of 8 mm Hg or more is considered positive. An asymmetric pressure rise between the 2 eyes with a corresponding degree of angle closure is also considered a positive sign. None of the provocative tests has been validated in a prospective study, however, and the predictive value of any provocative test has never been demonstrated. Thus, they are rarely used.

Ultimately, the decision to treat an asymptomatic patient with narrow angles rests on the clinical judgment of the ophthalmologist and the accurate assessment of the anterior chamber angle. Any patient with narrow angles, regardless of the results of provocative testing, should be advised of the symptoms of angle closure, of the need for immediate ophthalmic attention if symptoms occur, and of the value of long-term periodic follow-up. An iridectomy is not necessary in all patients with a suspicious or borderline narrow angle. If patients with a narrow angle have documented appositional or near appositional closure, PAS, increased segmental trabecular meshwork pigmentation, a history of previous angle closure, a positive provocative test, significant risk of angle closure (anterior chamber depth less than 2.0 mm, strong family history), then the angle should be felt to be occludable and an iridectomy performed.

Various factors that cause pupillary dilation may induce angle closure. These factors include a variety of drugs, as well as pain, emotional upset, or fright. In predisposed eyes with shallow anterior chambers, either mydriatic or miotic agents can precipitate acute angle closure. Mydriatic agents include not only dilating drops but also systemic medications that cause dilation. The effect of miotics is to pull the peripheral iris away from the chamber angle. However, miotics also cause the zonular fibers of the lens to relax, allowing the lens to come forward. Furthermore, their use results in an increase in the amount of iris–lens contact, thus potentially increasing pupillary block. For these reasons, miotics, especially the cholinesterase inhibitors, may also induce or aggravate angle closure. Gonioscopy should be repeated soon after miotic drugs are administered to patients with narrow angles.

A number of systemic medications, including allergy and cold medications, antidepressants, and anticholenergics, carry warnings against use by patients with glaucoma. Most of these drugs have the potential for precipitating angle closure in susceptible individuals because of anticholinergic or sympathomimetic activity. Although systemic administration generally does not raise intraocular drug levels to the same degree as does topical administration, even slight mydriasis in a patient with a critically narrow chamber angle can induce angle closure. For patients who require one of these medications and have significantly narrow angles, the ophthalmologist should strongly consider performing an iridectomy or warning the patient of their increased risk if they continue to take the medication.

Dapiprazole, available in a 0.5% solution, reverses phenylephrine-induced or tropicamide-induced pupillary dilation to baseline in 30 minutes compared with 3 hours when no alpha-adrenergic antagonist is used. The use of dapiprazole following pupillary dilation does not eliminate the possibility of precipitating angle closure; however, it does reduce the overall time that the pupil is dilated and the critical period when the pupil is middilated.

Foster PJ, Devereux JG, Alsbirk PH, et al. Detection of gonioscopically occludable angles and primary angle-closure glaucoma by estimation of limbal chamber depth in Asians: modified grading scheme. *Br J Ophthalmol.* 2000;84:186–192.

Plateau Iris

Plateau iris is an unusual type of PAC caused by anteriorly positioned ciliary processes that critically narrow the anterior chamber recess by pushing the peripheral iris forward. A component of pupillary block is often present. Following dilation of the pupil, the peripheral iris bunches up and obstructs the trabecular meshwork. Plateau iris may be suspected if the central anterior chamber seems unusually deep and the iris plane appears rather flat for an eye with angle closure. This suspicion can be confirmed with ultrasound biomicroscopy (Fig 5-2). The ophthalmologist should also suspect plateau iris if angle closure occurs in younger patients with myopia.

An iridectomy is performed to remove any component of pupillary block; this treatment is sufficient for eyes with *plateau iris configuration,* the more common manifestation. However, even after iridectomy, a few eyes with *plateau iris syndrome* will still be predisposed to develop chronic angle closure as a result of the peripheral iris anatomy. Acute angle closure can be precipitated in this syndrome with pupillary dilation. In this syndrome, the PAS have been reported to begin at Schwalbe's line and then extend in a posterior direction over the trabecular meshwork, scleral spur, and angle recess. The reverse is seen in pupillary-block–induced angle closure. These patients should be treated with long-term miotic therapy. Laser peripheral iridoplasty is also useful in individuals with this condition to flatten and thin the peripheral iris (Fig 5-3). Repeat gonioscopy is necessary, as the peripheral iris may bow anteriorly again over time, and the threat of chronic angle closure is always present.

Secondary Angle Closure With Pupillary Block

Lens-Induced Angle Closure

Phacomorphic glaucoma

As with primary angle closure, lens size and relative pupillary block play vital roles in this condition. The main difference is that primary angle closure tends to occur slowly

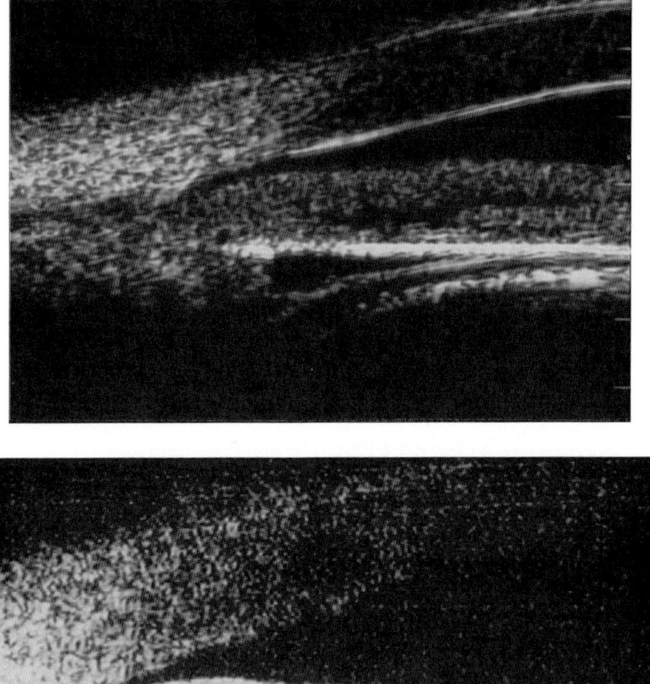

Figure 5-2 Ultrasound biomicroscopy images of a plateau iris. *(Photographs courtesy of Charles J. Pavlin, MD.)*

in patients with hyperopia who undergo progressive shallowing of the anterior chamber as a result of increasing anterior-posterior lens diameter. The process in phacomorphic glaucoma is much more rapid and is precipitated by marked lens swelling (intumescence) as a result of cataract formation and the development of pupillary block in an eye anatomically not disposed to closure (Figs 5-4, 5-5). As a result of the similarities, diagnosis is not always straightforward, but disparities between the 2 eyes in anterior chamber depth, gonioscopy, and degree of cataract should suggest a phacomorphic process (Fig 5-6). (See also BCSC Section 11, *Lens and Cataract.*) A laser iridectomy followed by cataract extraction in a quiet eye is the preferred treatment.

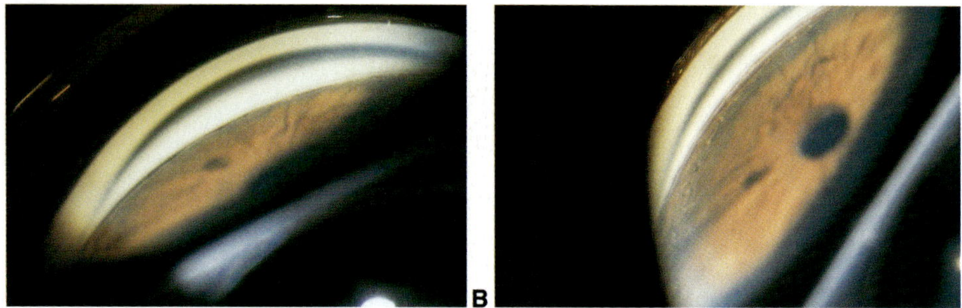

Figure 5-3 **A,** Plateau iris syndrome with a flat iris plane and closed angle. **B,** Plateau iris syndrome with an open angle following laser peripheral iridoplasty. *(Photographs courtesy of M. Roy Wilson, MD.)*

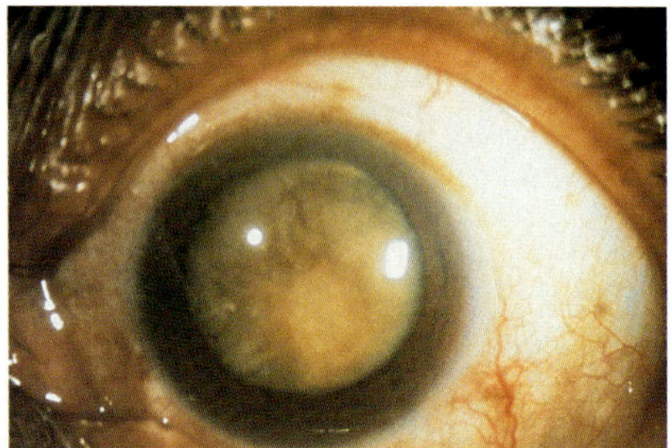

Figure 5-4 Phacomorphic glaucoma. Lens intumescence precipitates pupillary block and secondary angle closure in an eye not anatomically predisposed to angle closure. *(Photograph courtesy of Steven T. Simmons, MD.)*

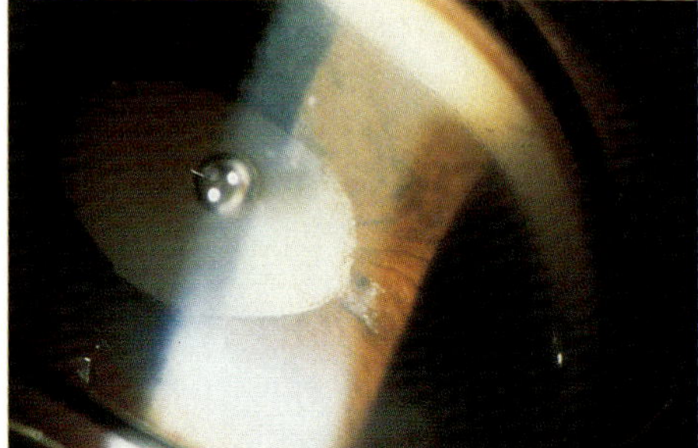

Figure 5-5 Phacomorphic glaucoma. Classic iris bombé develops as a result of a mature cataract and secondary posterior synechiae. *(Photograph courtesy of Steven T. Simmons, MD.)*

Ectopia lentis

Ectopia lentis is defined as displacement of the lens from its normal anatomic position. Anterior displacement of the lens can result in pupillary block by itself or in combination with the vitreous (Fig 5-7). The pupillary block causes iris bombé and shallowing of the anterior chamber angle to occur, with resultant secondary angle closure. This may present clinically as an acute event with pain, conjunctival hyperemia, and loss of vision or as a chronic angle-closure glaucoma with PAS formation secondary to repeated attacks. Laser iridectomy is the treatment of choice, as it is with PAC with pupillary block. Lens extraction is usually indicated to restore visual acuity and reduce recurrent lens block and the possible development of chronic angle closure. A list of conditions causing this entity is given in Table 5-2.

Microspherophakia, a congenital disorder in which the lens has a spherical or globular shape, may cause pupillary block and angle-closure glaucoma (Fig 5-8). Treatment with cycloplegia may flatten the lens and pull it posteriorly, breaking the pupillary block. Miotics may make the condition worse. Microspherophakia is often familial and may occur as an isolated condition or as part of either Weill-Marchesani or Marfan syndrome.

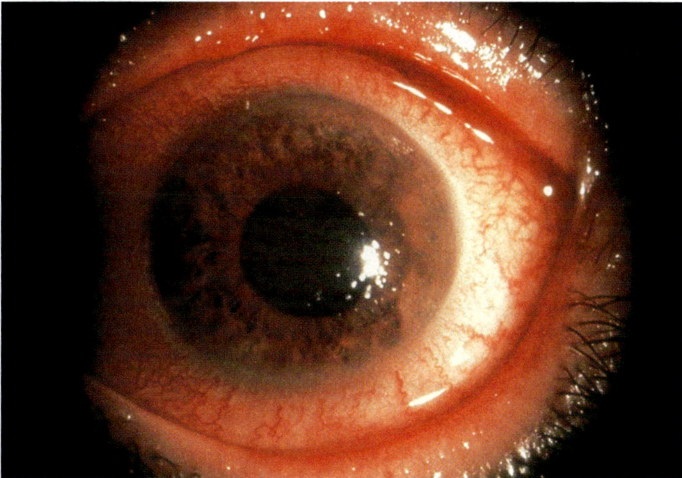

Figure 5-6 Phacomorphic glaucoma often presents clinically as acute angle-closure glaucoma. Disparities in the anterior chamber depths and degree of cataract between the 2 eyes can help the clinician distinguish between a phacomorphic process and primary angle-closure glaucoma. *(Photograph courtesy of Steven T. Simmons, MD.)*

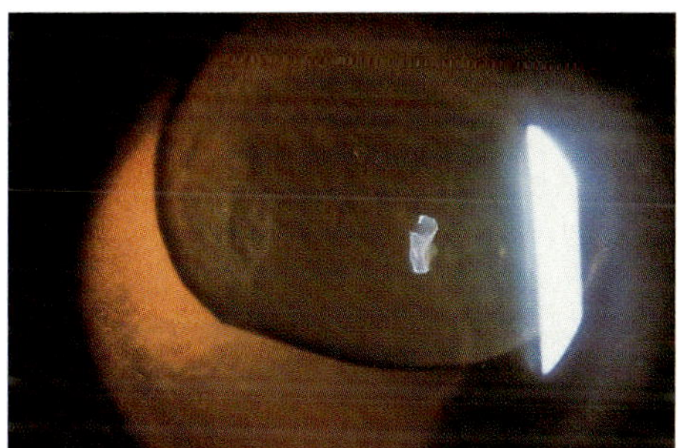

Figure 5-7 Ectopia lentis: dislocation of the lens into the anterior chamber through a dilated pupil. *(Photograph courtesy of Ron Gross, MD.)*

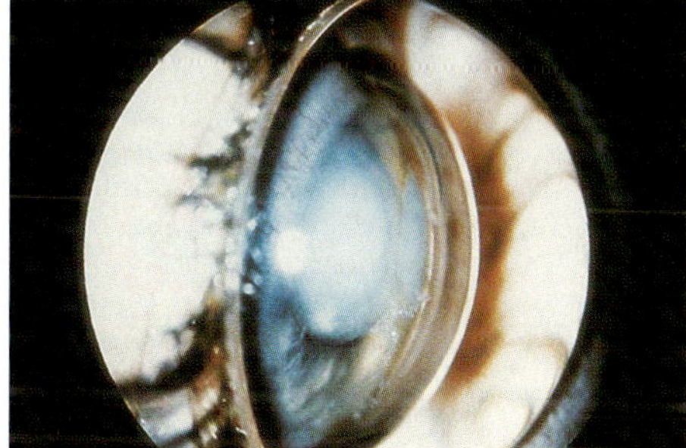

Figure 5-8 Ectopia lentis. In a case of microspherophakia, the lens is trapped anteriorly by the pupil, resulting in iris bombé and a dramatic shallowing of the anterior chamber. *(Photograph courtesy of G.L. Spaeth, MD.)*

Table 5-2 Common Causes of Ectopia Lentis

Trauma
Marfan syndrome
Homocystinuria
Microspherophakia
Weill-Marchesani syndrome

Aphakic or pseudophakic angle-closure glaucoma

Pupillary block may occur in *aphakic* and *pseudophakic* eyes. An intact vitreous face can block the pupil and/or an iridectomy in aphakic or pseudophakic eyes or in phakic eyes with dislocated lenses. Generally, the anterior chamber shallows and the iris demonstrates considerable bombé. Treatment with mydriatic and cycloplegic agents may restore the aqueous flow through the pupil but may also make the performing of a laser iridectomy difficult initially. Topical beta-adrenergic antagonists, alpha$_2$-adrenergic agonists, carbonic anhydrase inhibitors, and hyperosmotic agents can be effective in reducing IOP prior to the placement of an iridectomy. One or more laser iridectomies may be required.

A variant of this problem occurs with *anterior chamber intraocular lenses.* Pupillary block develops with apposition of the iris, vitreous face, and/or lens optic. The lens haptic or vitreous may obstruct the iridectomy or the pupil, and the peripheral iris bows forward around the anterior chamber IOL to occlude the chamber angle. The central chamber remains deep in this instance, because the lens haptic and optic prevent the central portions of the iris and vitreous face from moving forward. Laser iridectomies, often multiple, are required to relieve the block.

Pupillary block may occur after *extracapsular cataract extraction* when an iridectomy has not been performed at the time of surgery. Although not common, this complication can occur when the iris forms adhesions to a posterior chamber IOL or to the residual anterior or posterior capsule. Pupillary block may also occur following posterior capsulotomy when vitreous obstructs the pupil. A condition referred to as capsular block may also be seen whereby retained viscoelastic or fluid in the capsular bag pushes a posterior chamber IOL anteriorly, which may narrow the angle.

Secondary Angle Closure Without Pupillary Block

A number of disorders can lead to secondary angle closure without pupillary block, and several are discussed in this section. This form of secondary angle closure may occur through 1 of 2 mechanisms:

- contraction of an inflammatory, hemorrhagic, or vascular membrane, band, or exudate in the angle, leading to PAS
- forward displacement of the lens–iris diaphragm, often accompanied by swelling and anterior rotation of the ciliary body

Neovascular Glaucoma

This common, severe type of secondary angle-closure glaucoma is caused by a variety of disorders characterized by retinal or ocular ischemia or ocular inflammation (Table 5-3). The most common causes are diabetes mellitus, central retinal vein occlusion, and ocular ischemic syndrome. The disease is characterized by fine arborizing blood vessels on the surface of the iris and trabecular meshwork, which are accompanied by a fibrous membrane. The contraction of the fibrovascular membrane results in the formation of PAS, leading to the development of secondary angle-closure glaucoma.

Neovascularization of the anterior segment usually presents in a classic pattern that starts with fine vascular tufts at the pupil (Fig 5-9). As these vessels grow, they extend

Table 5-3 Disorders Predisposing to Neovascularization of the Iris and Angle

Systemic vascular disease	**Other ocular disease**
Carotid occlusive disease*	Chronic uveitis
Carotid artery ligation	Chronic retinal detachment
Carotid cavernous fistula	Endophthalmitis
Giant cell arteritis	Stickler syndrome
Takayasu (pulseless) disease	Retinoschisis
Ocular vascular disease	**Intraocular tumors**
Diabetic retinopathy*	Uveal melanoma
Central retinal vein occlusion*	Metastatic carcinoma
Central retinal artery occlusion	Retinoblastoma
Branch retinal vein occlusion	Reticulum cell sarcoma
Sickle cell retinopathy	**Ocular therapy**
Coats disease	Radiation therapy
Eales disease	**Trauma**
Retinopathy of prematurity	
Persistent hyperplastic primary vitreous	
Syphilitic vasculitis	
Anterior segment ischemia	

* most common causes

radially over the iris. The neovascularization crosses the ciliary body and scleral spur as fine single vessels that then branch as they reach and involve the trabecular meshwork (Figs 5-10, 5-11). Often the trabecular meshwork takes on a reddish coloration. With contraction of the fibrovascular membrane, PAS develop and coalesce, gradually closing the angle (Fig 5-12). Because the fibrovascular membrane cannot grow over healthy corneal endothelium, the PAS end at Schwalbe's line, distinguishing this condition from other secondary angle-closure glaucomas that result from an abnormal corneal endothelium such as ICE syndrome, which is discussed in the following section (Figs 5-13, 5-14).

Clinically, patients often present with an acute glaucoma associated with reduced vision, pain, conjunctival injection, microcystic corneal edema, and high IOP. If excessive pressure is applied during gonioscopy, fine neovascularization can be blanched, confusing this condition with acute angle closure, especially if corneal edema is present. While performing gonioscopy in patients suspected of having neovascularization, it is helpful to use a bright slit-lamp beam of light and high magnification in order to best visualize these fine vessels.

Rarely, anterior segment neovascularization may occur without demonstrable retinal ischemia, as in Fuchs heterochromic iridocyclitis and other types of uveitis, exfoliation syndrome, or isolated iris melanomas. When an ocular cause cannot be found, carotid artery occlusive disease should be considered. In establishing a correct diagnosis, it is important to distinguish dilated iris vessels associated with inflammation from newly formed abnormal blood vessels.

Because the prognosis for neovascular glaucoma is poor, prevention and early diagnosis is desirable. Gonioscopy is vitally important to the early diagnosis because angle neovascularization can occur without iris neovascularization. In central retinal vein

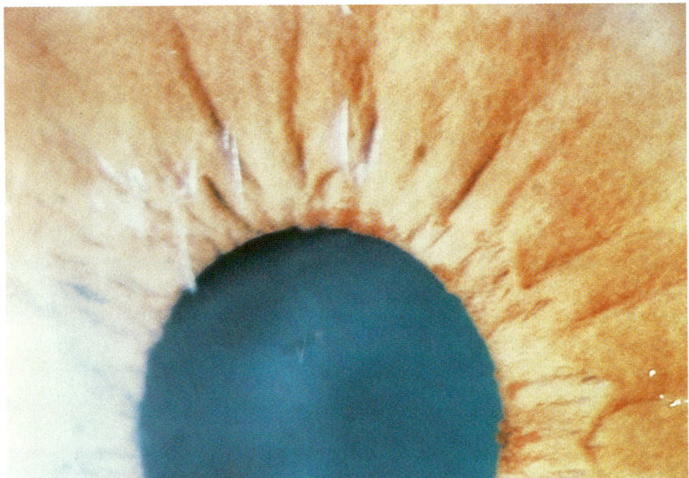

Figure 5-9 The initial presentation of iris neovascularization is usually small vascular tufts at the pupillary margin. *(Photograph courtesy of Steven T. Simmons, MD.)*

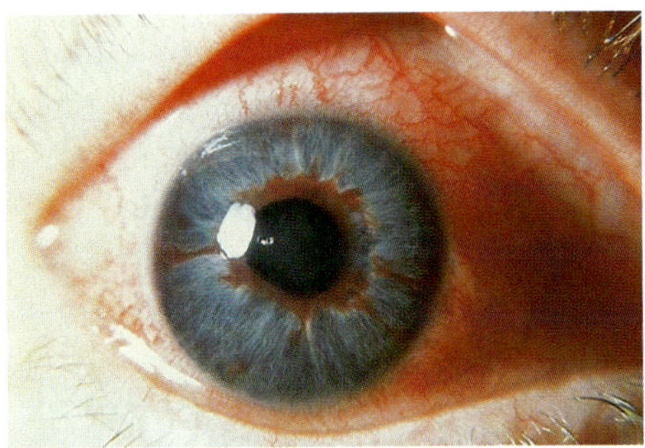

Figure 5-10 With growth, iris neovascularization extends from the pupillary margin radially toward the anterior chamber angle. *(Photograph courtesy of Steven T. Simmons, MD.)*

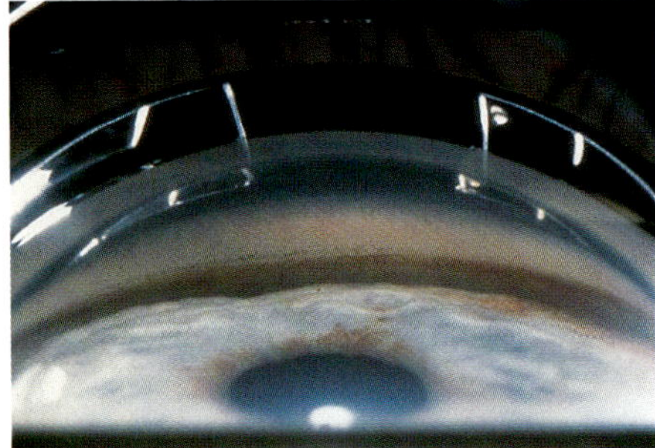

Figure 5-11 Initially, the iris neovascularization crosses the angle recess and scleral spur as single vessels that then branch over the trabecular meshwork. *(Photograph courtesy of Tom Richardson, MD.)*

occlusion (CRVO), approximately 10% of patients develop angle neovascularization alone. The most common cause of iris neovascularization is ischemic retinopathy, and retinal ablation should be performed whenever possible. The treatment of choice when the ocular media are clear is panretinal photocoagulation. When cloudy media prevent laser therapy, panretinal cryotherapy should be considered versus surgery to clear the media with endophotocoagulation or subsequent panretinal photocoagulation. Frequently, marked involution of the neovascularization occurs. The resulting decrease in neovascularization after retinal ablation may reduce or normalize the IOP, depending on the degree of synechial closure that has occurred. Even in the presence of total synechial angle closure, panretinal photocoagulation may improve the success rate of filtering surgery by eliminating the angiogenic stimulus and decrease the risk of hemorrhage at the time of surgery.

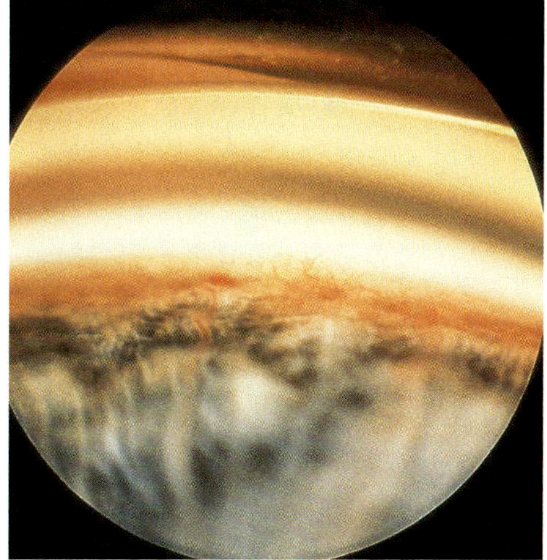

Figure 5-12 Iris neovascularization. With progressive angle involvement, peripheral anterior synechiae develop with contraction of the fibrovascular membrane, resulting in secondary neovascular glaucoma. *(Photograph courtesy of Steven T. Simmons, MD.)*

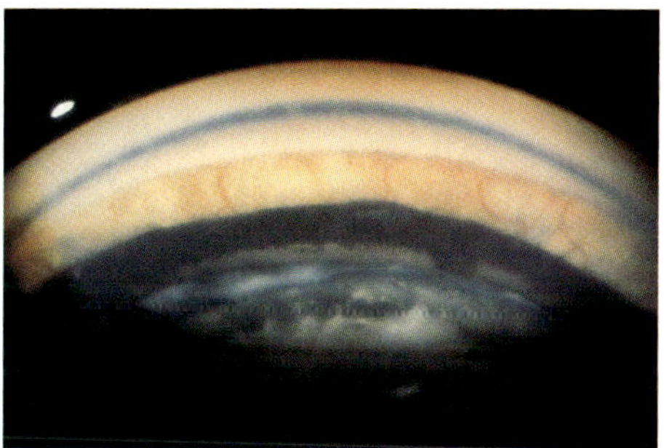

Figure 5-13 With endstage neovascular glaucoma, total angle closure occurs, obscuring the iris neovascularization. The PAS end at Schwalbe's line because the fibrovascular membrane does not grow over healthy corneal endothelium. *(Photograph courtesy of Steven T. Simmons, MD.)*

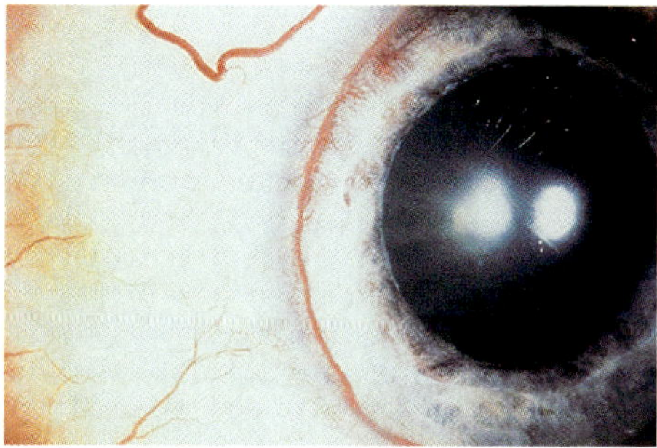

Figure 5-14 Often a large single vessel outlines the end of the PAS at the level of Schwalbe's line. *(Photograph courtesy of Steven T. Simmons, MD.)*

Medical therapy alone is usually not effective in controlling IOP when the outflow system has been occluded. Topical beta-adrenergic antagonists, alpha$_2$-adrenergic agonists, carbonic anhydrase inhibitors, cycloplegics, and corticosteroids may be useful in reducing IOP and decreasing inflammation prior to filtration surgery. Filtering surgery has a better chance of success once the neovascularization has regressed after panretinal photocoagulation. The use of the antimetabolites 5-fluorouracil and mitomycin C has been shown to increase the success rate and decrease the final IOP following trabeculectomy in patients with neovascular glaucoma. A variety of tube-shunt operations can also be effective in controlling the IOP in neovascular glaucoma and, in many cases, is the surgical procedure of choice. If these fail, a cyclodestructive procedure may help reduce the IOP.

Heuer DK, Lloyd MA. Management of glaucomas with poor surgical prognoses. *Focal Points: Clinical Modules for Ophthalmologists.* San Francisco: American Academy of Ophthalmology; 1995, module 1.

McGrath DJ, Ferguson JG, Sanborn GE. Neovascular glaucoma. *Focal Points: Clinical Modules for Ophthalmologists.* San Francisco: American Academy of Ophthalmology; 1997, module 7.

Sivak-Callcott JA, O'Day DM, Gass JD, et al. Evidence-based recommendations for the diagnosis and treatment of neovascular glaucoma. *Ophthalmology.* 2001;108:1767–1776.

Iridocorneal Endothelial (ICE) Syndrome

ICE syndrome is a group of disorders characterized by abnormal corneal endothelium that causes variable degrees of iris atrophy, secondary angle-closure glaucoma, and corneal edema. BCSC Section 8, *External Disease and Cornea,* discusses the corneal aspects of ICE syndrome. Three clinical variants have been described:

- Chandler syndrome
- essential/progressive iris atrophy
- iris nevus/Cogan-Reese syndrome

The condition is clinically unilateral, presents between 20 and 50 years of age, and occurs more often in women. No consistent association has been found with another ocular or systemic disease, and familial cases are very rare. Patients present complaining of decreased vision, pain secondary to corneal edema or secondary angle-closure glaucoma, or an abnormal iris appearance. In each of the 3 clinical variants, the corneal endothelium appears abnormal and takes on a beaten bronze appearance, similar to corneal guttae seen in Fuchs corneal endothelial dystrophy (Fig 5-15). Microcystic corneal edema may be present without elevated IOP, especially in Chandler syndrome. The unaffected eye may have subclinical irregularities of the corneal endothelium without other manifestations of the disease.

High PAS are characteristic of ICE syndrome, and these often extend anterior to Schwalbe's line (Fig 5-16). The PAS are caused by the contraction of the single or multiple

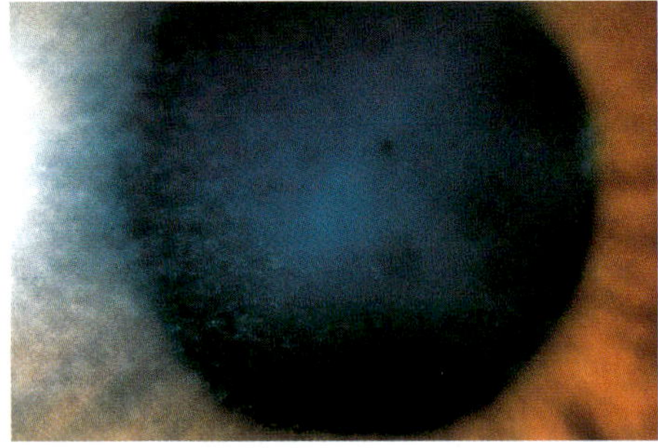

Figure 5-15 In all clinical varieties of iridocorneal endothelial syndrome, the corneal endothelium appears abnormal and takes on the appearance of beaten bronze, as demonstrated in this patient with Chandler syndrome. *(Photograph courtesy of Steven T. Simmons, MD.)*

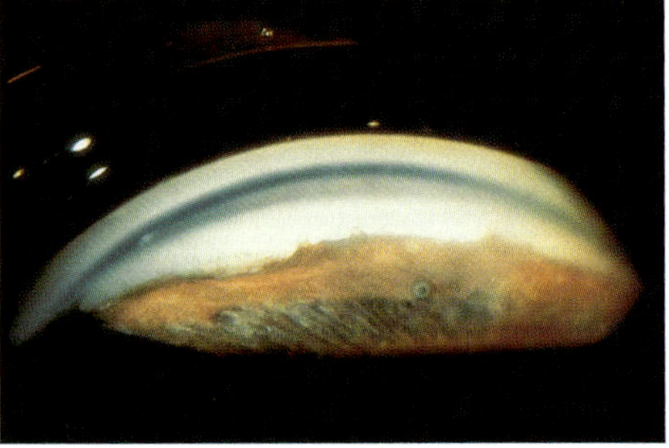

Figure 5-16 The classic high peripheral anterior synechiae seen in iridocorneal endothelial syndrome. These PAS extend anterior to Schwalbe's line in this patient with progressive iris atrophy. With angle closure, the secondary glaucoma occurs. *(Photograph courtesy of Steven T. Simmons, MD.)*

layers of endothelial cells and surrounding collagenous-fibrillar tissue that extend from the peripheral cornea over the trabecular meshwork and iris. These PAS result in synechial closure of the anterior chamber angle and lead to an angle-closure glaucoma. Similar to neovascular glaucoma, the degree of angle closure does not always correlate to the elevation in IOP, because some angles may be functionally closed by the endothelial membrane without synechial formation.

Various degrees of iris atrophy and corneal changes distinguish the specific clinical entities. Progressive iris atrophy is characterized by severe iris atrophy resulting in heterochromia, corectopia, ectropion uveae, iris stromal and pigment epithelial atrophy, and hole formation (Fig 5-17). In Chandler syndrome, minimal iris atrophy and corectopia occur, and the corneal and angle findings predominate (Figs 5-18, 5-19). Chandler syndrome is the most common of the clinical entities and makes up approximately 50% of the cases of ICE syndrome. The iris atrophy tends to be less severe in Cogan-Reese

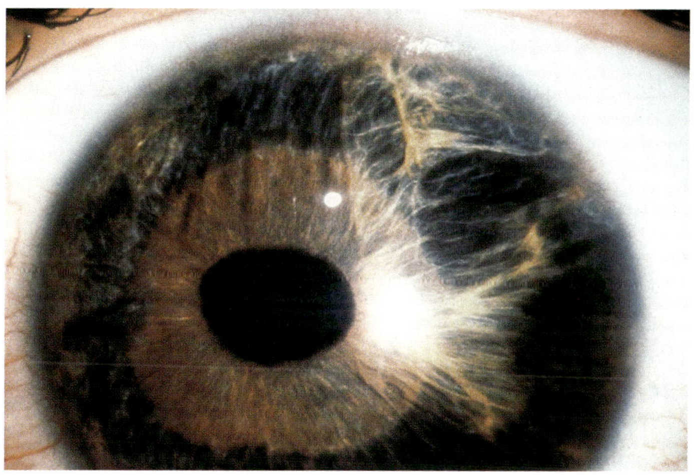

Figure 5-17 Iridocorneal endothelial syndrome. Corectopia and hole formation are typical findings in progressive iris atrophy. *(Photograph courtesy of Steven T. Simmons, MD.)*

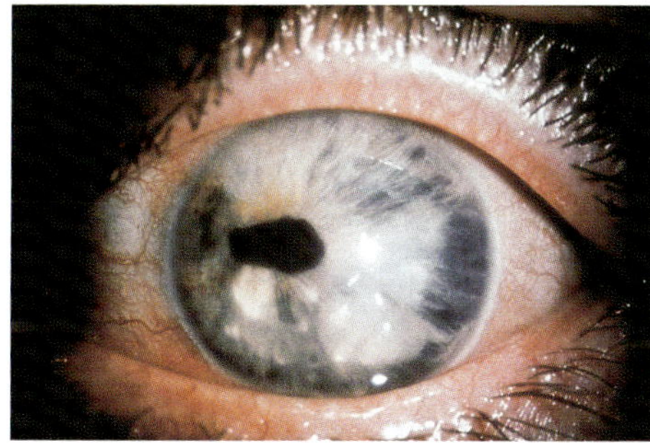

Figure 5-18 ICE syndrome. The iris atrophy is less severe in Chandler syndrome, but corectopia and bullous keratopathy are seen in this patient. *(Photograph courtesy of Steven T. Simmons, MD.)*

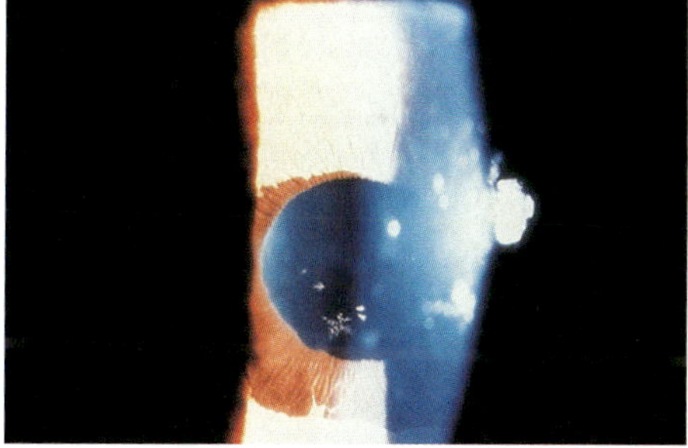

Figure 5-19 Ectropion uveae in a patient with Chandler syndrome. *(Photograph courtesy of Steven T. Simmons, MD.)*

syndrome. This condition is distinguished by tan pedunculated nodules or diffuse pigmented lesions on the anterior iris surface.

Glaucoma occurs in approximately 50% of patients with ICE syndrome, and the glaucoma tends to be more severe in progressive iris atrophy and Cogan-Reese syndrome. In the 3 clinical variations, corneal endothelial abnormalities are seen with a fine, hammered metal appearance to the posterior cornea. In this condition, the corneal endothelium migrates posterior to Descemet's membrane. Electron microscopy has shown this endothelial layer to vary in thickness, with areas of single and multiple endothelial layers, and to contain surrounding collagenous and fibrillar tissue. Unlike normal corneal endothelium, filopodial processes and cytoplasmic actin filaments are present, supporting the migratory nature of these cells. PAS are formed when this migratory endothelium and its surrounding collagenous, fibrillar tissue contracts. A viral cause was postulated for the mechanism of ICE syndrome after lymphocytes were seen on the corneal endothelium of affected patients. In serologic studies, both Epstein-Barr and herpes simplex viruses have been implicated.

The diagnosis of ICE syndrome must always be considered in young to middle-aged patients who present with unilateral angle-closure glaucoma. Specular microscopy can confirm the diagnosis by demonstrating an asymmetric loss of endothelial cells and atypical endothelial cell morphology in the involved eye. Therapy is directed toward the corneal edema and secondary glaucoma. Hypertonic saline solutions and medications to reduce the IOP, when elevated, can be effective in controlling the corneal edema. The angle-closure glaucoma can be treated medically with aqueous suppressants. Miotics are ineffective, and the role of hypotensive lipids remains uncertain. When medical therapy fails, filtering surgery (trabeculectomy or tube-shunt procedures) can be effective. Late failures have been reported with trabeculectomy secondary to endothelialization of the fistula. These can be reopened in some cases with an Nd:YAG laser.

Tumors

Tumors in the posterior segment of the eye or anterior uveal cysts may cause a unilateral secondary angle-closure glaucoma. Primary choroidal melanomas, ocular metastases, and retinoblastoma are the most common tumors to cause secondary angle closure. The mechanism of the angle-closure glaucoma is determined by the size, location, and pathology of the tumor. Choroidal and retinal tumors tend to shift the lens iris diaphragm forward as the tumors enlarge, causing secondary angle closure. Breakdown of the blood-aqueous barrier and inflammation from tissue necrosis can result in posterior and peripheral anterior synechiae formation, further exacerbating other underlying mechanisms of angle closure. Iris neovascularization can occur frequently with retinoblastomas, medulloepitheliomas, and choroidal melanomas, resulting in secondary angle closure and neovascular glaucoma.

Inflammation

Secondary angle-closure glaucoma can result from ocular inflammation. Fibrin and increased aqueous proteins from the breakdown of the blood–aqueous barrier predispose the eye to the formation of posterior synechiae (Fig 5-20) and PAS. If left untreated, these posterior synechiae can result in a secluded pupil, iris bombé, and secondary angle closure (Fig 5-21).

Inflammation may prompt PAS to form through peripheral iris edema, organization of inflammatory debris in the angle, and the bridging of the angle by large keratic precipitates (sarcoidosis). Unlike primary angle closure, where the PAS occur preferentially in the superior angle, they occur most frequently in inflammatory disease in the inferior angle (Fig 5-22). These PAS tend to be nonuniform in shape and height, which further differentiates inflammatory disease from primary angle closure (Fig 5-23). Ischemia secondary to inflammation may rarely cause rubeosis iridis and neovascular glaucoma.

Ocular inflammation can lead to the shallowing and closure of the anterior chamber angle by uveal effusion, resulting in anterior rotation of the ciliary body. Significant posterior uveitis causing massive exudative retinal detachment or choroidal effusions may lead to angle-closure glaucoma through forward displacement of the lens–iris diaphragm.

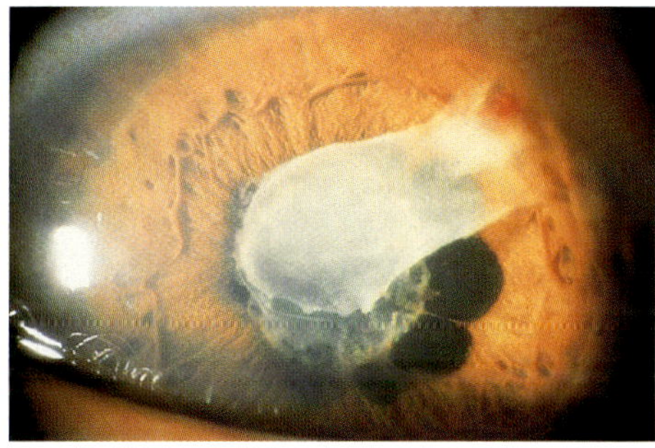

Figure 5-20 Inflammatory glaucoma. A fibrinous anterior chamber reaction and posterior synechiae formation are shown in a patient with ankylosing spondylitis. *(Photograph courtesy of Steven T. Simmons, MD.)*

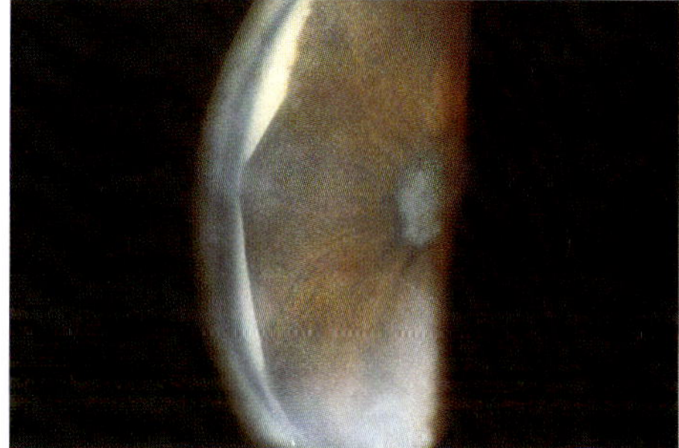

Figure 5-21 Inflammatory glaucoma. A secluded pupil is shown in a patient with long-standing uveitis with classic iris bombé and secondary angle closure. *(Photograph courtesy of Steven T. Simmons, MD.)*

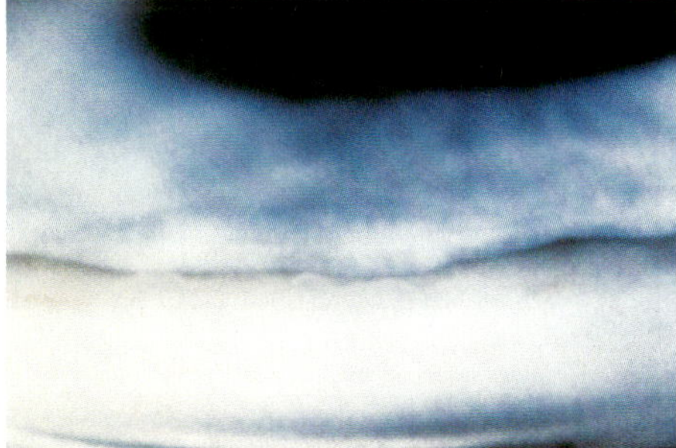

Figure 5-22 Inflammatory glaucoma. Keratic precipitates can be seen bridging the inferior anterior chamber angle in this patient with long-standing uveitis, resulting in the formation of PAS. *(Photograph courtesy of Joseph Krug, MD.)*

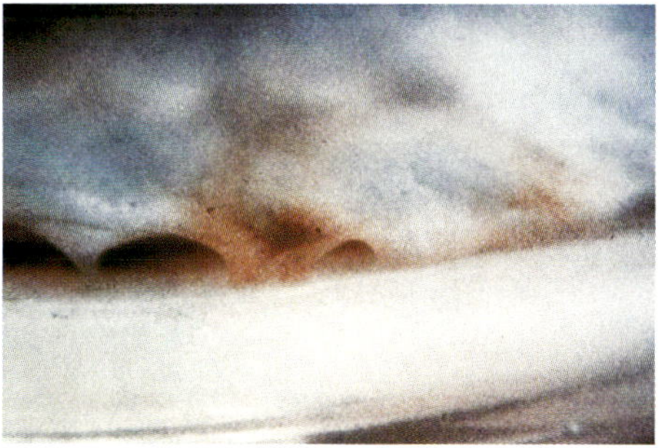

Figure 5-23 Inflammatory glaucoma. PAS in uveitis occur preferentially in the inferior anterior chamber angle and are nonuniform in height and shape, as demonstrated in this photograph. *(Photograph courtesy of Joseph Krug, MD.)*

Treatment is primarily directed at the underlying cause of uveitis. Aqueous suppressants and corticosteroids are the primary agents for reducing elevated IOP and preventing synechial angle closure.

Interstitial keratitis may be associated with open-angle or angle-closure glaucoma. The angle closure may be caused by chronic inflammation and PAS formation or by multiple cysts of the iris pigment epithelium.

Samples JR. Management of glaucoma secondary to uveitis. *Focal Points: Clinical Modules for Ophthalmologists.* San Francisco: American Academy of Ophthalmology; 1995, module 5.

Aqueous Misdirection

Aqueous misdirection is also known as *malignant glaucoma, ciliary block glaucoma,* and *posterior aqueous diversion syndrome.* This rare but potentially devastating form of glaucoma usually presents following ocular surgery in patients with a history of angle closure or PAS. It may also occur spontaneously in eyes with an open angle following cataract surgery or various laser procedures. The disease presents with uniform flattening of both the central and peripheral anterior chamber (Fig 5-24)—in contrast to iris bombé and acute angle-closure glaucoma, which predominately flatten the peripheral anterior chamber (Fig 5-25)—and an elevated IOP. The condition is thought to result from anterior rotation of the ciliary body and posterior misdirection of the aqueous, in association with a relative block to aqueous movement at the level of the lens equator, vitreous face, and ciliary processes.

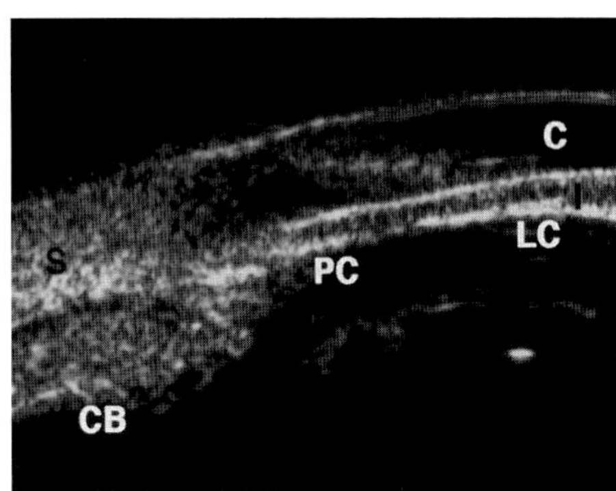

Figure 5-24 Ciliary block glaucoma, UBM. Expansion of the vitreous pushes the lens and ciliary body forward, causing a uniform shallowing of the anterior chamber. The central portion of the anterior lens capsule *(LC)* is nearly in contact with the cornea *(C)*. (*PC* = posterior chamber, *CB* = ciliary body) *(From Lundy, DC. Ciliary block glaucoma.* Focal Points: Clinical Modules for Ophthalmologists. *San Francisco: American Academy of Ophthalmology; 1999, module 3. Photograph courtesy of Jeffrey M. Liebmann, MD.)*

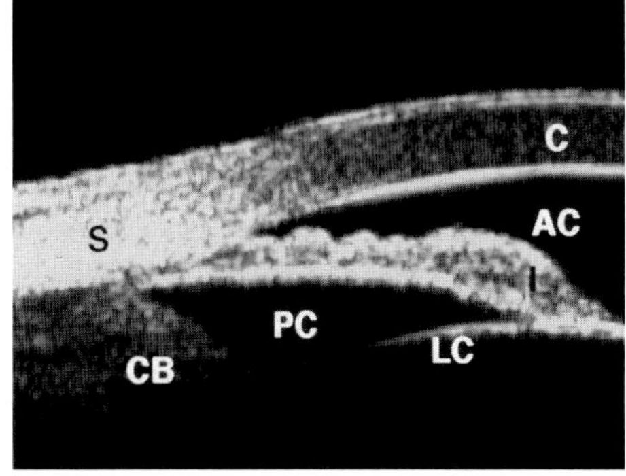

Figure 5-25 Acute angle closure, UBM. Pupillary block leads to forward bowing of the peripheral iris. The peripheral chamber is shallow, whereas the central chamber depth is relatively deep. (*C* = cornea, *AC* = anterior chamber, *PC* = posterior chamber, *LC* = lens capsule, *CB* = ciliary body). *(From Lundy, DC. Ciliary block glaucoma.* Focal Points: Clinical Modules for Ophthalmologists. *San Francisco: American Academy of Ophthalmology; 1999, module 3. Photograph courtesy of Jeffrey M. Liebmann, MD.)*

Clinically, the anterior chamber is shallow or flat with anterior displacement of the lens, pseudophakos, or vitreous face. Ciliary processes are seen to be rotated anteriorly and may be seen through an iridectomy to come in contact with the lens equator. Optically clear "aqueous" zones may be seen in the vitreous highlighting the underlying pathology. In the early postoperative setting, the diagnosis of aqueous misdirection is often difficult to distinguish from a choroidal effusion, pupillary block, or a suprachoroidal hemorrhage. Often the level of IOP, time frame following surgery, patency of an iridectomy, or presence of a choroidal effusion or suprachoroidal hemorrhage help the clinician make the appropriate diagnosis and initiate treatment. In some cases, unfortunately, the clinical picture is difficult to interpret and surgical intervention may be required to make the diagnosis.

Medical management includes intensive cycloplegic therapy, beta-adrenergic antagonists, $alpha_2$-adrenergic agonists, carbonic anhydrase inhibitors, and hyperosmotic agents. Miotics should not be used and can make aqueous misdirection worse. In aphakic and pseudophakic eyes, the anterior vitreous can be disrupted with the Nd:YAG laser. Argon laser photocoagulation of the ciliary processes has reportedly been helpful in treating this condition; this procedure may alter the adjacent vitreous face. Approximately 50% of patients will be controlled medically, whereas the remaining patients will require surgical intervention. The definitive surgical treatment is a vitrectomy combined with an anterior chamber deepening procedure. BCSC Section 12, *Retina and Vitreous,* discusses vitrectomy in greater detail.

Lundy DC. Ciliary block glaucoma. *Focal Points: Clinical Modules for Ophthalmologists.* San Francisco: American Academy of Ophthalmology, 199, module 3.

Nonrhegmatogenous Retinal Detachment and Uveal Effusions

A nonrhegmatogenous retinal detachment occurs as a result of subretinal fluid in which no retinal break is present. Retinoblastoma, Coats disease, metastatic carcinoma, choroidal melanoma, suprachoroidal hemorrhage, choroidal effusion/detachment, infections (HIV), and subretinal neovascularization in age-related macular degeneration with extensive effusion or hemorrhage can cause nonrhegmatogenous retinal detachments. See BCSC Section 12, *Retina and Vitreous,* for further discussion.

In a *rhegmatogenous retinal detachment,* the subretinal fluid can escape through the retinal tear and equalize the hydraulic pressure on both sides of the retina. In a nonrhegmatogenous retinal detachment, by contrast, the subretinal fluid accumulates, becomes a space-occupying lesion in the vitreous, and progressively pushes the retina forward against the lens like a hydraulic press. The fluid or hemorrhage may accumulate rapidly, and as it pushes the bullous retinal detachment forward to a retrolenticular position, it can flatten the anterior chamber completely. The retina may be dramatically visible behind the lens on slit-lamp examination.

Epithelial and Fibrous Downgrowth

Epithelial and fibrous proliferation are rare surgical complications that can cause devastating secondary glaucomas. Epithelial and fibrous downgrowth occurs when epithelium and/or connective tissue invades the anterior chamber through a defect in a wound site. Fortunately, improved surgical and wound closure techniques have greatly reduced the incidence of these entities (Fig 5-26). Fibrous ingrowth is more prevalent than epithelial downgrowth, progresses more slowly, and is often self-limited. Risk factors for the development of these entities include prolonged inflammation, wound dehiscence, delayed wound closure, or a Descemet's membrane tear.

Epithelial proliferation can be present in 3 forms: "pearl" tumors of the iris, epithelial cysts, and epithelial ingrowth. The latter 2 often cause secondary glaucoma. Epithelial cysts appear as translucent, nonvascular anterior chamber cysts that originate from the surgical or traumatic wound (Fig 5-27). Epithelial ingrowth presents as a grayish, sheetlike growth on the trabecular meshwork, iris, ciliary body, and posterior surface of the cornea. It is often associated with wound incarceration, wound gape, ocular inflammation, and corneal edema (Figs 5-28, 5-29). The epithelial downgrowth consists of nonkeratinized, stratified, squamous epithelium with an avascular subepithelial connective tissue layer. Underlying tissues undergo disorganization and destruction with epithelial contact.

The argon laser produces characteristic white burns on the epithelial membrane on the iris surface, which helps to confirm the diagnosis of epithelial downgrowth and to determine the extent of involvement. If the diagnosis remains in question, a cytologic examination of an aqueous aspirate can be performed. Radical surgery is recommended to remove the intraocular epithelial membrane and the affected tissues and to repair the fistula, but the prognosis remains poor.

Fibrovascular tissue may also proliferate into an eye from a penetrating wound. Unlike epithelial proliferation, fibrous ingrowth progresses slowly and is often self-limited. A common cause of corneal graft failure, fibrous ingrowth appears as a thick, gray-white, vascular, retrocorneal membrane with an irregular border. The ingrowth often involves the angle, resulting in PAS and the destruction of the trabecular meshwork (Fig 5-30). The resultant secondary angle-closure glaucoma is often difficult to control.

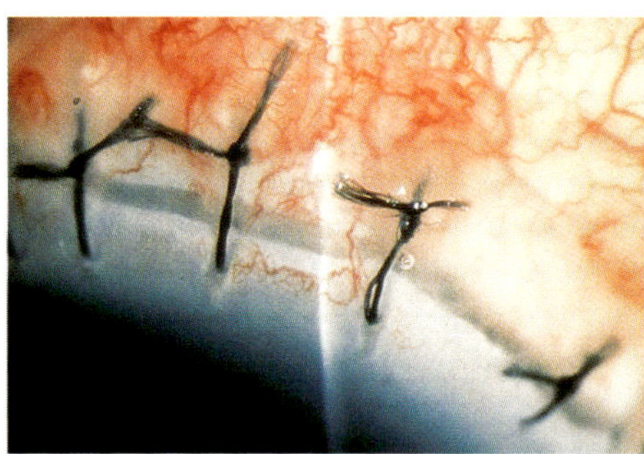

Figure 5-26 Epithelial and fibrous proliferation. This corneal scleral wound gape occurred following cataract extraction with silk closure of the incision. Improved surgical and wound closure techniques have greatly reduced the incidence of epithelial and fibrous proliferation. *(Photograph courtesy of Wills Eye Hospital slide collection, 1986.)*

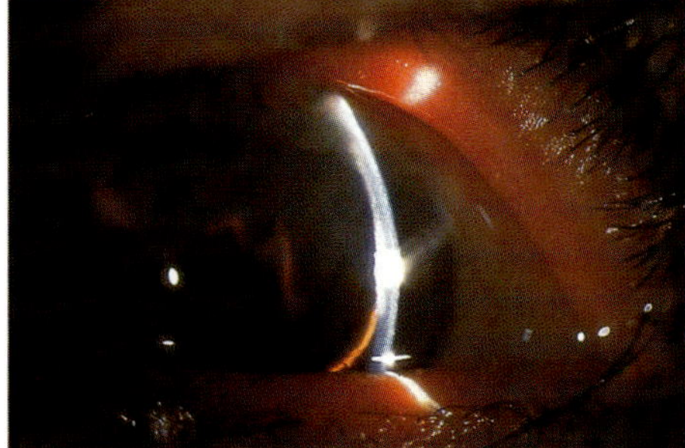

Figure 5-27 Epithelial cysts appear as translucent, nonvascular anterior chamber cysts that originate from a surgical or traumatic wound. The 2 large cysts shown in this photograph originated from a cataract incision. *(Photograph courtesy of Steven T. Simmons, MD.)*

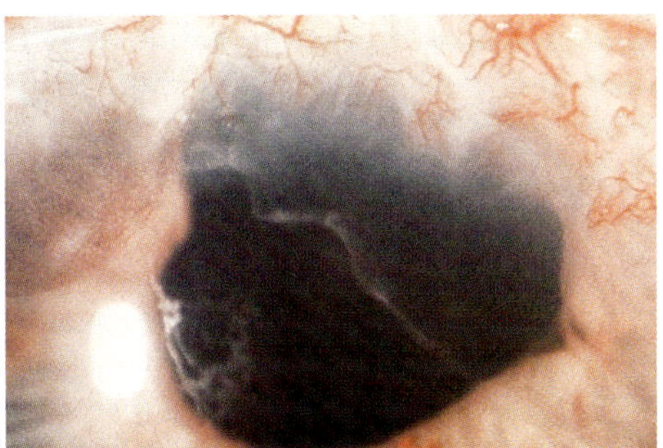

Figure 5-28 Epithelial ingrowth appears as a grayish, sheetlike growth on the endothelial surface of the cornea, usually originating from a surgical incision or traumatic wound. The epithelial ingrowth shown here originates from a cataract incision. *(Photograph courtesy of Steven T. Simmons, MD.)*

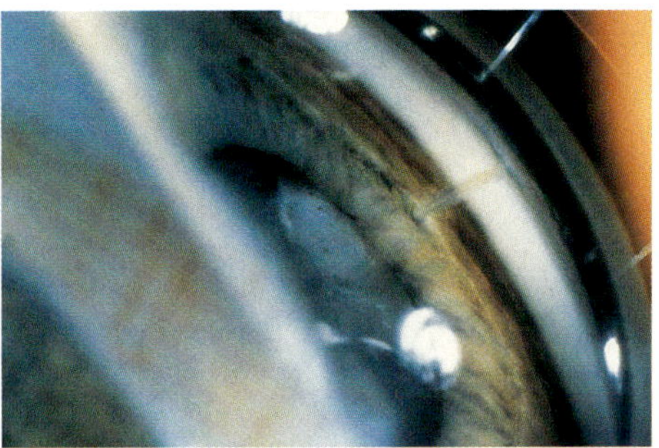

Figure 5-29 Epithelial ingrowth. The precipitating causes of epithelial ingrowth include vitreous incarceration in corneal and scleral wounds, as seen in this photograph, as well as wound gape, ocular inflammation, and hypotony secondary to choroidal effusions. *(Photograph courtesy of Steven T. Simmons, MD.)*

Medication is the preferred treatment of the secondary glaucoma, although surgical intervention may be required. See Chapter 7, Medical Management of Glaucoma, and Chapter 8, Surgical Therapy for Glaucoma, for detailed discussion.

Trauma

Angle-closure glaucoma without pupillary block may develop following ocular trauma from the formation of PAS associated with angle recession or from contusion, hyphema, and inflammation. See Chapter 4 for discussion of trauma.

Retinal Surgery and Retinal Vascular Disease

Angle-closure glaucoma may occur following treatment of retinal disorders, and it is important to measure IOP after retinal detachment surgery. Scleral buckling operations, especially encircling bands, can produce shallowing of the anterior chamber angle and frank angle-closure glaucoma, often accompanied by choroidal effusion and anterior rotation of the ciliary body, causing a flattening of the peripheral iris with a relatively deep central anterior chamber. Usually, the anterior chamber deepens with the opening of the anterior chamber angle over days to weeks with therapy of cycloplegics, anti-inflammatory agents, beta-adrenergic antagonists, carbonic anhydrase inhibitors, and hyperosmotic agents. If medical management is unsuccessful, argon laser iridoplasty, drainage of suprachoroidal fluid, or adjustment of the scleral buckle may be required. Iridectomy is usually of little benefit in this condition. The scleral buckle can impede venous drainage by compressing a vortex vein, increasing episcleral venous pressure and IOP. Only by shifting the scleral buckle or releasing the band can this elevation in IOP be treated permanently.

Following a pars plana vitrectomy, angle-closure glaucoma may result from the injection of air, long-acting gases such as sulfur hexafluoride and perfluorocarbons (perfluoropropane and perfluoroethane), or silicone oil. These substances are less dense than

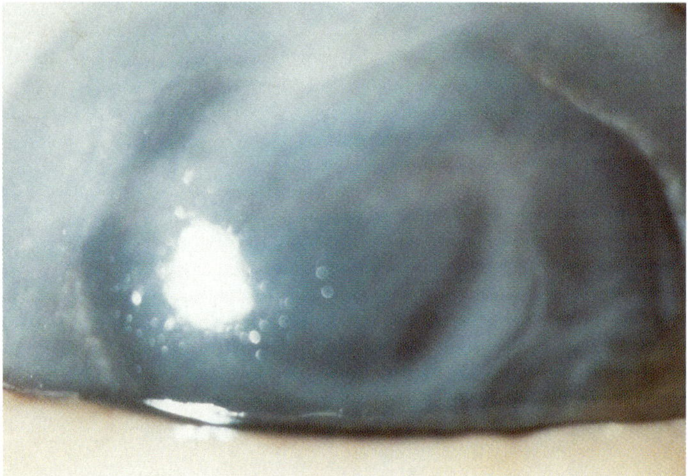

Figure 5-30 Fibrous ingrowth appears as a thick, grayish, vascular retrocorneal membrane that results in high PAS and destruction of the trabecular meshwork. *(Photograph courtesy of Steven T. Simmons, MD.)*

water and rise to the top of the eye, and an iridectomy may be beneficial. The iridectomy should be located inferiorly to prevent obstruction of the iridectomy site by the oil or gas. Eyes that have undergone complicated vitreoretinal surgery and have developed elevated IOP require individualized treatment plans. Treatment options include the following:

- removal of silicone oil
- release of the encircling element
- removal of expansile gases
- filtering surgery, including tube shunts
- cilioablation

Following panretinal photocoagulation, IOP may become elevated by an angle-closure mechanism. The ciliary body is thickened and rotated anteriorly, and often an anterior annular choroidal detachment occurs. Generally, this secondary glaucoma is self-limited, and therapy is directed at temporary medical management with cycloplegic agents, topical corticosteroids, and aqueous suppressants.

Central retinal vein occlusion (CRVO) sometimes causes early shallowing of the chamber angle, presumably because of swelling of the choroid and ciliary body. In rare cases, the angle becomes sufficiently compromised to cause angle-closure glaucoma. The chamber deepens and the glaucoma resolves over 1 to several weeks. Medical therapy treating the elevated IOP is usually preferred in combination with topical corticosteroids and cycloplegia. However, if the contralateral eye of a patient with CRVO has a potentially occludable anterior chamber angle, the ophthalmologist must consider an underlying pupillary-block mechanism and the possible need for bilateral iridectomy.

Nanophthalmos

A nanophthalmic eye is normal in shape but unusually small, with a shortened anteroposterior diameter (<20 mm), a small corneal diameter, and a relatively large lens for the eye volume. Thickened sclera may impede drainage from the vortex veins. These eyes are markedly hyperopic and highly susceptible to angle-closure glaucoma, which occurs at an earlier age than in primary angle closure. Intraocular surgery is frequently complicated by choroidal effusion and nonrhegmatogenous retinal detachment. Choroidal effusion may occur spontaneously, and it can induce angle-closure glaucoma. Laser iridectomy, argon laser peripheral iridoplasty, and medical therapy are the safest ways to manage glaucoma in these patients. Surgery should be avoided if possible because of the high rate of surgical complications.

Retinopathy of Prematurity/Persistent Hyperplastic Primary Vitreous

Contracting retrolental tissue seen in retinopathy of prematurity (retrolental fibroplasia) and persistent hyperplastic primary vitreous (PHPV) can cause progressive shallowing of the anterior chamber angle with subsequent angle-closure glaucoma. These conditions are discussed in more detail in BCSC Section 6, *Pediatric Ophthalmology and Strabismus,* and Section 12, *Retina and Vitreous.* In retinopathy of prematurity, the onset of this complication usually occurs at 3–6 months of age during the cicatricial phase of the disease. However, the angle-closure glaucoma may occur later in childhood.

PHPV is usually unilateral and often associated with microphthalmos and elongated ciliary processes. The contracture of the hyperplastic primary vitreous and swelling of a cataractous lens may result in subsequent angle-closure glaucoma.

Flat Anterior Chamber

A flat anterior chamber from any cause can result in the formation of PAS. Debate continues concerning how long a postoperative flat chamber should be treated conservatively before surgical intervention is undertaken. Hypotony in an eye with a postoperative flat chamber following cataract surgery often indicates a wound leak, and a Seidel test should be performed to locate the leak. Simple pressure patching or bandage contact lens application will often cause the leak to seal and the chamber to re-form. If the chamber does not re-form, it should be repaired surgically to prevent permanent synechial closure of the angle.

Some ophthalmologists repair the wound leak and re-form a flat chamber following cataract surgery within 24 hours. Others prefer corticosteroid therapy for several days to prevent synechiae formation. If the hyaloid face or an IOL is in contact with the cornea, the chambers should be re-formed without delay to minimize corneal endothelial damage. Early intervention should also be considered in the presence of corneal edema, excessive inflammation, or posterior synechiae formation.

Drug-Induced Secondary Angle-Closure Glaucoma

Topiramate (Topamax), a sulfamate-substituted monosaccharide, is an oral medication prescribed as an antiepileptic and antidepressant. In some patients using this medication, a syndrome characterized by acute myopic shift (>6 D) and acute bilateral angle-closure glaucoma can occur. Patients presenting with this syndrome experience bilateral, sudden loss of vision with acute myopia, bilateral ocular pain, and headache, usually within 1 month of initiating topiramate. Ocular findings of this syndrome include high myopia, a uniformly shallow anterior chamber with anterior iris and lens displacement, microcystic corneal edema, elevated IOP (40–70 mm Hg), a closed anterior chamber angle, and a ciliochoroidal effusion/detachment. The underlying mechanism of this syndrome is the ciliochoroidal effusion, which causes the relaxation of zonules and the profound anterior displacement of the lens–iris complex, causing the secondary angle-closure glaucoma and high myopia. Treatment of this syndrome is the immediate discontinuation of the topiramate and medical treatment of the elevated IOP. The secondary angle-closure glaucoma usually resolves within 24–48 hours with medical treatment, and the myopia resolves within 1 to 2 weeks of discontinuing the topiramate. Because pupillary block is not an underlying mechanism of this syndrome, a peripheral iridectomy is not indicated. Other sulfonamides, such as acetazolamide, have been reported to cause a similar clinical syndrome.

Epstein DL, Allingham RR, Schuman JS, eds. *Chandler and Grant's Glaucoma.* 4th ed. Baltimore: Williams & Wilkins; 1997.

Ritch R, Shields MB, Krupin T, eds. *The Glaucomas.* 2nd ed. St Louis: Mosby; 1996.

Shields MB. *Textbook of Glaucoma.* 4th ed. Philadelphia: Williams & Wilkins; 2000.

Stamper RL, Lieberman MF, Drake MV, eds. *Becker-Shaffer's Diagnosis and Therapy of the Glaucomas.* 7th ed. St Louis: Mosby; 1999.

CHAPTER 6

Childhood Glaucoma

BCSC Section 6, *Pediatric Ophthalmology and Strabismus,* in Chapter 21, Pediatric Glaucomas, also discusses the issues covered here.

Definitions and Classification

Primary congenital or *infantile glaucoma* is evident either at birth or within the first few years of life. These conditions are believed to be caused by dysplasia of the anterior chamber angle without other ocular or systemic abnormalities. *Secondary infantile glaucoma* is associated with inflammatory, neoplastic, hamartomatous, metabolic, or other congenital abnormalities of the eye. *Juvenile glaucoma* is recognized later in childhood (after 3 years of age) or in early adulthood.

The term *developmental glaucoma* includes primary congenital glaucoma and glaucoma associated with other developmental anomalies, either ocular or systemic. Glaucoma associated with other ocular or systemic abnormalities may be inherited or acquired. The term *buphthalmos* (cow's eye) refers to enlargement of the globe. This condition appears when the onset of elevated IOP occurs before the age of 3 in primary congenital or infantile glaucoma or in the pediatric glaucomas associated with other ocular and/or systemic abnormalities.

Epidemiology and Genetics

Glaucoma in the pediatric age group is heterogeneous. Primary congenital glaucoma, which accounts for approximately 50%–70% of the congenital glaucomas, occurs much less frequently than primary adult glaucoma, and primary infantile glaucoma is believed to be rare (1 in 10,000 births). Of pediatric glaucoma cases, 60% are diagnosed by the age of 6 months and 80% within the first year of life. Approximately 65% of patients are male, and involvement is bilateral in 70% of all cases.

Most cases of primary congenital glaucoma occur sporadically. Although some pedigrees suggest an autosomal dominant inheritance, more patients show a recessive pattern with incomplete or variable penetrance and possibly multifactorial inheritance. Two major loci of recessively inherited primary congenital glaucoma (*GLC3A* and *GLC3B*) have been identified on chromosome 2 (2p21) and chromosome 1 (1p36), respectively. Some types of juvenile glaucoma that have an autosomal dominant inheritance pattern have been mapped to chromosome 1q23–q25. Some cases of primary congenital glaucoma have been associated with chromosomal rearrangement. The natural history of this disorder is variable. Prior to effective surgical therapy, the worst cases of the disease almost always resulted in blindness.

Some patients with congenital, infantile, or juvenile glaucoma may also have Axenfeld-Rieger syndrome, aniridia, or a multisystem genetic disorder. All pediatric patients with glaucoma and adults who had glaucoma in childhood should be evaluated by a geneticist for counseling purposes.

Pathophysiology

Figure 6-1 shows the normal development, at 11 weeks, of the structures discussed here. Because histopathologic findings in infantile glaucoma vary, many theories of pathogenesis have been proposed; these fall into 2 main groups. Some investigators have proposed that a cellular or membranous abnormality in the trabecular meshwork is the primary pathologic mechanism. This abnormality is described as either an anomalous impermeable trabecular meshwork or a Barkan membrane covering the trabecular meshwork. Other investigators have emphasized a more widespread anterior segment anomaly, including abnormal insertion of the ciliary muscle.

Although the exact mechanism of primary infantile glaucoma remains unproven, there is little doubt that the disease represents a developmental anomaly of the angle structures. Many of its features suggest a developmental arrest in the late embryonic period. See also BCSC Section 2, *Fundamentals and Principles of Ophthalmology,* Part II, Embryology.

Clinical Features

Characteristic findings of infantile glaucoma include the classic triad of presenting symptoms in the newborn: *epiphora, photophobia,* and *blepharospasm.* Diagnosis of infantile glaucoma depends on careful clinical evaluation, including IOP measurement, measurement of corneal diameter, gonioscopy, measurement of axial length by ultrasonography and retinoscopy, and ophthalmoscopy. Optic nerve photography is helpful for future follow-up.

External eye examination may reveal buphthalmos with corneal enlargement greater than 12 mm in diameter during the first year of life. (The normal horizontal corneal diameter is 9.5–10.5 mm in full-term newborns and smaller in premature newborns.) Corneal edema may range from mild haze to dense opacification of the corneal stroma because of elevated IOP. Corneal edema is present in 25% of affected infants at birth and in more than 60% by the sixth month. Tears in Descemet's membrane called *Haab's striae* may occur acutely as a result of corneal stretching; these are typically oriented horizontally or concentric to the limbus.

Reduced visual acuity may occur as a result of optic atrophy, corneal clouding, astigmatism, amblyopia, cataract, lens dislocation, or retinal detachment. Amblyopia may be caused by the corneal opacity itself or by refractive error. The enlargement of the

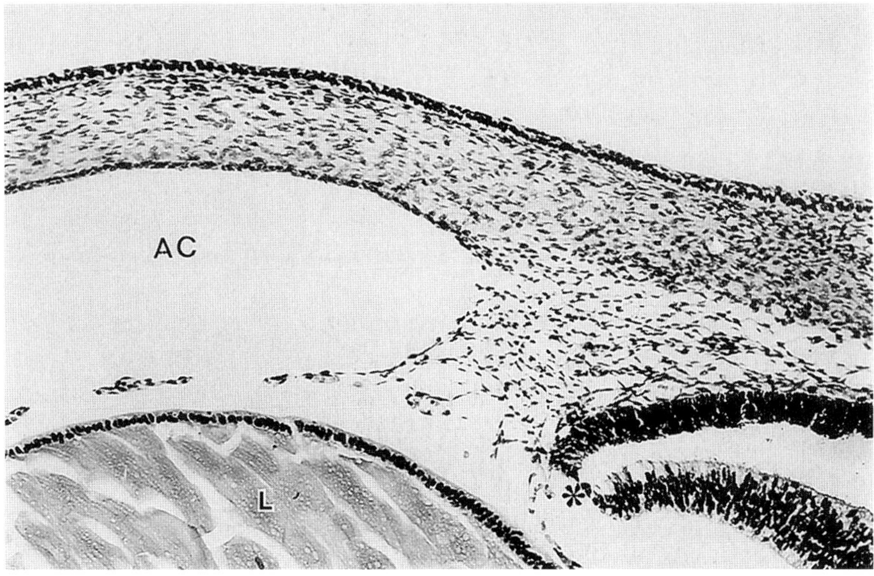

Figure 6-1 Light micrograph of the eye of an 11-week fetus in meridional section. The angular region is poorly defined at this stage and is occupied by loosely arranged, spindle-shaped cells. Schlemm's canal is unrecognizable, and ciliary muscles and ciliary processes are not yet formed; the latter are derived from neural ectodermal fold *(asterisk)*. Corneal endothelium appears continuous with cellular covering of primitive iris. *AC* = anterior chamber. *L* = lens. (Original magnification ×230.) *(Reproduced with permission from Tripathi RC, Tripathi BJ. Functional anatomy of the anterior chamber angle. In: Tasman W, Jaeger EA, eds.* Duane's Foundations of Clinical Ophthalmology. *Philadelphia: Lippincott; 1991.)*

eye causes myopia, whereas tears in Descemet's membrane can cause a large astigmatism. Appropriate measures to prevent or treat amblyopia should be initiated as early as possible.

It is possible for the clinician to measure the IOP in some infants under age 6 months without general anesthesia or sedation by performing the measurement while the infant is feeding or asleep following feeding. However, critical evaluation of infants requires an examination under anesthesia. Most general anesthetic agents and sedatives lower IOP. In addition, infants may become dehydrated in preparation for general anesthesia, also reducing the IOP. As anesthesia becomes deeper, IOP falls. The only exception to this rule is ketamine, which may raise IOP. The normal IOP in an infant under anesthesia may range from 10 to 15 mm Hg, depending on the tonometer.

Gonioscopy under anesthesia is recommended. In primary childhood glaucoma, the anterior chamber is characteristically deep with normal iris structure. Findings include a high and flat iris insertion, absence of angle recess, peripheral iris hypoplasia, tenting of the peripheral iris pigment epithelium, and thickened uveal trabecular meshwork. The angle is typically open, with a high insertion of the iris root that forms a scalloped line as a result of abnormal tissue with a shagreened, glistening appearance. This tissue holds the peripheral iris anteriorly. The angle is usually avascular, but loops of vessels from the major arterial circle may be seen above the iris root.

The normal anterior chamber angle in childhood is different from the adult angle. Many of the findings just listed are nonspecific, and it may be difficult to distinguish the gonioscopic findings in infantile glaucoma from a normal infant angle. If corneal edema prevents an adequate view of the angle, the epithelium may be removed with a scalpel blade or a cotton-tipped applicator soaked in 70% alcohol to improve visibility.

Visualization of the optic disc may be facilitated by using a direct ophthalmoscope and a direct gonioscopic or fundus lens on the cornea. The optic nerve head of a normal infant is pink with a small physiologic cup. Glaucomatous cupping in childhood resembles the cupping in adulthood, with preferential loss of neural tissue in the superior and inferior poles. In childhood, the scleral canal enlarges in response to elevated IOP, causing enlargement of the cup. Cupping may be reversible if IOP is lowered, and progressive cupping indicates poor control of IOP.

Photographic documentation of the optic disc is recommended. Ultrasonography may be useful in documenting progression of glaucoma by recording increasing axial length. Increase in axial length may be reversible following reduction of IOP, but corneal enlargement may not decrease following reduction of IOP.

Differential Diagnosis

Many other conditions with similar features are included in the differential diagnosis of infantile glaucoma (Table 6-1). Excessive tearing may be caused by an obstruction of the lacrimal drainage system. Ocular abnormalities associated with enlarged corneas include X-linked congenital megalocornea without glaucoma. Tears in Descemet's membrane resulting from birth trauma, often associated with forceps-assisted deliveries, are usually vertical or oblique. Corneal opacification and clouding have many possible causes:

- birth trauma
- dysgeneses (Peters anomaly and sclerocornea)
- dystrophies (congenital hereditary endothelial dystrophy and posterior polymorphous dystrophy)
- choristomas (dermoid and dermislike choristoma)
- intrauterine inflammation (congenital syphilis and rubella)
- inborn errors of metabolism (mucopolysaccharidoses and cystinosis)
- keratomalacia
- skin disorders that affect the cornea (congenital ichthyosis and congenital dyskeratosis)

Long-term Prognosis and Follow-up

Medications have limited long-term value for congenital and infantile glaucoma in most cases, and the preferred therapy is surgical. The initial procedures of choice are goniotomy or trabeculotomy if the cornea is clear, and trabeculotomy ab externo if the cornea is hazy. The success rates are similar for both procedures in patients with clear corneas.

Table 6-1 Diagnostic Considerations for Symptoms and Signs of Infantile Glaucoma

Excessive tearing
- Nasolacrimal duct obstruction
- Corneal epithelial defect or abrasion
- Conjunctivitis

Corneal enlargement or apparent enlargement
- X-linked megalocornea
- High myopia
- Exophthalmos
- Shallow orbits (eg, craniofacial dysostoses)

Corneal clouding
- Birth trauma
- Inflammatory corneal disease
- Congenital hereditary corneal dystrophies
- Corneal malformations (dermoid tumors, sclerocornea, Peters anomaly)
- Keratomalacia
- Metabolic disorders with associated corneal abnormalities (mucopolysaccharidoses, corneal lipidosis, cystinosis, and von Glerke disease)
- Skin disorders affecting the cornea (congenital ichthyosis and congenital dyskeratosis)

Optic nerve abnormalities
- Optic nerve pit
- Optic nerve coloboma
- Optic nerve hypoplasia
- Optic nerve malformation
- Physiologic cupping

Trabeculectomy and shunt procedures should be reserved for those cases where goniotomy or trabeculotomy has failed. Cyclophotocoagulation is necessary in some intractable cases.

Beta-adrenergic antagonists or carbonic anhydrase inhibitors may be used as temporizing therapy prior to surgery to control IOP and help clear a cloudy cornea. These drugs must be used with caution and at doses appropriate for the child's weight to prevent systemic side effects. The parents should be instructed in particular to occlude the nasolacrimal drainage system for at least 2 minutes immediately after administering topical beta-adrenergic antagonists and to be alert for apnea and hypotension. Young children on carbonic anhydrase inhibitors require assessment for possible acidosis, hypokalemia, and feeding problems. Alpha$_2$-adrenergic agonists should be avoided in children younger than 3 years of age because of the risk of CNS side effects such as apnea.

Long-term prognosis has greatly improved with the development of effective surgical techniques, particularly for patients who are asymptomatic at birth and present with onset of symptoms before 24 months of age. When symptoms are present at birth or when the disease is diagnosed after 24 months of age, the outlook for surgical control of IOP is more guarded. Even patients whose IOP is usually controlled by surgery may experience late complications such as amblyopia, corneal scarring, strabismus, anisometropia, cataract, lens subluxation, susceptibility of an eye with a thinned sclera to trauma, and recurrent glaucoma in the affected or unaffected eye many years later.

Developmental Glaucomas With Associated Ocular or Systemic Anomalies

Glaucoma may be associated with other ocular abnormalities, including the following conditions:

- microphthalmos
- corneal anomalies (microcornea, megalocornea, cornea plana, sclerocornea, corneal staphyloma)
- anterior segment dysgenesis (Axenfeld-Rieger syndrome, Peters anomaly, iridoschisis)
- aniridia
- lens anomalies (congenital cataracts, lens dislocation, microspherophakia)
- persistent hyperplastic primary vitreous
- congenital ectropion-uvea syndrome

Axenfeld-Rieger (A-R) Syndrome

Axenfeld-Rieger syndrome is a group of bilateral congenital anomalies that may include abnormal development of the anterior chamber angle, the iris, and the trabecular meshwork. It has an autosomal dominant inheritance pattern in most cases but can occur sporadically. Approximately 50% of cases are associated with glaucoma. Axenfeld-Rieger syndrome is the result of abnormal development of tissues derived from the neural crest.

Although this syndrome was initially separated into Axenfeld anomaly (posterior embryotoxon with multiple adherent peripheral iris strands), Rieger anomaly (Axenfeld anomaly plus iris hypoplasia and corectopia), and Rieger syndrome (Rieger anomaly plus developmental defects of the teeth or facial bones including maxillary hypoplasia, redundant periumbilical skin, pituitary abnormalities, or hypospadius), these disorders are now considered variations along the same clinical spectrum and are combined under the name Axenfeld-Rieger syndrome.

The typical corneal abnormality is a posterior embryotoxon (a prominent and anteriorly displaced Schwalbe's line), with the remainder of the cornea normal. Iridocorneal adhesions to Schwalbe's line range from threadlike to broad bands of iris tissue. The iris itself may range from normal to markedly atrophic with corectopia, hole formation, and ectropion uveae. Axenfeld-Rieger syndrome can be distinguished from other conditions that involve abnormalities of the iris, cornea, and anterior chamber as outlined in Table 6-2.

Peters Anomaly

Peters anomaly is typically a bilateral condition of central corneal opacity with adhesions between the central iris and posterior cornea. It is bilateral 80% of the time. The lens may be normal or abnormal. The condition is usually sporadic, although autosomal dominant and autosomal recessive forms have been reported. Approximately 50% of cases are associated with glaucoma.

In Peters anomaly, there is an annular corneal opacity (leukoma) in the central visual axis with iris strands extending from the collarette to the corneal opacity. This annular

Table 6-2 Differential Diagnosis of Axenfeld-Rieger Syndrome

Condition	Differentiating Features
Iridocorneal endothelial syndrome	Unilateral Middle age Corneal endothelial abnormalities
Isolated posterior embryotoxon	Lack of glaucoma, iris changes
Aniridia	Iris hypoplasia Associated corneal and macula changes
Iridoschisis	Lack of angle abnormalities, glaucoma
Peters' anomaly	Corneal changes
Ectopia lentis et pupillae	Lack of glaucoma
Oculodental digital dysplasia	Lack of angle changes, glaucoma

(Used with permission from Morrison JC, Pollack IP. *Glaucoma: Science and Practice.* New York: Thieme Medical Publishers; 2003:188).

corneal opacity corresponds to a central defect in the corneal endothelium and underlying Descemet's membrane. Patients with Peters anomaly may have defects in the posterior stroma, Descemet's membrane, and endothelium without extension of iris strands to the edge of the corneal leukoma. The lens may be in normal position, with or without a cataract, or the lens may be adherent to the posterior layers of the cornea. Patients with corneolenticular adhesions have a higher likelihood of ocular abnormalities such as microcornea and angle anomalies, and of systemic abnormalities, including those of the heart, genitourinary system, musculoskeletal system, ear, palate, and spine.

Aniridia

Aniridia is a bilateral condition characterized by variable iris hypoplasia that often appears as complete absence of the iris. Despite the name, there is always a rudimentary stump of iris visible on gonioscopy. Most cases are familial and are transmitted as an autosomal dominant form; however, about one third of cases are isolated sporatic mutations. Approximately 20% of sporadic cases are associated with Wilms tumor, although relatively few cases of Wilms tumor are seen in the familial form. The aniridia gene locus for both the familial and the sporadic forms is a mutation of the *PAX6* gene on the 11p13 chromosome. Approximately 50%–75% of patients with aniridia develop glaucoma. Although occasionally associated with congenital glaucoma, glaucoma in aniridia usually develops after the rudimentary iris stump rotates anteriorly to progressively cover the trabecular meshwork. This is a gradual process, and glaucoma may not occur until the second decade of life or later.

In aniridia, the iris appearance may vary greatly, from a rudimentary stump to a complete, or nearly complete but thin iris. Patients with aniridia may have limbal stem cell abnormalities that eventually result in a pannus that begins in the peripheral cornea and slowly extends centrally. Cataracts may be present at birth or develop later in life. Most patients with aniridia have foveal hypoplasia that leads to pendular nystagmus and reduced vision. Although 85% of patients with aniridia have an autosomal dominant form not associated with other systemic abnormalities, 2 other types have been described. WAGR syndrome is an autosomal dominant form seen in 13% of aniridia patients and may include *W*ilms tumor, *a*niridia, *g*enitourinary anomalies, and mental *r*etardation. An autosomal recessive form of aniridia, also called Gillespie syndrome, is associated with cerebellar ataxia and mental retardation and occurs in 2% of those with aniridia.

Other Anomalies and Syndromes

Developmental glaucoma with either an open or a closed angle may be associated with other anomalies and multisystem syndromes. Some important anomalies include syndromes with known chromosomal abnormalities, systemic disorders of unknown etiology, and ocular congenital disorders. Glaucomas associated with congenital systemic anomalies are summarized in Table 6-3.

A number of systemic disorders are also associated with pediatric glaucoma, including the following:

- Sturge-Weber syndrome
- neurofibromatosis
- Marfan syndrome
- homocystinuria
- Weill-Marchesani syndrome

With Sturge-Weber syndrome and neurofibromatosis in particular, upper eyelid involvement is associated with an increased risk of glaucoma. A number of these conditions have ocular findings similar to primary infantile glaucoma; in others, the glaucoma is secondary.

Sturge-Weber syndrome

Sturge-Weber sydrome is also known as *encephalotrigeminal angiomatosis, nevus flammeus,* or *port-wine stain.* It is usually a unilateral condition with ipsilateral facial cutaneous hemangioma (nevus flammeus or port-wine stain), ipsilateral cavernous hemangioma of the choroid, and ipsilateral leptomeningeal angioma. There is no race or gender predilection, and no inheritance pattern has been established. Glaucoma occurs in 30%–70% of patients. When glaucoma is seen in infants with this syndrome, it is thought to be due to congenital anterior chamber anomalies (similar to congenital glaucoma). Glaucoma developing after the first decade of life is believed to be the result of elevated episcleral venous pressure causing elevated IOP. Involvement of the central nervous system may be associated with seizures, focal neurologic defects, or mental retardation.

Neurofibromatosis

Neurofibromatosis (NF) is the most common phakomatosis. Two forms are recognized. Neurofibromatosis type 1 (NF-1), also known as *von Recklinghausen syndrome* or *peripheral neurofibromatosis,* is the most common type by far, with a prevalence of 1 in 3000–5000. NF-1 is localized to chromosome 17q11 and is inherited in an autosomal dominant fashion about half the time, with the other cases being sporadic. Ocular findings include Lisch nodules, optic nerve gliomas, eyelid neurofibromas, and glaucoma. Systemic findings include cutaneous café-au-lait spots, cutaneous neurofibromas, and axillary or

Table 6-3 Systemic Anomalies Associated With Childhood Glaucomas

GLAUCOMA ASSOCIATED WITH SYSTEMIC CONGENITAL SYNDROMES, WITH REPORTED CHROMOSOMAL ABNORMALITIES

Trisomy 21 (Down syndrome, trisomy G syndrome)
Mental deficiency, short stature, cardiac anomalies, hypotonia, atypical facies

Trisomy 13 (Patau syndrome)
Mental retardation, deafness, heart disease, motor seizures

Trisomy 18 (Edwards syndrome, trisomy E syndrome)
Low-set ears, high-arched hard palate, ventricular septal defects, rocker-bottom feet, short sternum, hypertonia

Turner (XO/XX) syndrome
Short stature, postadolescent females with sexual infantilism, webbed neck, mental retardation, congenital deafness, multiple systemic anomalies

GLAUCOMA ASSOCIATED WITH SYSTEMIC CONGENITAL DISORDERS

Lowe (oculocerebrorenal) syndrome
X-linked recessive disease, mental retardation, renal rickets, aminoaciduria, hypotonia, acidemia, cataracts

Stickler syndrome (hereditary progressive arthro-ophthalmopathy)
Autosomal dominant connective tissue dysprasia; ocular, oioiacia, and generalized skeletal abnormalities with high myopia; open-angle glaucoma; cataracts; vitreoretinal degeneration; retinal detachment

Zellweger (cerebrohepatorenal) syndrome
Congenital autosomal recessive syndrome, abnormal facies, cerebral dysgenesis, hepatic interstitial fibrosis, polycystic kidneys, central nervous system abnormalities
Ocular findings: nystagmus, corneal clouding, cataracts, retinal vascular and pigmentary abnormalities, optic nerve head lesions

Hallermann-Streiff syndrome (dyscephalic mandibulo-oculofacial syndrome, François dyscephalic syndrome)
Micrognathia, dwarfism, microphthalmos, cataract, aniridia, optic atrophy

Rubinstein-Taybi (broad-thumb) syndrome
Mental and motor retardation, typical congenital skeletal deformities of large thumbs and first toes
Ocular findings: bushy brows, hypertelorism, epicanthus, anti-mongoloid slant of eyelids, hyperopia, strabismus

Oculodentodigital dysplasia (Meyer-Schwickerath and Weyers syndrome)
Autosomal dominant inheritance, hypoplastic dental enamel, microdontia, bilateral syndactyly, thin nose, microcornea, microphthalmos

Prader-Willi syndrome
Chromosome 15 deletion, muscular hypotonia, hypogonadism, obesity, mental retardation
Ocular findings: ocular albinism, congenital ectropion uveae, iris stromal hypoplasia, angle abnormalities

Cockayne syndrome
Autosomal recessive disorder, dwarfism, mental retardation, progressive wasting, "bird-like" facies
Ocular findings: retinal degeneration, cataracts, corneal exposure, blepharitis, nystagmus, hypoplastic irides, irregular pupils

Fetal alcohol syndrome
Teratogenic effects of alcohol during gestation, facial abnormalities, mental retardation, anterior segment involvement resembling Axenfeld-Rieger syndrome and Peters anomaly, optic nerve hypoplasia

inguinal freckling. Neurofibromatosis type 2 (NF-2), or *central neurofibromatosis,* is localized to chromosome 22. The principal ocular finding with NF-2 is the development of posterior capsular cataracts in adolescence or young adulthood. NF-2 is not associated with glaucoma. NF-2 is defined by the presence of bilateral acoustic neuromas and is frequently accompanied by multiple other nervous system tumors including meningiomas, schwannomas, and ependymomas, typically involving cranial nerves and spinal cord or nerve roots. See also BCSC Section 6, *Pediatric Ophthalmology and Strabismus,* Chapter 27.

Secondary glaucoma

Secondary glaucoma may develop in infants and children from any cause seen in adults: trauma, inflammation, retinopathy of prematurity with secondary angle-closure glaucoma, lens-induced glaucoma, corticosteroid-induced glaucoma, pigmentary glaucoma, and glaucoma secondary to intraocular tumors. Retinoblastoma, juvenile xanthogranuloma, and medulloepithelioma are some of the intraocular tumors known to lead to secondary glaucoma in infants and children. Rubella and congenital cataract are also important associated conditions. Clinicians now realize that children often develop glaucoma within 3 years following surgery for congenital cataract but may develop glaucoma years later and require continued follow-up for this reason.

Beck AD. Diagnosis and management of pediatric glaucoma. *Ophthalmol Clin North Am.* 2001;14:501–512.

Higginbotham EJ, Lee DA, eds. *Management of Difficult Glaucoma: A Clinician's Guide.* Boston: Blackwell Scientific Publications; 1994.

Isenberg SJ, ed. *The Eye in Infancy.* 2nd ed. St Louis: Mosby; 1994.

Shields MB. *Textbook of Glaucoma.* 4th ed. Philadelphia: Williams & Wilkins; 2000.

Stamper RL, Lieberman MF, Drake MV, eds. *Becker-Shaffer's Diagnosis and Therapy of the Glaucomas.* 7th ed. St Louis: Mosby; 1999.

Tasman W, Jaeger EA, eds. *Duane's Clinical Ophthalmology.* Philadelphia: Lippincott; 2002.

CHAPTER 7

Medical Management of Glaucoma

Two decisions arise in choosing an appropriate glaucoma therapy: when to treat and how to treat. The risks of therapy must always be weighed against the anticipated benefits.

A patient with early open-angle glaucoma may be difficult to distinguish from a glaucoma suspect. Because the latter has a lower risk of ultimate ocular damage, the decision of when to treat the glaucoma suspect who has not demonstrated actual nerve damage remains an individual determination for each patient. The Ocular Hypertension Treatment Study (OHTS) has provided invaluable information to assist in this discussion. The first goal of OHTS was to determine the efficacy and safety of lowering IOP (from a baseline of 24–32 mm Hg) in decreasing the risk of development of primary open-angle glaucoma (POAG). A 20% decrease in IOP with medications decreased the risk of developing POAG from 9.5% in the observation group to 4.4% in the treatment group at 5 years. There were few safety concerns. The second goal was to identify baseline characteristics that increased the risk of POAG in patients with ocular hypertension. Higher IOP, older age, larger cup–disc diameter, and reduced central corneal thickness (CCT) were shown by multivariate analysis to be significant risk factors. Race and family history, as well as other factors, were not found to be independent risk factors. The recommendation was made that treatment should be considered in those with moderate or high risk of developing POAG.

The goal of currently available glaucoma therapy is to preserve visual function by lowering IOP below a level that is likely to produce further damage to the nerve. The treatment regimen that achieves this goal with the lowest risk, fewest side effects, and least disruption of the patient's life, taking into account the cost implications of treatment, should be the one employed. The so-called target pressure goal should actually be a range, with an upper IOP limit that is unlikely to lead to further damage of the nerve in a given patient. The range should be individualized, based on the IOP at which damage is thought to have occurred, severity of the damage, life expectancy, and associated risk factors.

The more advanced the glaucomatous process on initial presentation, the lower the target pressure generally needs to be to prevent further progression. This more aggressive target is to minimize the risk of progressive glaucoma damage. Once the optic nerve is damaged, it is more likely to incur more damage, and if severe visual loss is present, there is greater impact on the patient from any additional damage that may occur. An initial reduction in the IOP of 20% from baseline is suggested. However, reduction of IOP to the target pressure range does not guarantee that progression will not occur. *Therefore, the target pressure range needs to be constantly reassessed and changed as dictated by IOP fluctuations, optic nerve changes, and/or visual field progression.* Several recent studies have shown that a consistently lower IOP results in a reduced risk of progressive glaucoma damage.

The anticipated benefits of any therapeutic regimen should justify the risks, and regimens associated with substantial side effects should be reserved for patients with a high probability of progressive visual loss. For example, it is reasonable to expose a patient to the side effects of oral carbonic anhydrase inhibitors (CAIs) when significant damage to the visual field and optic nerve has occurred and the elevated IOP is not controlled by medications with fewer potential side effects. When progressive visual field loss or cupping has not been established, however, the physician should exercise caution in subjecting a patient to the risk of the significant side effects of these agents.

The interrelationship between medical and surgical therapy is also complex. The treatment of pupillary-block angle-closure glaucoma and infantile glaucoma is primarily surgical, either laser or incisional, with medical therapy taking a secondary role. Initial treatment of POAG has commonly been medical, with surgery undertaken only if medical treatment fails or is not well tolerated. The Glaucoma Laser Trial (GLT) found that as initial glaucoma therapy, argon laser trabeculoplasty was at least as effective as medications. The Collaborative Initial Glaucoma Treatment Study (CIGTS) reported that initial medical therapy or surgical therapy were essentially equally effective in preventing POAG progression. In fact, the rate of progression at 5 years was substantially less than anticipated. This has been attributed to the definition of progression used in the study and the aggressive IOP lowering obtained in both groups. Surgical therapy is discussed in detail in the following chapter.

The Advanced Glaucoma Intervention Study (AGIS): 4. Comparison of treatment outcomes within race: seven-year results. *Ophthalmology.* 1998;105:1146–1164.

The Advanced Glaucoma Intervention Study (AGIS): 7. The relationship between control of intraocular pressure and visual field deterioration. The AGIS Investigators. *Am J Ophthalmol.* 2000;130:429–440.

Kass MA, Heuer DK, Higginbotham EJ, et al. The Ocular Hypertension Treatment Study: a randomized trial determines that topical ocular hypotensive medication delays or prevents the onset of primary open-angle glaucoma. *Arch Ophthalmol.* 2002;120:701–713.

Leske MC, Heijl A, Hussein M, et al. Factors for glaucoma progression and the effect of treatment: the Early Manifest Glaucoma Trial. *Arch Ophthalmol.* 2003;121:48–56.

Lichter PR, Musch DC, Gillespie BW, et al. Interim clinical outcomes in the Collaborative Initial Glaucoma Treatment Study comparing initial treatment randomized to medications or surgery. *Ophthalmology.* 2001;108:1943–1953.

Treatment of secondary glaucoma is comparable to treatment of the primary glaucoma that it most closely resembles. Initially, the underlying cause of the glaucoma should be addressed, if possible. For example, panretinal photocoagulation (PRP) is probably the most vital part of the treatment of neovascular glaucoma and should be done in concert with the appropriate method of IOP reduction. In uveitic glaucoma, prostaglandin analogs are generally avoided—due to their potential for exacerbating intraocular inflammation—until other options have been tried.

In general, therapy should progress from the lowest risk to the highest risk, and then only when the initial therapy fails to reach the assigned target pressures and there is significant risk of progression. The efficacy of the therapeutic regimen should be reevaluated periodically. Specifically, a 1-eyed therapeutic trial should be considered to assess the efficacy of new medications; a reverse therapeutic trial can be performed to assess existing regimens. A reverse trial entails discontinuing a medication in only 1 eye and then comparing the effect in the treated versus the untreated eye. This allows assessment of the continued efficacy or side effects of a drug.

Medical Agents

Ocular hypotensive agents are divided into several groups based on chemical structure and pharmacologic action. The groups of agents in common clinical use include

- beta-adrenergic antagonists (nonselective and selective)
- parasympathomimetic (miotic) agents, including cholinergic and anticholinesterase agents
- carbonic anhydrase inhibitors (oral and topical)
- adrenergic agonists (nonselective and selective $alpha_2$ agonists)
- hypotensive lipids, including prostaglandin analogs, prostamides, and decosonoids
- combination medications
- hyperosmotic agents

The actions and side effects of the various glaucoma medications are listed in Table 7-1, along with dosage information and other concerns. The reader is referred back to this table throughout the discussions in this chapter. BCSC Section 2, *Fundamentals and Principles of Ophthalmology,* discusses and illustrates the mechanisms of action of these medications in Part V, Ocular Pharmacology.

Netland PA, Allen RC, eds. *Glaucoma Medical Therapy: Principles and Management.* Ophthalmology Monograph 13. San Francisco: American Academy of Ophthalmology; 1999.

Beta-Adrenergic Antagonists (Beta Blockers)

Topical beta-blocking agents lower IOP by inhibiting cyclic adenosine monophosphate (cAMP) production in ciliary epithelium, thereby reducing aqueous humor secretion 20%–50% (2.5 μL/min to 1.9 μL/min), with a corresponding IOP reduction of 20%–30%. The effect of beta blockers on aqueous production occurs within 1 hour of instillation and can be present for up to 4 weeks after discontinuation. Evidence suggests that beta blockers decrease aqueous production during the day but have much less effect during sleep. As systemic absorption occurs, a contralateral IOP-lowering effect in the untreated eye can also be observed. Most beta blockers are approved for twice-daily therapy. In many cases, once daily with the nonselective agents is possible. Generally, dosing first thing in the morning is preferred to effectively blunt an early morning pressure rise while minimizing the risk of systemic hypotension during sleep. Many nonselective beta blockers are available in more than 1 concentration. For example, timolol 0.25% is as effective in lowering IOP as timolol 0.5% in many patients.

Beta blockers are additive in combination with miotics, adrenergic agonists, CAIs (both topical and systemic), and hypotensive lipids. Combinations of beta blockers and

Table 7-1 Glaucoma Medications

Class/Compound	Brand Name	Strengths	Dosage	Method of Action	IOP Decrease	Side Effects: Ocular	Side Effects: Systemic	Comments, Including Time to Peak Effect and Washout
Beta-adrenergic antagonists (beta blockers)								
Nonselective								
Timolol maleate	Timoptic XE Timoptic Timolol gel	0.25, 0.5% 0.25, 0.5% 0.5%	qd qd, bid qd	Decrease aqueous production	20%–30%	Blurring, irritation, corneal anesthesia, punctate keratitis, allergy	Bradycardia, heart block, bronchospasm, decreased libido, CNS depression, mood swings	May be less effective if patient on systemic beta blockers, short-term escape, long-term drift Peak: 2–3 hours Washout: 1 month
Timolol hemihydrate	Betimol	0.5%	qd, bid	Same as above	Same as above	Same as above	Same as above	Less expensive
Levobunolol	Betagan	0.25, 0.5%	qd, bid	Same as above	Same as above	Same as above	Same as above	Peak: 2–6 hours
Metipranolol	OptiPranolol	0.3%	bid	Same as above	Same as above	Same as above	Same as above	Report of iritis Peak: 2 hours
Carteolol hydrochloride	Ocupress	1.0%	qd, bid				Intrinsic sympathomimetic	May have less effect on nocturnal pulse, blood pressure Peak: 4 hours Washout: 1 month
Selective								
Betaxolol	Betoptic (S)	0.25%	bid	Same as above	15%–20%	Same as above	Fewer pulmonary complications	Peak: 2–3 hours Washout: 1 month
Adrenergic agonists								
Nonselective								
Epinephrine	Epifrin	0.25, 0.5, 1.0, 2.0%	bid	Improve aqueous outflow	15%–20%	Irritation, conjunctival hyphema (rebound), eyelid retraction, mydriasis, adrenochrome deposits, follicular conjunctivitis (allergy), cystoid macular edema in aphakia, pseudophakia	Hypertension, headaches, extra systoles	Peak: variable, initial IOP rise followed by reduction lasting 12–24 hours Washout: 7–14 days

Class/Compound	Brand Name	Strengths	Dosage	Method of Action	IOP Decrease	Side Effects: Ocular	Side Effects: Systemic	Comments, Including Time to Peak Effect and Washout
Dipivefrin HCL	Propine	0.1%	bid	Same as above	Same as above	Same as above	Pro-drug makes systemic effects less likely	Peak/washout: same as epinephrine
Alpha$_2$-adrenergic agonists								
Selective								
Apraclonidine HCl	Iopidine	0.5, 1.0%	bid, tid	Decrease aqueous production, decrease episcleral venous pressure	20%–30%	Irritation, ischemia, allergy, eyelid retraction, conjunctival blanching, follicular conjunctivitis, puritis, dermatitis, ocular ache, photopsia, miosis	Hypotension, vasovagal attack, dry mouth and nose, fatigue	Useful in pre- or postlaser or cataract surgery, tachyphylaxis Peak: <1–2 hours Washout: 7–14 days
Highly selective								
Brimonidine tartrate 0.2%	Alphagan	0.2%	bid, tid	Decrease aqueous production, increase uveoscleral outflow	20%–30%	Blurring, foreign body sensation, eyelid edema, dryness, less ocular sensitivity/allergy than Iopidine	Headache, fatigue, hypotension, insomnia, depression, syncope, dizziness, anxiety	Primary adrenergic agent in current use, highly alpha$_2$ selective Peak: 2 hours Washout: 7–14 days
Brimonidine tartrate in Purite 0.15%	Alphagan P	0.15%	bid, tid	Same as above	Same as above	Same except less allergy than Alphagan	Same except less fatigue and depression than Alphagan	Same as above
Parasympathomimetic (miotic) agents								
Cholinergic agonists (direct acting)								
Pilocarpine HCl	Isopto Carpine Pilocar	0.2%–10.0% 0.5, 1.0, 2.0, 3.0, 4.0, 6.0%	bid–qid bid–qid	Increase trabecular outflow	15%–25%	Posterior synechiae, keratitis, miosis, brow ache, cataract growth, angle-closure potential, myopia, retinal tear/detachment, dermatitis, change in retinal sensitivity, color vision changes	Increased salivation, increased secretion (gastric), abdominal cramps	Exacerbation of cataract effect, more effective in lighter irides Peak: 1½–2 hours Washout: 48 hours

(Continues)

Table 7-1 Glaucoma Medications (Continued)

Class/Compound	Brand Name	Strengths	Dosage	Method of Action	IOP Decrease	Side Effects: Ocular	Side Effects: Systemic	Comments, Including Time to Peak Effect and Washout
Pilocarpine gel	Pilopine Gel HS	4.0%	qhs	Increase trabecular outflow	15%–25%	Same as above	Same as above	Same as above Peak: 2–3 hours Washout: 48 hours
Carbachol*	Isopto Carbachol	1.5, 3.0%	bid, tid	Same as above	15%–25%	May be useful in patients with pilocarpine sensitivity		Intraoperative carbachol useful to lower IOP
Anticholinesterase agents (indirect acting)								
Demecarium bromide	Humorsol	0.125, 0.25%	qd, bid	Same as above	15%–25%	Intense miosis, iris pigment cyst, myopia, cataract, retinal detachment, angle closure, punctal stenosis, pseudopemphigoid	Same as pilocarpine, more gastrointestinal difficulties	Increased inflammation with ocular surgery; may be helpful in aphakia, anesthesia risks (prolonged recovery); useful in eyelid-lash lice, postoperative cataract surgery
Carbonic anhydrase inhibitors								
Oral								
Acetazolamide	Diamox Diamox Sequels	62.5, 125, 250 mg 500 mg	bid–qid qd, bid	Decrease aqueous production	15%–20%	None	Poor tolerance of carbonated beverages, acidosis, depression, malaise, hirsutism, flatulence, paresthesias, numbness, lethargy, blood dyscrasias, diarrhea, weight loss, renal stones, loss of libido, bone marrow depression, hypokalemia, cramps, anorexia, altered taste, increased serum urate, enuresis	Sulfa allergy, caution to patients susceptible to ketoacidosis, hepatic insufficiency
Acetazolamide (parenteral)	Diamox	500 mg 5–10 mg/kg	Usually ≤1 qd q6–8 hrs	Same as above	Same as above	Same as above	Same as above	Same as above

Class/Compound	Brand Name	Strengths	Dosage	Method of Action	IOP Decrease	Side Effects: Ocular	Side Effects: Systemic	Comments, Including Time to Peak Effect and Washout
Dichlorphenamide	Daranide	50 mg	bid, tid	Same as above	Same as above	Same as above	Same as above	Same as above
Methazolamide	Neptazane	25, 50, 100 mg	bid, tid	Same as above	Same as above	Same as above	Same as above	Same as above
Topical								
Dorzolamide	Trusopt	2.0%	bid, tid	Same as above	15%–20%	Induced myopia, blurred vision, stinging, keratitis, conjunctivitis, dermatitis	Less likely to induce systemic effects of CAI, but may occur; bitter taste	Peak: 2–3 hours Washout: 48 hours
Brinzolamide	Azopt	1%	bid, tid	Same as above	Same as above	Less stinging when compared to Trusopt	Same as above	Same as above
Hypotensive lipids								
Prostaglandin analogues								
Latanoprost	Xalatan	.005%	qd	Increase uveoscleral outflow	25%–32%	Increased pigmentation of iris and lashes, hypertrichiasis, blurred vision, keratitis, CME, anterior uveitis, conjunctival hyperemia	Flulike symptoms, joint/muscle pain, headache	± IOP lowering effect with miotic Peak: 10–14 hours Washout: 4–6 weeks
Travoprost	Travatan	.004%	qd	Same as above	25%–32%	Same as above	Same as above	Same as above
Prostamides								
Bimatoprost	Lumigan	0.03%	qd	Increase uveoscleral and trabecular outflow	27%–33%	Same as above	Same as above	Same as above

(Continues)

* *Also has indirect actions*

Table 7-1 **Glaucoma Medications (Continued)**

Class/Compound	Brand Name	Strengths	Dosage	Method of Action	IOP Decrease	Side Effects: Ocular	Side Effects: Systemic	Comments, Including Time to Peak Effect and Washout
Decosanoids								
Unoprostone isopropyl	Rescula	0.15%	bid	Increase trabecular outflow	13%–18%	Same as above	Same as above	Peak: unknown Washout: unknown
Hyperosmotic agents								
Mannitol (parenteral)	Osmitrol	20%, 50% soln	2 g/kg body wt	Osmotic gradient dehydrates vitreous		IOP rebound, increased aqueous flare	Urinary retention, headache, congestive heart failure, expansion of blood volume, diabetic complications, nausea, vomiting, diarrhea, electrolyte disturbance, renal failure	Caution in heart failure; may precipitate diabetic ketoacidosis; useful in acute increased IOP; isosorbide less nausea, vomiting
Glycerin (oral)	Osmoglyn	50% soln	4–7 oz	Same as above		Similar to above	Can cause problems in diabetic patients; similar to above	
Fixed combinations								
Timolol/ Dorzolamide	Cosopt (Timoptic/ Trusopt)	0.5%/2%	bid	Decrease aqueous production	25%–30%	Same as nonselective oral beta blocker, topical CAI	Same as nonselective oral beta blocker, topical CAI	Peak: 2–3 hours Washout: 1 month

nonselective adrenergic agonists are only slightly additive, whereas more effect can be expected when beta blockers are combined with an alpha$_2$-adrenergic agonist. The magnitude of additional IOP lowering with hypotensive lipids remains indeterminate. Approximately 10%–20% of the patients treated with topical beta blockers fail to respond with significant lowering of the IOP. It should be noted that if a patient is on systemic beta-blocker therapy, then the addition of a topical beta blocker may be significantly less effective. Extended use of beta blockers may reduce their effectiveness, as the response of beta receptors is affected by constant exposure to an agonist (long-term drift, tachyphylaxis). Similarly, receptor saturation (drug-induced upregulation of beta receptors) may occur within a few weeks, with loss of effectiveness (short-term escape).

Six topical beta-adrenergic antagonists are approved for use for the treatment of glaucoma in the United States: betaxolol, carteolol, levobunolol, metipranolol, timolol maleate, and timolol hemihydrate. All except betaxolol are nonselective beta$_1$ and beta$_2$ antagonists. Beta$_1$ activity is largely cardiac and beta$_2$ activity is largely pulmonary. Because betaxolol is a selective beta$_1$ antagonist, it is safer than the nonselective beta blockers for use in patients with pulmonary, CNS, or other systemic conditions, but beta-blocker–related side effects can still occur. The IOP-lowering effect of betaxolol is less than that of the nonselective beta-adrenergic antagonists.

Carteolol demonstrates intrinsic sympathomimetic activity, which means that, while acting as a competitive antagonist, it also causes a slight to moderate activation of receptors. Thus, even though carteolol produces beta-blocking effects, these may be tempered, reducing the effect on cardiovascular and respiratory systems.

Both ocular and systemic side effects of beta-adrenergic antagonists are listed in Table 7-1. They include bronchospasm, bradycardia, increased heart block, lowered blood pressure, reduced exercise tolerance, and CNS depression. Patients with diabetes may experience reduced glucose tolerance and masking of hypoglycemic signs and symptoms. Abrupt withdrawal of ocular beta blockers can exacerbate symptoms of hyperthyroidism. Although betaxolol is somewhat less effective than the other beta-adrenergic antagonists in lowering IOP, it may be a safer alternative in some patients.

Before prescribing a beta-blocking agent, it is important to determine if the patient has ever had asthma, because beta blockers may induce severe bronchospasm in susceptible patients. The pulse should be measured and the beta blocker withheld if the pulse rate is slow or if more than first-degree heart block is present. Myasthenia gravis may be aggravated by these drugs. The use of a gel vehicle has been shown to decrease the plasma concentration of beta blockers compared to the solution modalities.

Other side effects of beta blockers include lethargy, mood changes, depression, altered mentation, light-headedness, syncope, visual disturbance, corneal anesthesia, punctate keratitis, impotence, reduced libido, allergy, and alteration of serum lipids. Beta blockers should be used with caution in children due to the relatively high systemic levels achieved. Although topical beta blockers have been shown to decrease HDL and increase cholesterol levels, there is no evidence that this translates into an actual increase in cardiovascular risk. However, this effect on the plasma lipid profile should be considered, particularly in those patients taking medications that affect plasma lipids.

The use of nasolacrimal occlusion or eyelid closure decreases systemic absorption and increases intraocular penetration of medications; the procedure is particularly important with the use of beta blockers. It may also facilitate a time interval between the instillation of different medications by patients using multiple medications.

Many of the beta blockers are available as generic agents. Although these may be less expensive, it is important to realize that in most cases few data are available to prove or disprove equivalent efficacy or similar side effect profiles between branded and generic medications. In addition, because multiple generics are available for a given agent, the possibility that differences exist among generic agents could affect patient care.

Novack GD. Ophthalmic beta blockers since timolol. *Surv Ophthalmol.* 1987;31:307–327.

Van Buskirk, EM. Adverse reactions from timolol administration. *Ophthalmology.* 1980;87: 447–450.

Parasympathomimetic Agents

Parasympathomimetic agents, commonly called miotics, have been used in the treatment of glaucoma for more than 100 years. They are divided into 2 groups:

- direct-acting cholinergic agonists
- indirect-acting anticholinesterase agents

Direct-acting agents affect the motor endplates in the same way as acetylcholine, which is transmitted at postganglionic parasympathetic junctions, as well as at other autonomic, somatic, and central synapses. Indirect-acting agents inhibit the enzyme acetylcholinesterase, thereby prolonging and enhancing the action of naturally secreted acetylcholine. *Pilocarpine* is the most commonly prescribed direct-acting agent. *Carbachol* has both direct and indirect actions, although its primary mechanism is direct. The only indirect-acting agent still available is *echothiophate iodide* (see Table 7-1), although the availability is limited.

Both direct- and indirect-acting agents reduce IOP by causing contraction of the longitudinal ciliary muscle, which pulls the scleral spur to tighten the trabecular meshwork, increasing the outflow of aqueous humor. These agents can reduce the IOP by 15%–25%. The currently accepted indications for miotic therapy include chronic treatment of increased IOP in patients with some filtering angle open and prophylaxis for angle-closure glaucoma prior to iridectomy.

The parasympathomimetic agents have been shown to reduce uveoscleral outflow in animals, and it is possible that this action may actually worsen the glaucoma if miotics are used in patients with little to no trabecular outflow, although the effects on the uveoscleral outflow system in humans remain speculative. In addition, these agents cause the pupillary sphincter to contract (hence their common name, *miotics*), stimulate secretory activity in the lacrimal and salivary glands, and disrupt the blood-aqueous barrier. These actions have little bearing on the IOP-lowering effect, except in angle-closure glaucoma, where the mechanical action of the contracting pupillary sphincter may pull the iris away from the trabecular meshwork, and in pigment dispersion syndrome, where the peripheral iris configuration is altered.

Miotic agents have been associated with retinal detachment in some patients; use of stronger direct-acting miotics as opposed to weaker miotic agents leads to increased risk. A peripheral retina evaluation is suggested prior to the initiation of miotic therapy. If possible, an alternate medication may be considered in patients with peripheral retinal disease that predisposes them to retinal detachment. In view of the plethora of other ocular hypotensive agents now available, miotic therapy has become less commonly employed in general.

Induced myopia resulting from ciliary muscle contraction is a side effect common to all cholinergic agents. The short-acting drugs may produce varying refractive changes, especially in young patients. Brow ache may accompany the ciliary spasm, and the miosis interferes with vision in dim light and in patients with lens opacities. Starting with a weak concentration and gradually increasing the dose to optimal therapeutic benefit will decrease these side effects.

Pilocarpine adsorbed to a polymer gel is administered once daily at bedtime (pilocarpine gel). Although the IOP-lowering effect may last 24 hours in some patients, other individuals show loss of drug effect after 18–20 hours. Induced myopia and miosis are less prominent with the gel than with drops, but they may still interfere with vision. The miosis may be visually disabling in patients with a central lens opacity such as a posterior subcapsular cataract. If the gel has not dissipated by morning, the patient may have blurred vision on awakening. Pilocarpine gel may be useful in some younger patients, in patients bothered by variable myopia or intense miosis, in older patients with lens opacities, and in patients who have difficulty complying with more frequent dosing regimens.

Indirect-acting miotics or the stronger direct-acting agents may induce a paradoxical angle closure, because contraction of the ciliary muscle leads to forward movement of the lens–iris diaphragm, an increase in the anteroposterior diameter of the lens, and a very miotic pupil. These effects may increase pupillary block.

The indirect-acting miotics are cataractogenic, and evidence suggests that the direct-acting agents may also be weakly cataractogenic. In adults, indirect-acting miotics may induce generalized cataract formation in addition to anterior subcapsular opacity. In children, they may also induce the formation of iris pigment epithelial cysts. The strong miotics may cause epiphora by both direct lacrimal stimulation and punctal stenosis. These agents may also cause ocular surface changes resulting in drug-induced pseudopemphigoid.

Reports of increased inflammation following surgery associated with the use of stronger miotics suggest that these agents should be discontinued prior to surgery. In addition, the anticholinesterase agents should be discontinued and other agents substituted at least 2–4 weeks prior to ocular surgery, because they cause increased bleeding during surgery and severe fibrinous iridocyclitis postoperatively. Because miotics can break down the blood–aqueous barrier, their use in treating uveitic glaucoma should be limited.

Although direct-acting miotics rarely induce systemic side effects, indirect-acting medications may be responsible for systemic parasympathetic stimulation. Diarrhea, abdominal cramps, increased salivation, bronchospasm, and even enuresis may result. Pseudocholinesterase activity in the red blood cells is depressed for 6 weeks after cessation of eyedrops. Because cholinesterase is suppressed throughout the body, depolarizing agents such as succinylcholine should be avoided while the patient is using these eyedrops and for 6 weeks after discontinuation.

Although this class of agents effectively lowers IOP, it is often so poorly tolerated due to ocular side effects, including miosis and induced myopia, that other classes of agents are often preferred. In addition, particularly the weaker miotics require frequent instillation, 3 or 4 times daily, further limiting their usefulness. However, pilocarpine is among the most affordable of agents, and the miotics are much better tolerated in eyes that are not phakic. Because of the potential for significant ocular and systemic side effects, indirect-acting parasympathomimetic agents are used less commonly than the direct-acting agents. Indeed, indirect-acting agents are usually reserved for treatment of glaucoma in aphakic and pseudophakic eyes when IOP is not controlled by less toxic agents and in phakic eyes when filtering surgery has failed.

Hoskins HD, Jr, Kass MA. Cholinergic drugs. In: Hoskins HD Jr, Kass MA, eds. *Becker-Shaffer's Diagnosis and Therapy of the Glaucomas.* 6th ed. St. Louis: Mosby; 1989:420–434.

Sherwood MB, Grierson I, Millar L, et al. Long-term morphologic effects of antiglaucoma drugs on the conjunctiva and Tenon's capsule in glaucoma patients. *Ophthalmology.* 1989;96:327–335.

Carbonic Anhydrase Inhibitors

CAIs decrease aqueous humor formation by direct antagonist activity on ciliary epithelial carbonic anhydrase and perhaps, to a lesser extent only with systemic administration, by producing a generalized acidosis. The enzyme carbonic anhydrase is also present in many other tissues, including corneal endothelium, iris, retinal pigment epithelium, red blood cells, brain, and kidney. Over 90% of the ciliary epithelial enzyme activity must be abolished to decrease aqueous production and lower IOP.

The systemic agents are most useful in acute situations (eg, acute angle-closure glaucoma). They can be given orally, intramuscularly, and intravenously. Because of the side effects of systemic CAIs, however, chronic therapy with these agents should be reserved for patients whose glaucoma cannot be controlled by alternative topical therapy.

Systemic acetazolamide and methazolamide are the oral CAI agents most commonly used; another agent in this group is dichlorphenamide (see Table 7-1). Methazolamide has a longer duration of action and is less bound to serum protein than acetazolamide. Methazolamide and sustained-release acetazolamide are the best tolerated of the systemic CAIs. Methazolamide is metabolized by the liver, thereby decreasing some of the risk of systemic side effects. Acetazolamide is not metabolized and is excreted in urine.

Side effects of systemic CAI therapy are usually dose-related. Many patients develop paresthesias of the fingers or toes and complain of lassitude, loss of energy, and anorexia. Weight loss is common. Abdominal discomfort, diarrhea, loss of libido, impotence, and an unpleasant taste in the mouth, as well as severe mental depression, may also occur. There is an increased risk of the formation of calcium oxylate and calcium phosphate renal stones. Because methazolamide has greater hepatic metabolism and causes less acidosis, it may be less likely to cause renal lithiasis than acetazolamide.

CAIs are chemically derived from sulfa drugs, and this may cause similar allergic reactions and cross reactivity. Aplastic anemia is a rare but potentially fatal idiosyncratic reaction to CAIs. Thrombocytopenia and agranulocytosis can also occur. Although routine complete blood counts have been suggested, they are not predictive of this idiosyncratic reaction and are not routinely recommended. Hypokalemia is a potentially serious complication that is especially likely when oral CAIs are used concurrently with another drug that causes potassium loss (eg, a thiazide diuretic). Serum potassium should be monitored regularly in such patients.

Oral CAIs are potent medications with significant side effects. Therefore, the lowest dose that reduces the IOP to an acceptable range should be used. Methazolamide is often effective in doses as low as 25–50 mg given 2 to 3 times daily. Acetazolamide may be started at 62.5 mg every 6 hours, and higher doses may be used, if tolerated. Sustained-release formulations such as Diamox Sequels may have fewer side effects.

Topical CAI agents are also available for chronic treatment of IOP elevation. Dorzolamide and brinzolamide are sulfonamide derivatives that reduce aqueous formation by direct inhibition of carbonic anhydrase in the ciliary body with fewer systemic side effects than the oral agents. Dorzolamide and brinzolamide are currently available for use 3 times daily, although reduction of IOP is only slightly greater when compared to twice-daily therapy. Both agents are equally efficacious and reduce IOP (monotherapy) by 14%–17%, not as great a reduction as the oral CAIs. For patients on an adequate oral CAI dose, there is no advantage to also using a topical CAI.

Common adverse effects of topical CAIs include bitter taste, blurred vision, and punctate keratopathy. Ocular surface irritation with dorzolamide may be a result of the drug's relative greater acidity (lower pH) when compared with that of brinzolamide. Eyes with compromised endothelial cell function may also be at risk for corneal decompensation. The brinzolamide suspension may cause more blurring than the dorzolamide solution. Systemic lassitude is a side effect as well.

Fraunfelder FT, Fraunfelder FW, eds. *Drug-Induced Ocular Side Effects.* Boston: Butterworth-Heinemann; 2001.

Strahlman E, Tipping R, Vogel R. A double-masked, randomized 1-year study comparing dorzolamide (Trusopt), timolol, and betaxolol. International Dorzolamide Study Group. *Arch Ophthalmol.* 1995;113:1009–1016.

Adrenergic Agonists

The nonselective adrenergic agonists epinephrine and dipivefrin increase conventional trabecular and uveoscleral outflow. The latter appears to be influenced by epinephrine-induced stimulation of prostaglandin synthesis. Interestingly, epinephrine-related agents may initially increase aqueous production; with chronic use, however, they decrease it. Adding nonselective adrenergic agonists to beta antagonists usually produces modest additional pressure lowering.

Epinephrine, a mixed alpha and beta agonist, and related compounds have a lesser hypotensive effect in eyes with dark irides. The IOP-lowering effect begins at 1 hour and is maximal at 2–6 hours. Individual responses to epinephrine used as a single drug therapy may vary from a 10% to a 20% decrease in IOP. Tolerance, or *tachyphylaxis*, is common with long-term use, although in some individuals, epinephrine may become more effective over time. In addition, many patients become intolerant due to extraocular reactions.

Dipivefrin is a *pro-drug* that is chemically transformed into epinephrine by esterase enzymes in the cornea. Dipivefrin has greater corneal penetration than epinephrine salt, and the activity of this drug prior to its alteration by the esterase enzymes is relatively low. These qualities give it 2 major advantages over epinephrine salt:

- A lower topical concentration of dipivefrin has an intraocular effect similar to a higher dosage of epinephrine salt.
- Therapeutic effectiveness in the eye can be achieved with fewer topical and systemic side effects.

Table 7-1 lists potential ocular and systemic side effects of both epinephrine and dipivefrin. Important systemic side effects include headache, increased blood pressure, tachycardia, arrhythmia, and nervousness. Epinephrine causes adrenochrome deposits from oxidized metabolites in the conjunctiva, cornea, and lacrimal system, and it may stain soft contact lenses (Fig 7-1). The use of these agents often causes pupillary dilation as a consequence of alpha-agonist action that stimulates norepinephrine receptors, and thus may precipitate or aggravate angle closure in susceptible individuals. Allergic blepharoconjunctivitis occurs in approximately 20% of patients over time. Cystoid macular edema may be precipitated or exacerbated in aphakic and pseudophakic eyes without intact posterior capsules. This maculopathy is usually reversible if recognized early; however, epinephrine or dipivefrin should be used with caution in these eyes. Rebound conjunctiva hyperemia is common when these drugs are discontinued. Although this condition is harmless, patients may be disturbed by the appearance and usually need reassurance. Clinically, the nonselective adrenergic agents have been essentially completely replaced with the selective alpha$_2$-adrenergic agonists due to the improved efficacy and side effect profiles.

Alpha$_2$-adrenergic agonists

Ocular alpha$_1$ effects include vasoconstriction, pupillary dilation, and eyelid retraction, whereas ocular alpha$_2$ effects are primarily IOP reduction and possible neuroprotection. Apraclonidine and brimonidine are relatively selective alpha$_2$ agonists that have been developed for glaucoma therapy. Brimonidine is much more highly selective for the alpha$_2$ receptor than apraclonidine.

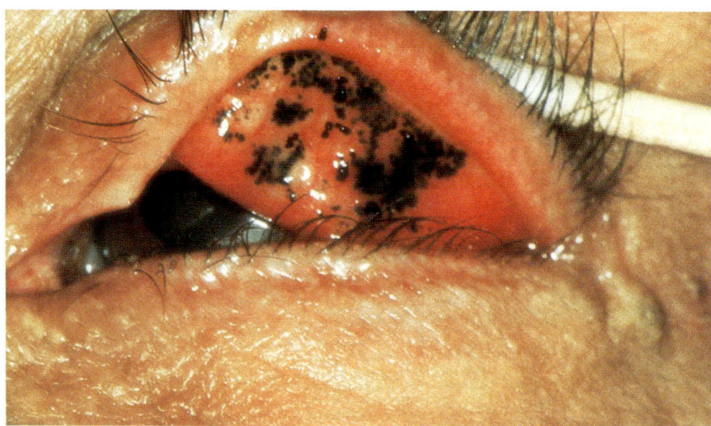

Figure 7-1 Conjunctiva with adrenochrome deposits following chronic epinephrine use. *(Photograph courtesy of Elizabeth A. Hodapp, MD.)*

Apraclonidine hydrochloride (para-aminoclonidine) is an alpha$_2$-adrenergic agonist and a clonidine derivative that prevents release of norepinephrine at nerve terminals. It decreases aqueous production as well as episcleral venous pressure and improves trabecular outflow. However, its true ocular hypotensive mechanism is not fully understood. When administered pre- and postoperatively, the drug is effective in diminishing the acute IOP rise that follows argon laser iridectomy, argon laser trabeculoplasty, Nd:YAG laser capsulotomy, and cataract extraction. Apraclonidine hydrochloride may be effective for the short-term lowering of IOP, but development of topical sensitivity and tachyphylaxis often limits long-term use.

Use of brimonidine tartrate encounters less tachyphylaxis than apraclonidine, and allergenicity such as follicular conjunctivitis and contact blepharitis-dermatitis is also lower (up to 40% for apraclonidine, less than 15% for brimonidine 0.2%, and less than 10% for brimonidine-Purite 0.15%). Brimonidine-Purite 0.15% has been shown to be as efficacious as brimonidine 0.2% but with a lower incidence of all side effects. It contains a lower concentration without benzalkonium chloride as the preservative at a neutral pH. Cross sensitivity to brimonidine in patients with known hypersensitivity to apraclonidine is minimal. Systemic side effects include dry mouth and lethargy. The use of brimonidine in infants and young children should be avoided due to an increased risk of somnolence, hypotension, seizures, apnea, and serious derangements of neurotransmitters in the CNS, presumably due to increased CNS penetration of the drug. Brimonidine lowers IOP by decreasing aqueous production and increasing uveoscleral outflow. As with beta blockers, a peripheral mechanism may account for part of the IOP reduction from brimonidine 0.2%, as a 1-week, single-eye treatment trial caused a statistically significant reduction of 1.2 mm Hg in the fellow eye.

Brimonidine's peak IOP reduction is approximately 26% (2 hours postdose). At peak, it is comparable to a nonselective beta blocker and superior to the selective beta blocker betaxolol, although at trough (12 hours postdose), the reduction is only 14%–15%, or less effective than the nonselective beta blockers but comparable to betaxolol during the first 6–12 months of therapy. Although approved for therapy 3 times daily, brimonidine is commonly used twice daily, particularly when used as an adjunctive agent.

Caution is recommended when using either apraclonidine or brimonidine in patients on a monoamine oxidase inhibitor (MAOI) or tricyclic antidepressant therapy. Apraclonidine has a much greater affinity for alpha$_1$ receptors than does brimonidine and is therefore more likely to produce vasoconstriction in the eye.

Robin AL. Argon laser trabeculoplasty medical therapy to prevent the intraocular pressure rise associated with argon laser trabeculoplasty. *Ophthalmic Surg.* 1991;22:31–37.

Schuman JS, Horwitz B, Choplin NT, et al. A 1-year study of brimonidine twice daily in glaucoma and ocular hypertension: a controlled, randomized, multicenter clinical trial. *Arch Ophthalmol.* 1997;115:847–852.

Hypotensive Lipids (Prostaglandin Analogs, Prostamide, Decosanoid)

Hypotensive lipids are a relatively new class of ocular hypotensive agents. Currently, 4 hypotensive lipids have been approved for clinical use. Two are prostaglandin analogs: travoprost and latanoprost. Latanoprost has the most extensive clinical experience and is approved for initial therapy for glaucoma. Two other hypotensive lipids, bimatoprost (prostamide) and unoprostone isopropyl (decosanoid) are also available. Unlike latanoprost and travoprost, which lower IOP by increasing uveoscleral outflow by 50%, bimatoprost decreases IOP by increasing uveoscleral outflow by 50% and increasing trabecular outflow by 25%–30%. All of these drugs work by increasing aqueous outflow. All have a component of pressure-independent outflow (usually thought of as uveoscleral outflow). The effects of these drugs on pressure-dependent outflow (usually thought of as trabecular outflow) is controversial, with some studies demonstrating an effect (bimatoprost and latanoprost) and others showing no effect (latanoprost and travoprost). The exact mechanism by which these drugs increase outflow is not known; however, it has been shown that latanoprost results in increased spaces between the muscle fascicles within the ciliary body, presumably increasing aqueous flow and uveoscleral outflow.

Latanoprost and travoprost are pro-drugs that penetrate the cornea and become biologically active after being hydrolyzed by corneal esterase. Both latanoprost and travoprost reduce IOP by 25%–32%. Bimatoprost lowers IOP by 27%–33%; unoprostone is less effective, lowering IOP 13%–18%. Latanoprost, travoprost, and bimatoprost are used once a day, usually at night, and are less effective when used twice daily; unoprostone is used twice daily.

An ocular side effect unique to this class of drugs is the darkening of the iris and periocular skin as a result of increased numbers of melanosomes (increased melanin content—melanogenesis) within the melanocytes. The risk of iris pigmentation is permanent and correlates with baseline iris pigmentation. Blue irides may experience increased pigmentation in 10%–20% of eyes in the initial 18–24 months of therapy, whereas nearly 60% of eyes that are light brown, blue-green, or two-toned may experience increased pigmentation over the same time period. The long-term sequelae of this side effect is unknown, but there are no data to suggest any additional risk. Other side effects reported in association with the use of a topical hypotensive lipid include conjunctival hyperemia, hypertrichosis, trichiasis, distichiasis, hyperpigmentation of the eyelid skin, and hair growth around the eyes. These effects appear to be reversible with drug discontinuation. Exacerbations of underlying herpes keratitis, cystoid macular edema, and uveitis have been reported. The latter 2 side effects are more common in eyes with preexisting risk factors for either macular edema or uveitis. Studies to date have demonstrated that the incidence of these side effects varies among these 4 agents. Hyperemia is more common with bimatoprost and travoprost, whereas the incidence of the other side effects among the 4 drugs, if present, has not been definitively demonstrated. Because bimatoprost, latanoprost, and travoprost reach peak effectiveness 10–14 hours after administration, bedtime application is recommended to maximize efficacy and decrease patient symptoms related to vascular dilation.

Camras CB, Alm A, Watson P, et al. Latanoprost, a prostaglandin analog, for glaucoma therapy: efficacy and safety after 1 year of treatment in 198 patients. Latanoprost Study Group. *Ophthalmology.* 1996;103:1916–1924.

Higgingotham EJ, Schuman JS, Goldberg I, et al. One-year, randomized study comparing bimatoprost and timolol in glaucoma and ocular hypertension. *Arch Ophthalmol.* 2002;120:1286–1293.

Netland PA, Landry T, Sullivan EK, et al. Travoprost compared with latanoprost and timolol in patients with open-angle glaucoma or ocular hypertension. *Am J Ophthalmol.* 2001;132:472–484.

Combined Medications

Medications that are combined and placed in a single bottle have the potential benefits of improved efficacy, convenience, and compliance, as well as reduced cost. Adrenergic agonists and parasympathomimetic agents (epinephrine and pilocarpine) have been available for many years as a combined agent. They are weakly additive in IOP-lowering effect, thus satisfying FDA guidelines that the fixed combination be more efficacious than either agent given alone

Cosopt, the fixed combination of a beta blocker (timolol maleate 0.5%) and topical carbonic anhydrase inhibitor (dorzolamide 2%), demonstrates similar efficacy compared with the 2 agents given separately: timolol maleate 0.5% twice daily and Trusopt 2% given 3 times daily. The advantage of this combined therapy may be the convenience and lessened confusion of 1 bottle rather than 2, which may increase the likelihood of greater compliance. However, the twice-daily dosing may create greater exposure to the potential beta-blocker systemic side effects, as beta blockers alone are generally equally effective when given only once daily. The ocular side effects are the same as for both drugs individually. The indications for this combined medication may be as a substitute for both a beta blocker and topical carbonic anhydrase inhibitor. If Cosopt is used as monotherapy, a monocular trial of timolol should be tried first. If timolol is effective in significantly, but not sufficiently, lowering the IOP, then a monocular trial of dorzolamide should be used with timolol. An alternative trial could involve Cosopt in 1 eye twice daily and timolol in the opposite eye. It is important to prove that both the timolol component and the dorzolamide component each have an effect on IOP before choosing the combined medication, except in emergent situations.

Strohmaier K, Snyder E, DuBiner H, et al. The efficacy and safety of the dorzolamide-timolol combination versus the concomitant administration of its components. Dorzolamide-Timolol Study Group. *Ophthalmology.* 1998;105:1936–1944.

Hyperosmotic Agents

Hyperosmotic agents are used to control acute episodes of elevated IOP. Common hyperosmotic agents include oral glycerin and intravenous mannitol.

When given systemically, hyperosmotic agents lower the IOP by increasing the blood osmolality, which creates an osmotic gradient between the blood and the vitreous humor, drawing water from the vitreous cavity and reducing IOP. The larger the dose and the more rapid the administration, the greater the reduction in IOP because of the increased gradient. The substance distributed only in extracellular water (eg, mannitol) is more effective than a drug distributed in total body water (eg, urea). When the blood–aqueous barrier is disrupted, the osmotic agent enters the eye faster than when the barrier is intact, thus reducing both the effectiveness of the drug and its duration of action.

Hyperosmotic agents are rarely administered for longer than a few hours because their effects are transient as a result of the rapid reequilibration of the osmotic gradient.

They become less effective over time, and a rebound elevation in IOP may occur if the agent penetrates the eye and reverses the osmotic gradient.

Side effects of these drugs include headache, mental confusion, backache, and acute congestive heart failure and myocardial infarction. The rapid increase in extracellular volume and cardiac preload caused by hyperosmotic agents may precipitate or aggravate congestive heart failure. Intravenous administration is more likely than oral dosage to cause this problem. In addition, subdural and subarachnoid hemorrhages have been reported after treatment with hyperosmotic agents. Glycerin can produce hyperglycemia or even ketoacidosis in patients with diabetes, because it is metabolized into sugar and ketone bodies. Hypoglycemic agents, as well as oral CAIs, are contraindicated in patients in renal failure or on dialysis.

General Approach to Medical Treatment

Open-Angle Glaucoma

The clinician should tailor therapy for open-angle glaucoma to the individual needs of the patient. As noted previously, a target IOP range is established as a goal. However, the effectiveness of therapy can only be established by careful repeated scrutiny of the patient's optic nerve and visual field status.

Characteristics of the medical agents available for the treatment of glaucoma are summarized in Table 7-1. The clinician making management decisions should keep efficacy and compliance in mind. Treatment is usually initiated with a single topical medication, unless the starting IOP is extremely high, in which case 2 or more medications may be indicated. The selection of the agent for initial medical therapy should be individualized based on the efficacy, safety, and tolerability of the drug and the patient's status and needs. A brief discussion of treatment options with the patient can be effective in determining the optimal choice. Hypotensive lipids, beta blockers, $alpha_2$ agonists, and topical CAIs are all reasonable choices for first-line therapy. The once-daily lipids are the most effective agents to lower IOP and have the best systemic safety profile. Thus, they are commonly the first class of medications used in most patients. Beta blockers are the best tolerated in and about the eye. Because of the variability of IOP, it is best (unless the IOP is extremely high) to test the medication in 1 eye until the effectiveness of therapy has been established. At that point, both eyes can be treated.

Patients should be taught how to space their medications, and instructional charts should be given. It may be useful to coordinate the administration of medication with a part of the daily routine such as meals. Patients should be shown how to administer eyedrops properly. Eyedrops to be given at the same time should be separated by at least 5 minutes to prevent washout of the first by the second. Instructions on nasolacrimal occlusion or gentle eyelid closure to reduce the systemic effects from topical eye medications should be given. Teaching the patient to close the eyes for 1 full minute after instillation of the drop helps promote corneal penetration and reduce systemic absorption. An assistive drop device may be considered, especially for patients who live alone or are unable to successfully instill drops.

If one drug is not adequate to reduce IOP to the estimated desired safe level, the initial agent may be discontinued and another agent tried, preferably as a therapeutic trial in 1 eye. If no single agent controls the pressure, a combination of topical agents should be used. Again, individualizing the choice of agent is helpful in selecting the next best choice. These choices include miotic therapy in nonphakic patients, and, rarely, systemic CAIs may be used for short periods of time when the clinical situation warrants the risk of side effects. Clearly, when the individual requires 3 or more medications, compliance becomes more difficult and the potential for local ocular and systemic side effects increases.

Patients who are intolerant of multiple topical glaucoma agents secondary to local ocular side effects may be experiencing reactions to the preservatives. Benzalkonium chloride is the most commonly used agent and is present in nearly all available topical ophthalmic drops. If this is suspected, alternatives include preservative-free timolol maleate (unit dose) and brimonidine 0.15% with Purite (an alternative preservative). If the level of glaucoma damage permits, it may be beneficial, for rehabilitating the ocular surface, to stop all topical medications and use nonpreserved artificial tears frequently. The temporary use of oral CAIs may be useful to lower IOP during this period, if clinically warranted.

Patients rarely associate systemic side effects with topical drugs and, consequently, seldom volunteer symptoms. The ophthalmologist must inquire about these symptoms. Communication with the primary care physician is important not only to let the family doctor know the potential side effects of antiglaucoma medication but also to discuss the interactions of any other systemic medications with the glaucoma process. Modification of systemic beta blocker therapy for hypertension, for example, may affect glaucoma control. Physicians should be aware that compliance may decline as the complexity and expense of the medical regimen increase.

Patients with open-angle glaucoma require careful monitoring. IOP, although important, is only one of the factors to monitor, and optic nerve photographs or drawings and visual fields must be compared periodically to determine the stability of the disease (see Chapter 3). The condition of the patient and the severity of the disease determine how often each of these parameters must be checked. If the cupping or visual field damage shows evidence of progression despite apparent control of acceptable IOP, other diseases should be considered (see the discussion of normal-tension glaucoma in Chapter 4). Other possible explanations include an IOP level too high for the particular patient's optic nerve, IOP that may be spiking at times when the patient is not in the office, thin central corneal thickness, sleep apnea, concomitant angle closure, and poor patient compliance.

Angle-Closure Glaucoma

Medical treatment for acute angle-closure glaucoma is aimed at preparing the patient for laser iridectomy. The goals of medical treatment are to reduce IOP rapidly to prevent further damage to the optic nerve, to clear the cornea, to reduce intraocular inflammation, to allow pupillary constriction, and to prevent formation of posterior and peripheral anterior synechiae (see Chapter 5). Treatment of chronic angle closure is the same as that for POAG, although miotics play a greater role; however, miotics may induce a paradoxical increase in IOP if the angle is closed and the trabecular meshwork is nonfunctional.

Use of Glaucoma Medications During Pregnancy or by Nursing Mothers

Unfortunately, there is little definitive information concerning the use of glaucoma medications in pregnant women or nursing mothers. The FDA has designated brimonidine as a class B agent; all other agents are class C. The CAIs have been shown to be teratogenic in rodents, and prostaglandins increase uterine contractility. Thus, although human information is lacking, CAIs should not be used by women in their child-bearing years or by those who are pregnant. Beta blockers are concentrated fivefold in breast milk. Because of the effects on infants, beta blockers, as well as brimonidine, should be avoided in nursing mothers. In general, it is prudent to minimize the use of medications in these patients whenever possible.

Compliance

Prescribing medications for patients does no good if they do not use them. The first step in improving compliance is to educate patients. The patient who understands the importance and benefits of treatment is more likely to comply. Education also includes a discussion of treatment alternatives such that the patient can participate in the selection of specific therapies. When patients are aware of the possible side effects, compliance is enhanced. It is also vital to teach patients how to instill medications and confirm that they or someone else will be successful in instilling drops. The next step in enhancing compliance is to design the treatment regimen so that it is as simple as possible. The fewest number of medications, instilled with the least frequency is optimal. When multiple drugs and doses are needed, make sure the patient understands the regimen and coordinate the schedule to daily events. A written schedule is very helpful.

Future Therapy

(This section contributed by John R. Samples, MD.)

Genetic therapy for ocular disease has already been successfully applied to the murine retinal degeneration model of retinitis pigmentosa. The genetic approaches for treating trabecular cells are limited because trabecular cell division is slow. This makes infecting the meshwork cells with retrovirus unlikely to be effective because retrovirus requires actively replicating cells for infection. Herpesvirus, which can transfect neurons, may be useful for directly treating the retina and optic nerve. Adenovirus is advantageous because it does not require cell mitosis and can deliver reporter genes to the trabecular meshwork. In fact, the high uptake of the virus by the trabecular meshwork cells, possibly aided by their high phagocytic capacity, indicates that this tissue may be one of the easiest targets for this form of gene delivery. Although viral vector therapy has much potential, it has not yet been done in humans due to concern that the viruses may have dangerous side effects, such as insertional mutagenesis. This has had the effect of making nonvector therapies more attractive. Nonvector therapies have more potential and versatility and are more likely to be readily accepted. They can replace defective genes, inhibit transcription, correct mutant RNA, and directly replace needed protein. In this regard, cationic liposomes are an attractive alternative to viral transfer because they have lower immunogenicity and no DNA size constraints. However, the liposome transfection efficiency of nondividing cells is very low. Targeting liposomes with directive antibodies or binding proteins specific for the surface of the trabecular cells may overcome this disadvantage.

Human artificial chromosomes (HACs) present another intriguing possibility because cell replication is not required. Given that both the gene and its regulation sequence are inserted, the gene is turned off and on appropriately. Once in the nucleus, the artificial chromosome is replicated along with the host chromosomes, providing a permanent, 1-time therapy.

Ribozymes are RNA molecules with enzymatic activity. They bind to a specific RNA sequence and cleave it at a unique site, thereby replacing the mutant with normal mRNA and restoring the wild-type gene production. Ribozymes and antisense oligonucleotides are both potential treatments for *GLC1A* through *GLC1F* because all of these open-angle glaucoma loci demonstrate autosomal dominant inheritance. Antisense therapy involves using either vectors or liposomes to add a complementary sequence of RNA or DNA to the cytoplasm. This sequence binds to the mutant mRNA, targets it for rapid destruction by nucleases, and blocks production of the abnormal protein. Antisense oligonucleotides express both the normal and the mutant copy of the gene. If some form of POAG is shown to result from similar dominant negative interactions, antisense therapy is probably the simplest and most effective method for inhibiting synthesis of the resulting mutant peptide. Ultimately, the effectiveness of antisense therapy relies on the molecular biology of the defective molecule.

CHAPTER 8

Surgical Therapy for Glaucoma

Surgical therapy for glaucoma is usually undertaken when medical therapy is not appropriate, not tolerated, not effective, or not properly utilized by a particular patient, and the glaucoma remains uncontrolled with either documented progressive damage or a very high risk of further damage. Surgery is usually the primary approach for infantile and pupillary-block glaucoma. In patients with primary open angle glaucoma (POAG), surgery has traditionally been considered when medical therapy has failed. Caution is especially important because of the potential side effects of surgery, including bleb-associated problems, cataracts, and infection. Early studies of trabeculectomy as initial therapy for glaucoma, which were performed before the introduction of some contemporary antiglaucoma medications, suggested that trabeculectomy might offer some advantages—reduction of patient visits to the doctor and possibly better visual field preservation, for example. The results of the Collaborative Initial Glaucoma Treatment Study (CIGTS), however, showed that both initial medical or initial surgical therapy result in similar visual field outcome after 5 years of follow-up. In both groups, there was a low incidence of visual field progression. Based on this study and current practice, most clinicians defer incisional surgery until after an attempt is made to treat with medical therapy.

Lichter PR, Musch DC, Gillespie BW, et al. Interim clinical outcomes in the Collaborative Initial Glaucoma Treatment Study comparing initial treatment randomized to medications or surgery. *Ophthalmology.* 2001;108:1943–1953.

Migdal C, Gregory W, Hitchings R. Long-term functional outcome after early surgery compared with laser and medicine in open-angle glaucoma. *Ophthalmology.* 1994;101:1651–1657.

When surgery is indicated, the clinical setting must guide the selection of the appropriate procedure. Each of the many possible procedures is appropriate in specific conditions and clinical situations. Many different glaucoma surgical procedures are performed to lower IOP. Among these are trabeculectomy and its variations, nonpenetrating filtration procedures, glaucoma drainage tube implants, angle surgery for congenital and angle-closure glaucoma, and ciliary body ablation. Other procedures, such as iridectomy and gonioplasty, address the problems of aqueous access to the angle. For each condition, it is necessary to understand the indications, contraindications, and preoperative evaluation necessary for surgical planning. Understanding the pathophysiology of the disease, as discussed throughout this volume, is essential to generating an appropriate surgical plan.

Glaucoma surgery can be accomplished with laser or incisional surgical techniques. The discussion in this chapter follows a systematic approach to help the clinician in decision making. Each surgical procedure is described in terms of indications, contraindications, techniques, and complications and other considerations.

Surgery for Open-Angle Glaucoma

Laser Trabeculoplasty

Indications

Historically, the indication for laser trabeculoplasty (LTP) could be simply expressed as a patient with glaucoma on maximum tolerated medical therapy who requires lower IOP and in whom the angle is open on gonioscopy. At present, most clinicians still initiate some form of medical therapy before advancing to LTP, but LTP may be considered as an initial or next step in the management of glaucoma. Patients who are intolerant or noncompliant with initial medical therapy may be candidates for LTP. The question the surgeon and patient must address is when, in the course of glaucoma therapy, it is appropriate to employ LTP.

The Glaucoma Laser Trial (GLT) Research Group conducted a multicenter, randomized clinical trial to assess the efficacy and safety of LTP as an alternative to treatment with topical medication in patients with newly diagnosed, previously untreated POAG. Within the first 2 years of follow-up, LTP as initial therapy appeared to be as effective as medication. However, more than half of the eyes treated initially with laser required the addition of 1 or more medications to control IOP over the course of the study. Further, the medication protocols used in the study no longer resemble the medical regimens commonly employed for the treatment of POAG.

The Glaucoma Laser Trial (GLT). 2. Results of argon laser trabeculoplasty versus topical medicines. Glaucoma Laser Trial Research Group. *Ophthalmology.* 1990;97:1403–1413.

The Glaucoma Laser Trial (GLT) and glaucoma laser trial follow-up study. 7. Results. Glaucoma Laser Trial Research Group. *Am J Ophthalmol.* 1995;120:718–731.

Laser trabeculoplasty effectively reduces IOP in patients with POAG, pigmentary glaucoma, and exfoliation syndrome. Aphakic and pseudophakic eyes may respond less favorably than phakic eyes. IOP control does not seem to be diminished by subsequent cataract extraction. When effective, LTP is expected to lower IOP 20%–25%.

Mechanism

Several possible mechanisms of action have been proposed for the increased outflow facility following successful LTP. The treated area of trabecular meshwork may shrink, causing stretching of adjacent areas. Chemical mediators, specifically interleukin 1 beta and tumor necrosis factor alpha, are released from trabecular meshwork cells, increasing outflow facility through induction of specific matrix metalloproteinases. It has been suggested that there is a different mechanism for selective laser trabeculoplasty (SLT) involving selective effects on pigmented endothelial cells and possible activation of macrophages.

Contraindications

There are few contraindications to LTP in POAG when the angle is accessible. It is not advised in patients with inflammatory glaucoma, iridocorneal endothelial (ICE) syndrome, neovascular glaucoma, or synechial angle closure, or in patients with developmental glaucoma. LTP can be tried in angle recession, but the underlying tissue alterations may cause it to be ineffective. Another relative contraindication of LTP is the lack of effect in the fellow eye. If the eye has advanced damage and high IOP, LTP is unlikely to achieve the required low target pressure.

Preoperative evaluation

As with all ocular surgery, the preoperative evaluation for LTP should include a detailed medical and ocular history and a comprehensive eye examination. Particular attention must be paid to visual field examination, gonioscopy, and optic nerve evaluation. The angle must be open gonioscopically. Whereas eyes require some visible pigment in the angle for effective laser trabeculoplasty, the degree of pigmentation in the angle will determine the power setting. The more pigmented the trabecular meshwork, the less energy is required for both argon and Selecta lasers to create the necessary effect.

Technique

In the argon laser procedure, a 50-μm laser beam of 0.1 second duration is focused through a goniolens at the junction of the anterior nonpigmented and the posterior pigmented edge of the trabecular meshwork (Fig 8-1). Application to the posterior trabecular meshwork tends to produce inflammation, pigment dispersion, prolonged elevation of IOP, and peripheral anterior synechiae (PAS). The power setting (300–1000 mW)

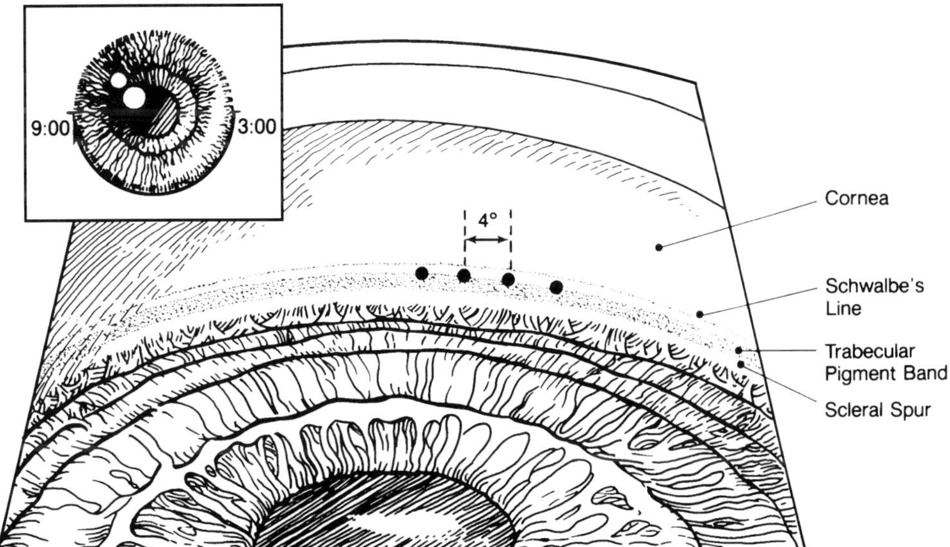

Figure 8-1 Position of argon laser trabeculoplasty treatment in the trabecular meshwork. Inset shows 180° application of laser treatment. *(After Solish AM, Kass MA. Laser trabeculoplasty. In: Waltman SR, Keates RH, Hoyt CS, eds.* Surgery of the Eye. *New York: Churchill Livingstone; 1988:1.)*

should be titrated to achieve the desired endpoint: blanching of the trabecular meshwork or production of a tiny bubble. If a large bubble appears, the power is reduced and titrated to achieve the proper effect. As LTP was originally described, laser energy was applied to the entire circumference (360°) of the trabecular meshwork. Evidence suggests that many patients have a satisfactory IOP reduction with less risk of short-term pressure elevation when only one half of the circumference (180°) is treated, using approximately 40–50 applications over 180°.

The procedure with the diode laser is similar; a 75-μm laser beam is focused through a goniolens with a power setting of 600–1000 mW and duration of 0.02 second.

Selective laser trabeculoplasty

SLT is an FDA-approved procedure in which the laser targets intracellular melanin. A frequency-doubled (532-nm) Q-switched Nd:YAG laser with a 400 μm spot size is used to deliver 0.4–1.0 mJ of energy for 0.3 ns to perform the procedure. Early results suggest that the procedure is safe and effective, with IOP results similar to those achieved with argon LTP. Preliminary evidence also suggests that this procedure may be repeated, although multiple retreatment studies have not yet been reported. Histologic studies have shown no coagulative damage after SLT and less structural changes of the trabecular meshwork after SLT compared with argon laser therapy (ALT). Long-term and retreatment studies are being conducted to clarify and validate these preliminary findings.

Damji KF, Shah KC, Rock WJ, et al. Selective laser trabeculoplasty v argon laser trabeculoplasty: a prospective randomised clinical trial. *Br J Ophthalmol.* 1999;83:718–722.

Kramer TR, Noecker RJ. Comparison of the morphologic changes after selective laser trabeculoplasty and argon laser trabeculoplasty in human eye bank eyes. *Ophthalmology.* 2001;108:773–779.

Latina MA, Sibayan SA, Shin DH, et al. Q-switched 532-nm Nd:YAG laser trabeculoplasty (selective laser trabeculoplasty): a multicenter, pilot, clinical study. *Ophthalmology.* 1998; 105:2082–2090.

Weinreb RN, Ruderman J, Juster R, et al. Influence of the number of laser burns administered on the early results of argon laser trabeculoplasty. *Am J. Ophthlamol.* 1983;95:287–292.

Complications

The most significant complication of laser trabeculoplasty is a transient rise in IOP, which occurs in approximately 20% of patients. IOP has been reported to reach 50–60 mm Hg and may cause additional damage to the optic nerve. This rise is less common when only 180° of the angle is treated per session.

IOP elevations are of particular concern in patients with advanced cupping. Rises in IOP are usually evident within the first 1–4 hours after treatment, and all patients should be monitored closely for this complication. The adjunctive use of topical apraclonidine 1% or brimonidine 0.2% has been shown to blunt postoperative pressure elevation. Other topical medications shown to blunt the IOP spikes include beta blockers, pilocarpine, and topical carbonic anhydrase inhibitors (CAIs). Hyperosmotic agents and oral CAIs may be helpful in eyes with IOP spikes not responsive to topical medications.

Low-grade iritis may follow LTP. Some surgeons routinely treat with topical anti-inflammatory drugs for 4–7 days; others use them only if inflammation develops. Other complications of LTP include the rare persistent elevation of IOP requiring filtering surgery, hyphema, and the formation of PAS.

Results and long-term follow-up

From 4 to 6 weeks should be allowed before evaluating the full effect of the first treatment and making a decision about additional treatment. Approximately 80% of patients with medically uncontrolled open-angle glaucoma experience a drop in IOP for a minimum of 6–12 months following LTP. Longer-term data have shown that 50% of patients with an initial response maintain a significantly lower IOP 3–5 years after treatment. Success at 10 years is approximately 30%. Highest success rates are seen in older patients with POAG and pseudoexfoliative glaucoma. Eyes with pigmentary glaucoma may show a good initial decrease in IOP, but with continued pigment shedding, this decrease may not be sustained.

Elevation of IOP may recur in some patients after months or even years of control. Additional laser treatment may be helpful in some patients, especially if the entire angle has not been treated previously. Retreatment of an angle that has been fully treated (approximately 80–100 spots over 360°) has a lower success rate and a higher complication rate than does primary treatment. If initial LTP fails to bring IOP under control, a trabeculectomy should be considered.

Chung PY, Schuman JS, Netland PA, et al. Five-year results of a randomized, prospective, clinical trial of diode vs argon laser trabeculoplasty for open-angle glaucoma. *Am J Ophthalmol.* 1998;126:185–190.

Mitrev PV, Schuman JS. Lasers in glaucoma management. *Focal Points: Clinical Modules for Ophthalmologists.* San Francisco: American Academy of Ophthalmology; 2001, module 9.

Ritch R, Shields MB, Krupin T, eds. *The Glaucomas.* 2nd ed. St Louis: Mosby; 1996.

Wise JB, Witter SL. Argon laser therapy for open-angle glaucoma: a pilot study. *Arch Ophthalmol.* 1979;97:319–322.

Incisional Surgery for Open-Angle Glaucomas

Incisional surgery is indicated in open-angle glaucoma when IOP cannot be maintained by nonsurgical therapies at a level considered low enough to prevent further pressure-related damage to the optic nerve or visual field loss. The glaucoma may be uncontrolled for various reasons:

- Maximal tolerated medical therapy fails to adequately reduce IOP.
- The amount of medical therapy necessary to control IOP is not well tolerated or places the patient at unacceptable risk.
- Glaucomatous optic neuropathy or visual field loss is progressing despite apparent "adequate" reduction of IOP with medical therapy.
- The patient cannot comply with the necessary medical regimen.

Although incisional procedures to lower IOP are traditionally referred to as *filters,* it would be more correct physiologically and anatomically to refer to them as *fistulizing procedures.* However, this discussion uses the traditional terminology, which remains in widespread use. The goal of filtering surgery is to create a new pathway (fistula) for the bulk flow of aqueous humor from the anterior chamber through the surgical defect in the sclera into the subconjunctival and sub-Tenon's spaces. The filtering procedure most commonly used is guarded trabeculectomy. Full-thickness procedures have largely fallen into disuse because of the high complication rate, especially since the introduction of antifibrotic agents.

Indications

The indication for incisional surgery for glaucoma has been expressed as: "A patient with glaucoma on maximum tolerable medical therapy who has had maximal laser benefit and whose optic nerve function is failing or is likely to fail."

This statement raises several important considerations. The presence of glaucoma and a high probability of optic nerve damage is a clear indication. With the potential complications of glaucoma surgery, however, it is not reasonable to perform a trabeculectomy in an ocular hypertensive eye with a low risk of developing damage. In less clear-cut situations—for example, when 1 eye has sustained significant damage and the IOP is high in the fellow eye despite maximum tolerated medical therapy—some surgeons will recommend surgery prior to unequivocal detection of damage.

Weinreb RN, Mills RP, eds. *Glaucoma Surgery: Principles and Techniques.* 2nd ed. Ophthalmology Monograph 4. San Francisco: American Academy of Ophthalmology; 1998:20.

The concept of "maximum tolerated medical therapy" merits discussion. The physician can determine that the patient is at maximum tolerable medical therapy only by advancing therapy beyond the tolerated level and documenting intolerance. This process can be frustrating for the physician and patient alike. An alternative concept is *core therapy,* in which treatment consists of those medications likely to work well in combination. If a patient does not have a satisfactory IOP response, a few alterations may be made, but it is likely that further medical intervention will simply delay indicated surgery.

Failure of medical therapy may be a result of noncompliance, which is a relative indication for surgery. Sometimes patients use their medications only around the time of an office visit. Thus, there may be progression despite apparent acceptable IOP. It is difficult to elicit an accurate history in this situation.

Although the hallmark of glaucoma is progressive optic nerve damage, it is actually relatively uncommon to make a surgical decision based on the detection of progressive change in the optic nerve or retinal nerve fiber layer. Progression of visual field damage is a far more common clinical indication for surgery, even though multiple field examinations may be required to determine with certainty that a damaged field has become more damaged. Many decisions to operate are based on a clinical judgment that the IOP is too high considering the stage of the disease. Thus, whereas an IOP of 25 mm Hg is not an indication for surgery in an eye with ocular hypertension, surgery may be indicated to lower this IOP in the setting of advanced glaucomatous optic neuropathy with only a small central field remaining. It is not always necessary to perform LTP before proceeding to trabeculectomy. Certain conditions tend not to respond well to LTP. Eyes with very high IOP and advanced damage are unlikely to achieve substantial and sufficient IOP lowering with LTP.

Contraindications

Relative contraindications for glaucoma filtering surgery can be ocular or systemic. A blind eye should not be considered for incisional surgery. Ciliary body ablation is a better alternative for lowering IOP in such eyes if necessary for pain control, although even this procedure is not without risk. The risk of sympathetic ophthalmia should always be kept in mind when any procedure on a blind eye or an eye with poor visual potential is considered. Conditions that predispose to trabeculectomy failure such as active anterior segment neovascularization (rubeosis iridis) or active iritis are relative contraindications. The underlying problem should be addressed first, or a surgical alternative such as glaucoma drainage implant surgery should be considered. It may be extremely difficult to perform a successful trabeculectomy in an eye that has sustained extensive conjunctival injury or has an extremely thin sclera from extensive prior surgery or necrotizing scleritis. This is sometimes the case following trauma or retinal detachment surgery.

Filtering surgery is less successful in younger or aphakic/pseudophakic patients. A lower success rate is also found in patients with uveitic glaucoma or in patients who have had previously failed filtration procedures. Black patients have a higher failure rate with filtering surgery.

Preoperative evaluation

The patient must be medically stable for an invasive ocular procedure under local anesthesia. Preoperative evaluation should determine and document factors that may affect surgical planning, as well as those that determine the structural and functional status of the eye.

Control of preoperative inflammation with corticosteroids helps to reduce postoperative iritis and scarring of the filtering bleb. In the rare instances when they are used, anticholinesterase agents should be discontinued if possible and replaced temporarily by alternative medications at least 3–6 weeks before surgery to reduce bleeding and iridocyclitis. Systemic CAIs should be discontinued postoperatively, using topical CAIs in the fellow eye, if needed.

In preparation for surgery, IOP should be reduced as closely as possible to normal levels to minimize the risk of expulsive choroidal hemorrhage. Antiplatelet medications should be discontinued, and systemic hypertension should be controlled.

Patients should be informed of the purpose and expectations of surgery: to arrest or delay progressive visual loss caused by their glaucoma. They should understand that glaucoma surgery alone rarely improves vision and that glaucoma medications may still be required postoperatively, that surgery may fail completely, that vision could be lost as a result of surgery, and that glaucoma may progress despite successful surgery.

It is important to note that patients with far advanced visual field loss or field loss that is impinging on fixation are at risk for loss of central acuity following a surgical procedure. The most common cause of loss of visual acuity after trabeculectomy is cataract. Hypotony maculopathy and cystoid macular edema may also cause vision loss. Loss of central visual field in the absence of other explanations ("wipe-out") may occur, but rarely. Advanced age, preoperative visual field with macular splitting, and early postoperative hypotony are risk factors for "wipe-out." Early, undetected, postoperative elevation of IOP may also be associated with "wipe-out." Bleb infections and endophthalmitis may occur long after filtration surgery and may also cause vision loss.

Costa VP, Smith M, Spaeth GL, et al. Loss of visual acuity after trabeculectomy. *Ophthalmology.* 1993;100:599–612.

Trabeculectomy technique

Knowledge of both the internal and external anatomy of the limbal area is essential for successful incisional surgery results. Trabeculectomy is a guarded partial-thickness filtering procedure performed by removing a block of limbal tissue beneath a scleral flap. The scleral flap provides resistance and limits the outflow of aqueous, thereby reducing the complications associated with early hypotony such as flat anterior chamber, cataract, serous and hemorrhagic choroidal effusion, macular edema, and optic nerve edema.

Because of the lower incidence of postoperative complications, trabeculectomy is the most commonly performed filtering operation. The use of antifibrotic agents such as mitomycin C and 5-fluorouracil, combined with techniques of releasable sutures or laser suture lysis, enhances the longevity of guarded procedures, offers lower IOPs, and avoids some of the complications associated with full-thickness procedures.

Successful trabeculectomy surgery involves reducing IOP and avoiding or managing complications. Unlike cataract surgery, the success of trabeculectomy often depends on appropriate and timely postoperative intervention to influence the functioning of the filter. Complete healing of the epithelial and conjunctival wound with incomplete healing of the scleral wound is the goal of this procedure.

A trabeculectomy can be broken down into several basic steps:

- *Preoperative evaluation:* As discussed earlier, before contemplating a surgical procedure, the ophthalmologist must consider factors such as the patient's general health, presumed life expectancy, and status of the fellow eye.
- *Exposure:* A corneal traction suture or superior rectus bridle suture can rotate the globe down, giving excellent exposure of the superior sulcus and limbus, which can be very helpful for a limbus-based conjunctival flap (Fig 8-2). The speculum should be adjusted to keep pressure off the globe.
- *Conjunctival wound:* A fornix-based or limbus-based conjunctival flap can be used (Figs 8-3, 8-4). Each technique has advantages and disadvantages. The fornix-based flap provides better exposure at the limbus, and it is easier to do when a skilled assistant is not available. However, it is more difficult to achieve a watertight closure with this incision. The limbus-based conjunctival flap is technically more challenging but allows for a secure closure well away from the limbus. The incision should be positioned 8–10 mm posterior to the limbus, and care should be taken to avoid the tendon of the superior rectus muscle. The conjunctival flap may be dissected either superiorly at 12 o'clock or in either superior quadrant, depending on surgeon preference.
- *Scleral flap:* The exact size and shape of the scleral flap does not seem critical. Rather, it is the relationship of the flap to the underlying sclerostomy that provides resistance to outflow. Although flap design will vary by surgeon preference, a common technique involves creating a 3- to 4-mm triangular, trapezoidal, or rectan-

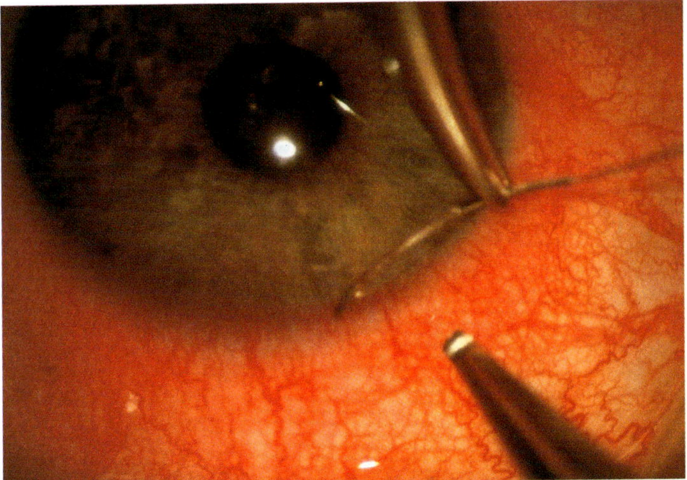

Figure 8-2 Exposure for trabeculectomy: A corneal traction suture (shown) or superior rectus bridle suture (see Figure 8-3) is inserted. *(Photograph courtesy of Robert D. Fechtner, MD.)*

gular flap (Fig 8-5). It is important to dissect the flap anteriorly into clear cornea. The term *trabeculectomy* may have become a misnomer, as most surgeons prefer to remove a peripheral corneal block. When the flap is too far posterior, the risk of bleeding from iris root and ciliary body is greater.

- *Paracentesis* (Fig 8-6): To enable the surgeon to control the anterior chamber, a paracentesis should be performed. This procedure allows for gradual lowering of IOP, control of the anterior chamber through installation of basic saline solution (BSS) or viscoelastic, and intraoperative testing of the patency of the filtration site as well as of the integrity of the conjunctival closure. BSS is instilled through the paracentesis, and sutures are added to the scleral flap until the flow is judged to be satisfactory. When a postoperative flat chamber occurs, the paracentesis already in place is used to re-form the chamber, which is much safer than trying to create a paracentesis in an eye with a flat chamber.
- *Sclerostomy:* The sclerostomy can be created with a punch or with sharp dissection (Fig 8-7). The size of the ostomy is determined by the scleral flap and the amount of overlap desired by the surgeon. A small amount of tissue should remain at the edges of the ostomy to allow for resistance to outflow from the flap. More overlap is generally associated with less flow, whereas less overlap is usually associated with more flow.
- *Iridectomy:* Most surgeons perform an iridectomy in order to lessen the risk of iris occluding the ostomy and to reduce the risk of pupillary block (see Figure 8-7C). Care should be taken to avoid amputating ciliary processes or disrupting the zonular fibers or hyaloid face.
- *Closure of scleral flap:* With the advent of laser suture lysis and releasable sutures, many surgeons close the flap relatively tightly to avoid early shallow chambers. After a few days or weeks, flap sutures may be released to promote filtration. Flow should be tested around the flap before the conjunctiva is closed (Fig 8-8). Leakage

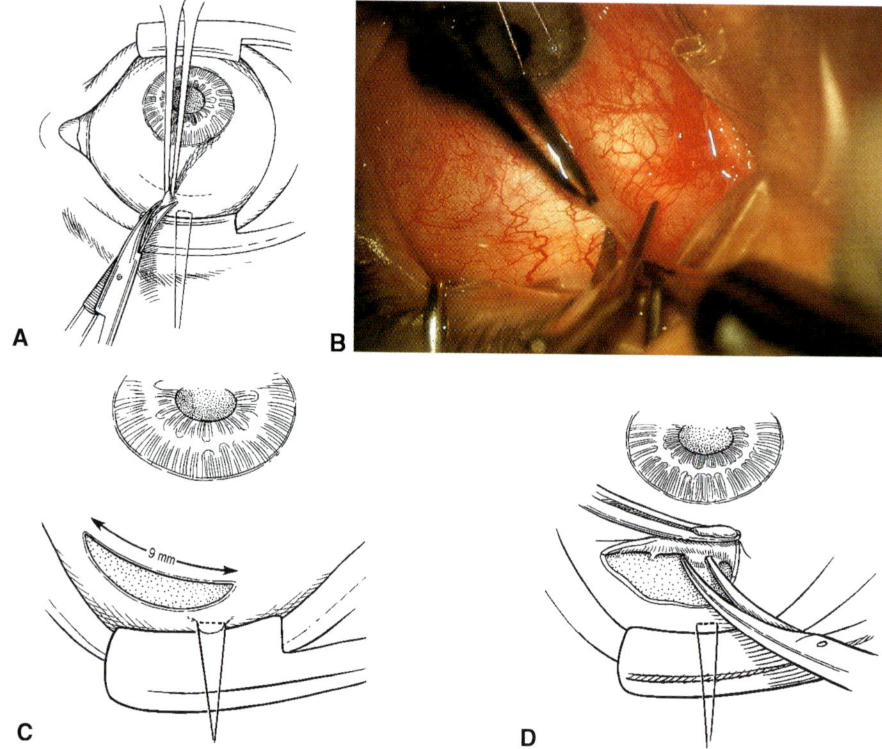

Figure 8-3 Limbus-based conjunctival flap. **A,** Drawing shows initial incision through conjunctiva and Tenon's capsule. **B,** Clinical photograph corresponding to *A* shows the initial incision for the creation of a limbus-based conjunctival flap. **C,** Completion of conjunctiva–Tenon's incision 8–9 mm posterior to limbus. **D,** Anterior dissection of conjunctiva-Tenon's flap with excision of Tenon's episcleral fibrous adhesions. *(Parts A, C, and D reproduced with permission from Weinreb RN, Mills RP, eds.* Glaucoma Surgery: Principles and Techniques. *2nd ed. Ophthalmology Monograph 4. San Francisco: American Academy of Ophthalmology; 1998:29–31. Part B courtesy of Robert D. Fechtner, MD.)*

around the flap may be adjusted intraoperatively by the placement of additional sutures, removal of sutures, or application of cautery to shrink the wound edges. The flap must, at a minimum, be sufficiently tight that the anterior chamber is maintained at the end of the procedure.

- *Closure of conjunctiva:* Many techniques have been developed for conjunctival closure (Fig 8-9). For a fornix-based flap, conjunctiva is secured at the limbus. For a limbus-based flap, conjunctiva and Tenon's capsule are closed separately or in a single layer.

Antifibrotic agents

The application of antifibrotic agents such as 5-fluorouracil and mitomycin C results in greater success and lower IOP following trabeculectomy; however, the rate of serious postoperative complications may increase, and these agents must not be used indiscriminantly. Antifibrotic agents should be used with caution in primary trabeculectomies on young patients with myopia because of an increased risk of hypotony.

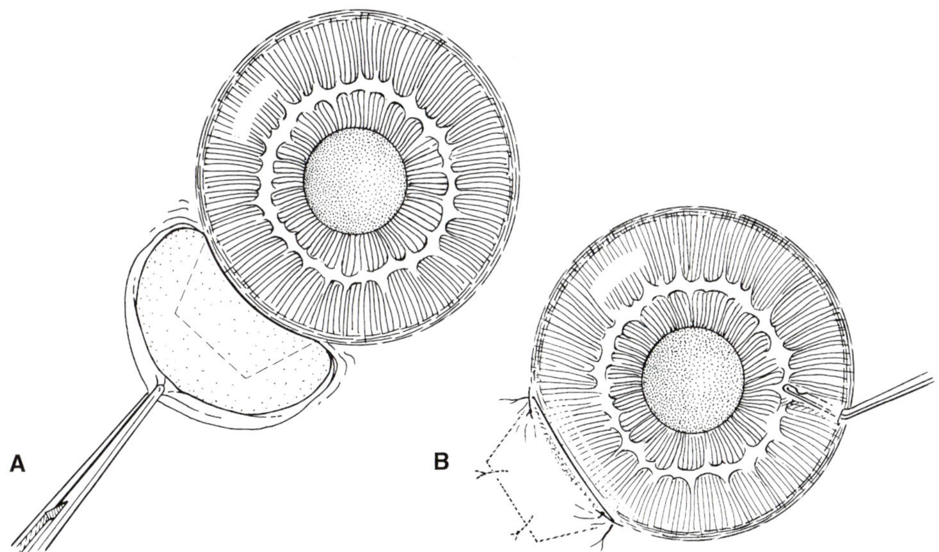

Figure 8-4 Fornix-based conjunctival flap (alternative to limbus-based flap). **A,** Drawing shows initial incision through conjunctiva and the insertion of Tenon's capsule. The arch length of the initial incision is approximately 6–7 mm. The tissue adjacent to the incision is undermined with blunt scissors before the scleral flap is prepared. **B,** The flap is closed either at both ends with interrupted sutures or with a running mattress suture. *(Reproduced with permission from Weinreb RN, Mills RP, eds.* Glaucoma Surgery: Principles and Techniques. *2nd ed. Ophthalmology Monograph 4. San Francisco: American Academy of Ophthalmology; 1998:43.)*

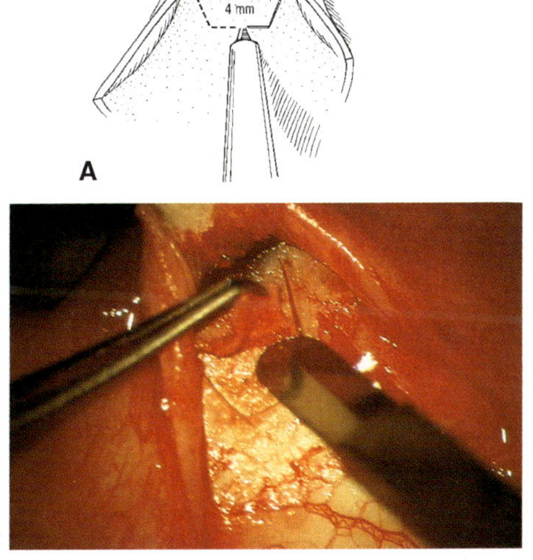

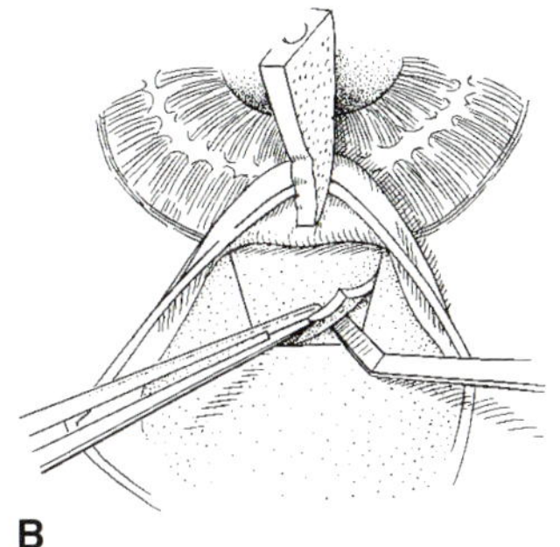

Figure 8-5 Creation of the scleral flap. **A,** Preparation of split-thickness scleral flap 4 mm wide at base and 2.5 mm wide at apex. Flap is 2.5 mm in height. **B,** Dissection of scleral flap from scleral bed with spatula blade. **C,** Clinical photograph corresponding to **B** shows trapezoidal scleral flap. *(Parts A and B reproduced with permission from Weinreb RN, Mills RP, eds.* Glaucoma Surgery: Principles and Techniques. *2nd ed. Ophthalmology Monograph 4. San Francisco: American Academy of Ophthalmology; 1998:33. Part C courtesy of Robert D. Fechtner, MD.)*

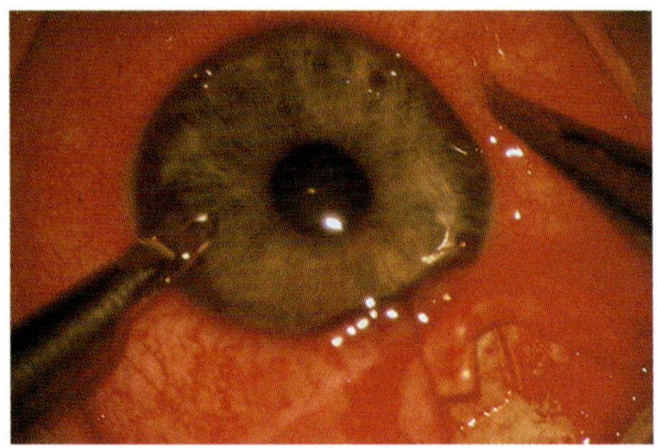

Figure 8-6 Paracentesis is created through clear cornea. *(Photograph courtesy of Robert D. Fechtner, MD.)*

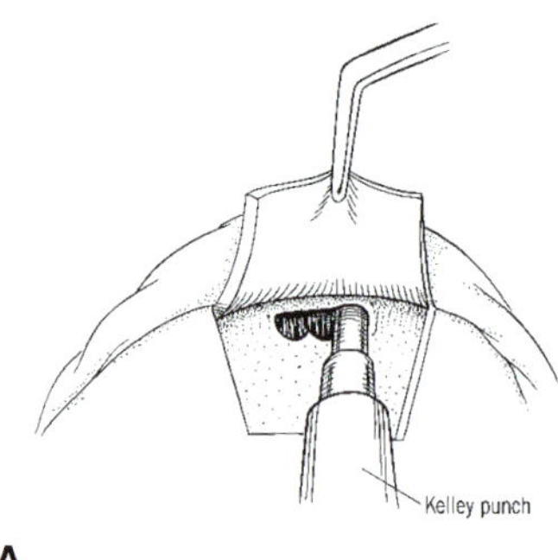

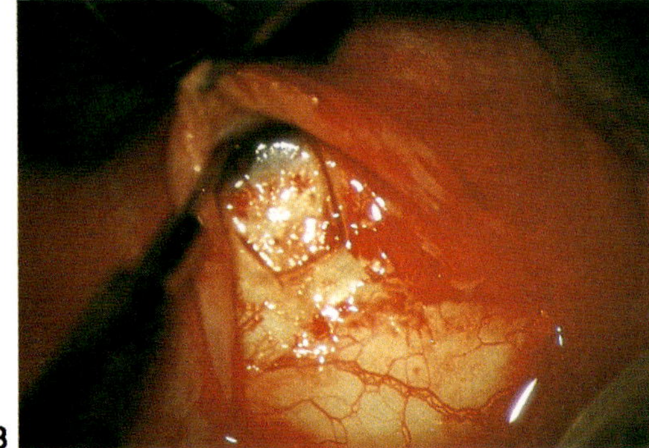

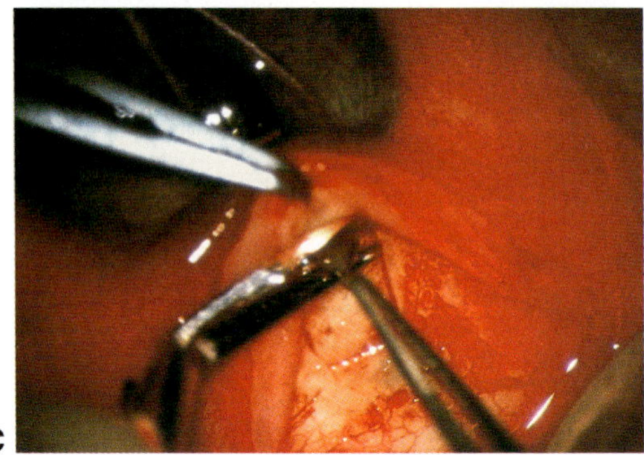

Figure 8-7 Sclerostomy and iridectomy created with a punch or with sharp dissection. **A,** Schematic shows a sclerostomy created with a Kelley punch. **B,** Clinical photograph corresponds to **A. C,** Peripheral iridectomy is made with iridectomy scissors. *(Part A reproduced with permission from Weinreb RN, Mills RP, eds.* Glaucoma Surgery: Principles and Techniques. *2nd ed. Ophthalmology Monograph 4. San Francisco: American Academy of Ophthalmology; 1998:34. Parts B and C courtesy of Robert D. Fechtner, MD.)*

Five-fluorouracil, a pyrimidine analog, inhibits fibroblast proliferation and has proven useful in reducing scarring after filtering surgery. The agent undergoes intracellular conversion to the active deoxynucleotide 5-fluoro-2′-deoxyuridine 5′-monophosphate (FdUMP), which interferes with DNA synthesis through its action on thymidylate synthetase.

Although it was originally advocated for high-risk groups such as patients with aphakic or pseudophakic eyes, neovascular glaucoma, or a history of previous failed operations, this agent is now used on a routine basis by many surgeons. Five-fluorouracil (50 mg/mL on a surgical sponge) may be used intraoperatively in a fashion similar to that described below for mitomycin C. Regimens for postoperative administration vary according to the observed healing response. A total of 5 mg in 0.1–0.5 cc can be injected

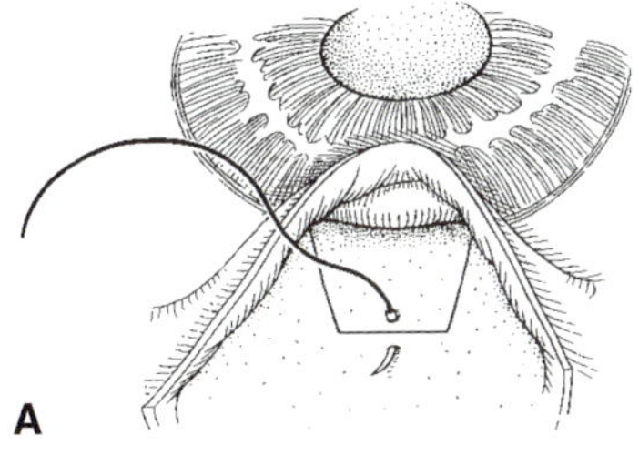
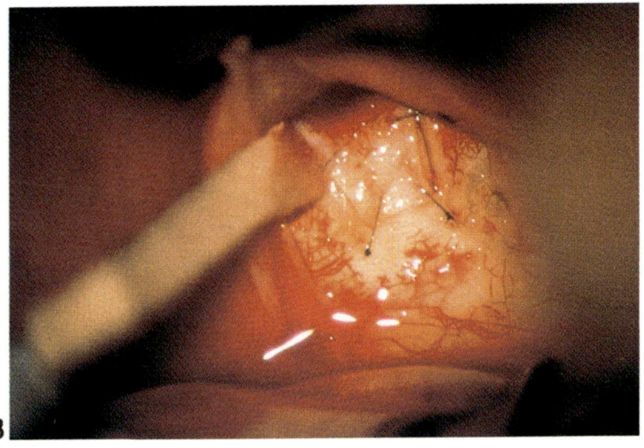

Figure 8-8 Closure of scleral flap. **A,** Schematic illustration. **B,** Flap closure is tested for flow with a surgical spear. *(Part A reproduced with permission from Weinreb RN, Mills RP, eds.* Glaucoma Surgery: Principles and Techniques. *2nd ed. Ophthalmology Monograph 4. San Francisco: American Academy of Ophthalmology; 1998:36. Part B courtesy of Robert D. Fechtner, MD.)*

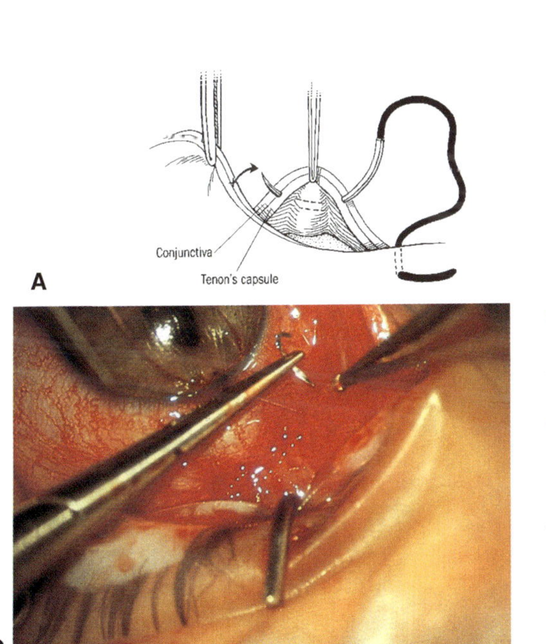

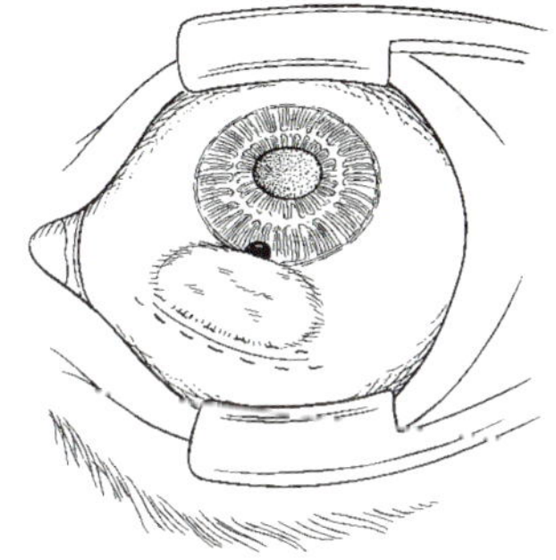

Figure 8-9 Conjunctival closure. **A,** Surgeon's view shows loops through conjunctiva and Tenon's capsule. **B,** Finished closure with distended bleb. **C,** Clinical photograph of conjunctival suturing corresponds to **A.** *(Parts A and B reproduced with permission from Weinreb RN, Mills RP, eds.* Glaucoma Surgery: Principles and Techniques. *2nd ed. Ophthalmology Monograph 4. San Francisco: American Academy of Ophthalmology; 1998:37. Part C courtesy of Robert D. Fechtner, MD.)*

with relatively mild discomfort. The total dose can be titrated to the observed healing response and corneal toxicity. Complications such as corneal epithelial defects commonly occur and require discontinuation of 5-fluorouracil injections. The site of injection can be varied from 180° away to adjacent to the bleb.

Mitomycin C is a naturally occurring antibiotic-antineoplastic compound that is derived from *Streptomyces caespitosus.* It acts as an alkylating agent after enzyme activation resulting in DNA cross-linking. Mitomycin C is a potent antifibrotic agent. It is most commonly administered intraoperatively by placing a surgical sponge soaked in mitomycin C within the subconjunctival space in contact with sclera at the planned trabeculectomy site. Concentrations in current usage are typically between 0.1 and 0.5 mg/mL with a duration of application from 1 to 5 minutes. Few data are available to compare regimens, and most surgeons increase concentration or duration based on risk factors for trabeculectomy failure. Mitomycin C is toxic, and intracameral exposure must be avoided.

Flap management

Techniques allowing tighter initial wound closure of the scleral flap help to prevent early postoperative hypotony. The use of releasable flap sutures or the placement of additional sutures that can be cut postoperatively to facilitate outflow following trabeculectomy are 2 of these techniques. In laser suture lysis, the conjunctiva is compressed with either a Zeiss goniolens or a lens designed for suture lysis (such as the Hoskins, Ritch, or Mandelkorn lenses), and the argon laser (set at 300–600 mW, 50–100 μm, and 0.02–0.1 second) can usually lyse the selected nylon suture with one application. It is important to avoid creating a full-thickness conjunctival burn. Shorter duration of laser energy and avoidance of pigment or blood are helpful. Most surgeons wait at least 48 hours before performing laser suture lysis. Filtration is best enhanced if lysis or suture release is completed within 2 weeks or before the flap has fibrosed. This period may be lengthened to several months when antifibrotic agents have been used.

Postoperative considerations in filtering surgery

The success of glaucoma surgery depends on careful postoperative management. Topical corticosteroids are typically administered 4–6 times daily initially and tapered as the clinical course dictates. Topical antibiotics, cycloplegic agents (atropine), or mydriatics (phenylephrine) may also be used. Topical corticosteroids should be tapered according to the degree of conjunctival hyperemia, which may continue for weeks, rather than in response to the visible anterior chamber reaction, which usually resolves more quickly. Long-term use of prophylactic antibiotics is generally not recommended. The postoperative course after filtration surgery is rarely uneventful, and much of the care is aimed at preventing or managing complications.

Complications of filtering surgery

Early and late complications of filtering surgery are listed in Table 8-1. Bleb-related complications may occur early (within 3 months of surgery) or late (after 3 months postoperatively). Early complications include wound leakage and hypotony, shallow or flat anterior chamber, and serous or hemorrhagic ciliochoroidal effusions. Late complications include bleb-related endophthalmitis, bleb leakage, ocular hypotony, bleb failure, overhanging blebs, painful blebs, and hypotony maculopathy. The filtering bleb can leak, produce dellen, or expand so as to interfere with eyelid function or extend onto the cornea and interfere with vision or cause irritation. Blebs may also encapsulate or fibrose, causing an increased IOP. Filtering blebs are dynamic. They evolve over time and must be monitored. All patients must be informed of the warning signs of endophthalmitis and instructed to seek ophthalmic care immediately should any signs develop.

Late-onset bleb-related endophthalmitis is a potentially devastating complication of filtering surgery. The incidence of postoperative endophthalmitis associated with glaucoma surgery with or without antifibrosis drugs has been reported to range from 0.06% to 13.2%. Risk factors for bleb-related endophthalmitis include blepharitis or conjunctivitis, ocular trauma, nasolacrimal duct obstruction, contact lens use, chronic bleb leak, male gender, and young age. Trabeculectomy performed at the inferior limbus has been associated with a higher risk of bleb-related endophalmitis compared with trabeculectomy at the superior limbus. Use of adjunctive antifibrosis drugs such as 5-fluorouracil or mitomycin C has been associated with increased risk for bleb-related endophthalmitis, perhaps because these blebs are often thin-walled and avascular. Patients may present with blebitis or with blebitis and endophthalmitis (Fig 8-10).

Causes of hypotony after filtration surgery include overfiltration and bleb leakage. Aqueous leakage from a filtering bleb may occur as an early or late complication after surgery. Early-onset bleb leaks are usually related to wound closure. The techniques of

Table 8-1 Complications of Filtering Surgery

Early Complications	Late Complications
Infection	Leakage or failure of the filtering bleb
Hypotony	Cataract
Flat anterior chamber	Blebitis
Aqueous misdirection	Endophthalmitis/bleb infection
Hyphema	Symptomatic bleb (dysesthetic bleb)
Formation or acceleration of cataract	Bleb migration
Transient IOP elevation	Hypotony
Cystoid macular edema	
Hypotony maculopathy	
Choroidal effusion	
Suprachoroidal hemorrhage	
Persistent uveitis	
Dellen formation	
Loss of vision	

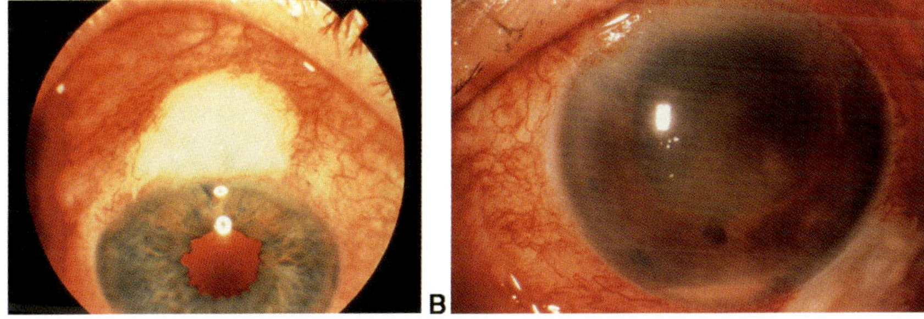

Figure 8-10 Bleb-related infection. Patients may present with blebitis, which is characterized by mucopurulent infiltrate within the bleb, localized conjunctival hyperemia, and minimal intraocular inflammation **(A)**. More severe infections include both blebitis and endophthalmitis **(B)**, characterized by diffuse bulbar conjunctival hyperemia, purulent material within the bleb, hypopyon formation, and marked vitritis. Location of the bleb at the inferior limbus **(B)** may be associated with an increased risk of bleb-related infection. *(Reproduced with permission from Greenfield DS. Dysfunctional glaucoma filtration blebs.* Focal Points: Clinical Modules for Ophthalmologists. *San Francisco: American Academy of Ophthalmology; 2002, module 4.)*

choroidal drainage and anterior chamber re-formation should be familiar to any surgeon who performs filtering surgery, which incurs the risk of flat chamber associated with choroidal detachment. Suprachoroidal fluid is drained through one or more posterior sclerotomies, as the chamber is deepened through a paracentesis. Late-onset leaks occur more frequently after full-thickness filters such as posterior lip sclerectomy or after use of antifibrosis drugs. Untreated bleb leaks may lead to vision-threatening complications, including shallowing of the anterior chamber, PAS formation, cataract, corneal decompensation, choroidal effusion suprachoroidal hemorrhage, endophthalmitis, and hypotony maculopathy. Clinical manifestations of hypotony maculopathy include decreased vision, hypotony, optic nerve and retinal edema, and radial folds of the macula.

Failure of the bleb may occur following filtration surgery. Eyes with failing blebs may have reduced bleb height, increased bleb-wall thickness, vascularization of the bleb, loss of conjunctival microcysts, and increased IOP. Risk factors for bleb failure include anterior segment neovascularization, African-American race, aphakia, prior failed filtering procedures, uveitis, prior cataract surgery, and young age. Initial management of failing blebs often includes antiglaucoma medications and digital massage. In eyes that do not respond to this initial therapy, transconjunctival needle revision may restore aqueous flow.

The use of contact lenses with a filtering bleb presents special problems. Contact lenses may be difficult to fit in the presence of a filtering bleb, or the lens may ride against the bleb, causing discomfort and increasing the risk of infection. Several options can be considered for the patient with high myopia needing trabeculectomy who prefers not to wear spectacles. Refractive surgery options include PRK, LASIK, or intracorneal ring segments prior to trabeculectomy. Clear lens extraction (either before or after or combined with trabeculectomy) is controversial. In some circumstances, hard or soft contact lens use under close supervision may be considered after trabeculectomy. Contact lens use is often more feasible in patients treated with glaucoma drainage implants compared with posttrabeculectomy patients. When an initial filtering procedure is not adequate to control the glaucoma and resumption of medical therapy is not successful, revision of original surgery, repeat filtering surgery at a new site, or tube-shunt and possibly cyclodestructive procedures may be indicated.

Camras CB. Diagnosis and management of complications of glaucoma filtering surgery. *Focal Points: Clinical Modules for Ophthalmologists.* San Francisco: American Academy of Ophthalmology; 1994, module 3.

Greenfield DS. Dysfunctional glaucoma filtration blebs. *Focal Points: Clinical Modules for Ophthalmologists.* San Francisco: American Academy of Ophthalmology; 2002, module 4.

Haynes WL, Alward WL. Control of intraocular pressure after trabeculectomy. *Surv Ophthalmol.* 1999;43:345–355.

Full-Thickness Sclerectomy

Full-thickness filtering operations are performed by removing a block of limbal tissue with a punch, trephine, laser, or cautery (Fig 8-11). The advantage of full-thickness filtering procedures is that they lower IOP and can maintain the lowered level for long periods of time. Also, using this procedure, average postoperative IOP in the low teens

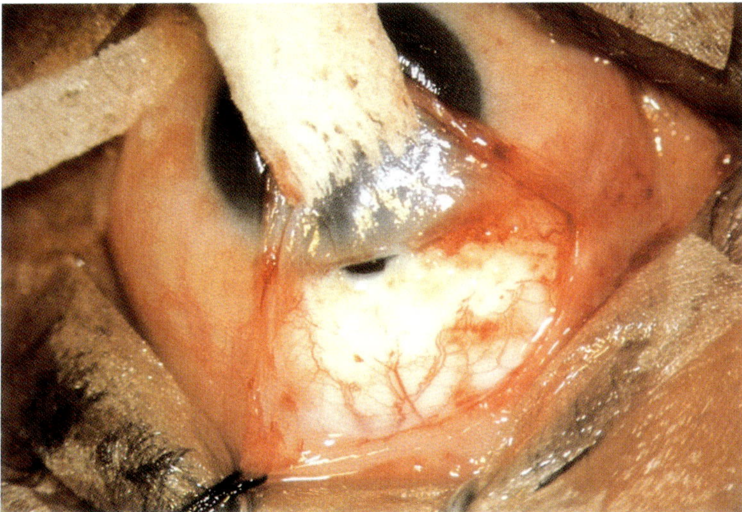

Figure 8-11 Intraoperative photograph of full-thickness sclerectomy performed with Descemet's punch.

can be achieved without antifibrosis drugs. Historically, ophthalmic surgeons performed these procedures on patients in whom a postoperative IOP lowered to the mid to high teens would not be considered adequate. Currently, the use of concurrent or subsequent antifibrotic agents such as mitomycin C or 5-fluorouracil equalize the IOP outcomes for full-thickness and guarded filtering procedures. The disadvantages of full-thickness compared with partial-thickness techniques include a higher incidence of postoperative flat anterior chamber, cataract, hypotony, choroidal effusion, leakage of filtering blebs, and endophthalmitis. Thus, trabeculectomy with antifibrosis drugs is generally preferred by surgeons compared with full-thickness sclerectomy.

Combined Cataract and Filtering Surgery

Both cataract and glaucoma are conditions that show increasing prevalence with aging. It is not surprising that many patients with glaucoma eventually develop cataracts either naturally or as a result of the effects of glaucoma therapy.

Indications

Indications for combining glaucoma surgery (usually trabeculectomy) with cataract extraction include the following:

- glaucoma that is uncontrollable either medically or after laser trabeculoplasty when visual function is significantly impaired by a cataract
- cataract requiring extraction in a glaucoma patient who has advanced cupping and visual field loss
- cataract requiring extraction in a glaucoma patient requiring medications to control IOP in whom medical therapy is poorly tolerated
- cataract requiring extraction in a glaucoma patient who requires multiple medications to control IOP

The precise number of medications representing "multiple medications" varies depending on the surgeon and the individual patient. Many surgeons perform trabeculectomy with cataract surgery when patients have stable IOP but are using 2 to 3 medications. The goal in these cases is to avoid perioperative problems with elevated IOP and to achieve long-term control of IOP without antiglaucoma medications. Many surgeons would perform cataract surgery alone in a patient who has controlled IOP using 1 medication, with mild to moderate cupping and little or no visual field loss.

Relative contraindications

Combined cataract and filtering surgery should be avoided in the following situations, in which glaucoma surgery alone is preferred:

- glaucoma that requires a very low target IOP
- advanced glaucoma with uncontrolled IOP and immediate need for successful reduction of IOP

Considerations

A combined procedure may prevent a postoperative rise in IOP. Combined procedures are generally less effective than filtering procedures alone in controlling IOP over time, although combined procedures using small-incision phacoemulsification techniques with an antifibrotic agent appear to have improved success rates that more closely mirror those of trabeculectomy alone. For patients in whom glaucoma is the greatest immediate threat to vision, filtering surgery alone may be performed first. The postoperative discontinuation of miotics, if used, is often enough to increase visual acuity so that cataract extraction and IOL implantation may be delayed.

Several clinical challenges are common in patients with coexisting cataract and glaucoma. Medical therapy for glaucoma may create chronic miosis, and the surgeon must deal with a small pupil. Patients with exfoliation syndrome often have fragile zonular support of the lens, and vitreous loss is therefore more common in such complicated eyes. As with all surgery, the risks, benefits, and alternatives should be discussed with the patient.

Technique

Several surgical approaches to coexisting cataract and glaucoma are now in use, and a debate has surfaced with the development of successful small-incision clear corneal cataract extraction. Single-site combined surgery with phacoemulsification had been the commonly accepted approach when a scleral tunnel technique was used. Two-site surgery with a clear corneal cataract extraction and a standard trabeculectomy has recently gained in popularity. Long-term control of IOP is better with combined glaucoma and cataract operations compared with cataract surgery alone. For patients who have IOP controlled medically, clear corneal cataract surgery alone may be the appropriate choice. As no violation of conjunctiva or sclera occurs, there is little reason to perform an incidental trabeculectomy. Rather, standard trabeculectomy can be performed when dictated by independent indications. Although little evidence exists to compare long-term outcomes with these different approaches, it makes sense for the surgeon to perform his or her best cataract procedure, as the primary indication for surgery is the presence of cataract.

Balyeat HD. Cataract surgery in the glaucoma patient. Part 1: A cataract surgeon's perspective. *Focal Points: Clinical Modules for Ophthalmologists.* San Francisco: American Academy of Ophthalmology; 1998, module 3.

Friedman DS, Jampel HD, Lubomski LH, et al. Surgical strategies for coexisting glaucoma and cataract: an evidence-based update. *Ophthalmology.* 2002;109:1902–1913.

Skuta GL. Cataract surgery in the glaucoma patient. Part 2: A glaucoma surgeon's perspective. *Focal Points: Clinical Modules for Ophthalmologists.* San Francisco: American Academy of Ophthalmology; 1998, module 4.

Weinreb RN, Mills RP, eds. *Glaucoma Surgery: Principles and Techniques.* 2nd ed. Ophthalmology Monograph 4. San Francisco: American Academy of Ophthalmology; 1998:65–85.

Surgery for Angle-Closure Glaucoma

The first clinical decision point following the diagnosis of angle-closure glaucoma is to distinguish between angle closure based on a pupillary-block mechanism and angle closure based on another mechanism. Laser iridectomy is the procedure of choice to relieve pupillary block, but this is of no use in an eye with complete synechial closure as a result of neovascularization or chronic inflammation. It is sometimes necessary, however, to perform the iridectomy as much for diagnostic purposes as for therapeutic ones. For example, the diagnosis of plateau iris can be definitely confirmed only when a patent iridectomy fails to change peripheral iris configuration and relieve angle closure.

The treatment of pupillary-block glaucoma, whether primary or secondary, is a laser or an incisional iridectomy. These procedures provide an alternative route for aqueous trapped in the posterior chamber to enter the anterior chamber, which allows the iris to recede from its occlusion of the trabecular meshwork (Fig 8-12). Laser surgery has become the preferred method in almost all cases. Both the argon laser and Nd:YAG laser are effective, but the Nd:YAG laser has become the more popular instrument used. Following the successful resolution of pupillary block, IOP may return to normal or may remain elevated. At this point, the indications for surgery become similar to those for POAG, except for possible surgical goniosynechialysis.

For eyes with secondary angle closure not caused by pupillary block, an attempt should be made to identify and treat underlying conditions. For example, an eye with rubeosis iridis from diabetic retinopathy should have retinal ablation prior to glaucoma surgery. In early cases, the IOP elevation may be reversible. Even in the presence of complete synechial angle closure from rubeosis, the neovascularization may regress following retinal ablation, allowing subsequent successful filtering surgery.

Laser Iridectomy

Indications

The indications for iridectomy include the presence of pupillary block and the need to determine the presence of pupillary block. Laser iridectomy is also indicated to prevent pupillary block in an eye considered at risk, as determined by gonioscopic evaluation or because of an angle-closure attack in the fellow eye.

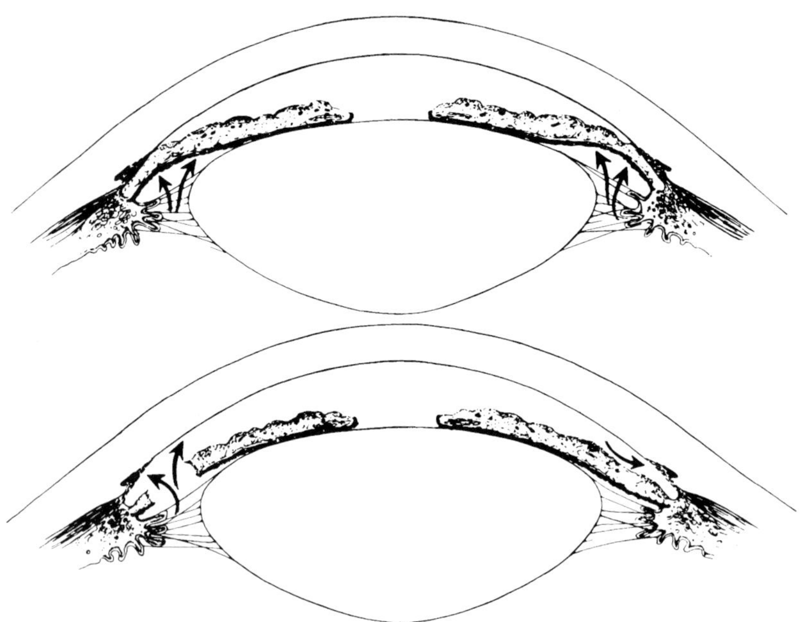

Figure 8-12 Angle-closure glaucoma. Laser or surgical iridectomy breaks the pupillary block and results in opening of the entire peripheral angle if no permanent peripheral anterior synechiae are present. *(Reproduced and modified with permission from Kolker AE, Hetherington J, eds.* Becker-Shaffer's Diagnosis and Therapy of the Glaucomas. *5th ed. St Louis: Mosby; 1983.)*

Contraindications

An eye with active rubeosis iridis may bleed following laser iridectomy. The risk of bleeding is also increased in a patient taking systemic anticoagulants, including aspirin. The argon laser may be more appropriate than the Nd:YAG should laser iridectomy be performed in such an individual. Although laser iridectomy is not helpful for angle closure not caused by a pupillary block mechanism, it is sometimes necessary to perform the laser iridectomy to ensure that pupillary block is not present.

Preoperative consideration

In the setting of acute angle closure, it is often difficult to perform laser iridectomy because of the cloudy cornea, shallow chamber, and engorged iris. The clinician should attempt to break the attack medically and then proceed to surgery. Corneal edema may be improved prior to laser by pretreatment with topical glycerin. It is easiest to penetrate the iris in a crypt. Care should be taken to keep the iridectomy peripheral and covered by eyelid, if possible, to avoid monocular diplopia. Pretreatment with pilocarpine may be helpful by stretching and thinning the iris. Pretreatment with apraclonidine can help blunt IOP spikes.

Technique

The argon laser may be used to produce an iridectomy in most eyes, but very dark and very light irides present technical difficulties. Using a condensing contact lens, the typical initial laser settings are 0.02–0.1 second of duration, 50-µm spot size, and 800–1000 mW of power. There are a number of variations in technique, and iris color dictates which technique is chosen. Complications include localized lens opacity, acute rise in IOP (which may damage the optic nerve), transient or persistent iritis, early closure of the iridectomy, posterior synechiae, and corneal and retinal burns.

The Q-switched Nd:YAG laser generally requires fewer pulses and less energy than an argon laser to create a patent iridectomy and has become the preferred technique for most eyes. Also, the effectiveness of this laser is not affected by iris color, and the iridectomy created by this laser does not close as often over the long term as one created by argon laser. With a condensing contact lens, the typical initial laser setting is 2–8 mJ. Potential complications include corneal burns, disruption of the anterior lens capsule or corneal endothelium, bleeding (usually transient), postoperative IOP spike, inflammation, and delayed closure of the iridectomy. To prevent damage to the lens, the surgeon must use caution with the Q-switched Nd:YAG laser in performing further enlargement of the opening once patency is established. The location should be as peripheral as possible, at the point where the distance between the iris and lens is greatest.

Postoperative care

Bleeding may occur from the iridectomy site, particularly with the Nd:YAG laser. Often, compression of the eye with the laser lens will tamponade the vessel, thereby slowing bleeding until coagulation can occur. In rare cases when this does not work, it may be helpful to use the argon laser to coagulate the vessel. Postoperative pressure spikes may occur, as with LTP, and they are treated as described in the section on LTP. Inflammation is treated as necessary with topical corticosteroids.

Complications

The complications associated with a particular laser mode were listed earlier in discussion of that laser. In general, potential complications from laser iridectomy include focal lens or corneal damage, retinal detachment, bleeding, visual symptoms, and IOP spike. Lens damage can be avoided by ceasing the procedure as soon as the iris is penetrated and by placing the iridectomy in the periphery of the superior iris. Retinal detachment is very rare but has been associated with Nd:YAG laser iridectomy. Bleeding and IOP spikes are discussed in the preceding section.

Murphy PH, Trope GE. Monocular blurring: a complication of YAG laser iridotomy. *Ophthalmology.* 1991;98:1539–1542.

Ritch R, Shields MB, Krupin T, eds. *The Glaucomas.* 2nd ed. St Louis: Mosby; 1996.

Shields MB. *Textbook of Glaucoma.* 4th ed. Philadelphia: Williams & Wilkins; 2000.

Laser Gonioplasty, or Peripheral Iridoplasty

Indications

Gonioplasty, or iridoplasty, is a technique to deepen the angle that is occasionally useful in angle-closure glaucoma resulting from plateau iris. Stromal burns are created with the argon laser in the peripheral iris to cause contraction and flattening. It is difficult to diagnose plateau iris unless an iridectomy has been created and the angle configuration has not changed and, therefore, remains occludable.

Contraindications

The contraindications are the same as those for laser iridectomy.

Preoperative considerations

An angle that is closed from plateau iris will not open with creation of a laser iridectomy, as the underlying mechanism is not pupillary block. This is often a difficult condition to diagnose accurately.

Technique

Typical laser settings are 0.1–0.5 second duration, 200- to 500-µm spot size, and 200–500 mW of power. This procedure can be used to open the angle temporarily, in anticipation of a more definitive laser or incisional iridectomy, or in other types of angle closure such as plateau iris syndrome and nanophthalmos. Argon laser gonioplasty may be useful to treat synechial angle closure, in patients with angle closure of months' to even years' duration (laser goniosynechialysis). A gonioscopy lens with a diameter smaller than the corneal diameter may be used, which allows simultaneous compression gonioscopy if necessary. A spot size of 100 to 200 µm is used, but otherwise the settings are the same as for gonioplasty.

Wand M. Argon laser gonioplasty for synechial angle closure. *Arch Ophthalmol.* 1992;110:363–367.

Incisional Surgery for Angle Closure

Peripheral iridectomy

Incisional surgical iridectomy may be required if a patent iridectomy cannot be achieved with a laser. Such situations include a cloudy cornea, a flat anterior chamber, and insufficient patient cooperation.

Cataract extraction

When pupillary block is associated with a visually significant cataract, lens extraction might be considered as a primary procedure. However, laser iridectomy may stop an acute attack of pupillary block, so that cataract surgery may be performed more safely at a later time.

Chamber deepening and goniosynechialysis

When peripheral anterior synechiae (PAS) develop in cases of angle-closure glaucoma, iridectomy alone may not relieve the glaucoma adequately. Chamber deepening through a paracentesis with intraoperative gonioscopy may break PAS of relatively recent onset. A viscoelastic agent and/or an iris or cyclodialysis spatula may be useful, in a procedure known as *goniosynechialysis*, to break synechiae.

Campbell DG, Vela A. Modern goniosynechialysis for the treatment of synechial angle-closure glaucoma. *Ophthalmology.* 1984;91:1052–1060.

Shingleton BJ, Chang MA, Bellows AR, et al. Surgical goniosynechialysis for angle-closure glaucoma. *Ophthalmology.* 1990;97:551–556.

Other Procedures to Lower IOP

Incisional and nonincisional procedures to control IOP include tube-shunt surgery, ciliary body ablation, cyclodialysis, and viscocanalostomy and other nonpenetrating procedures.

Glaucoma Tube Shunt

Many different types of devices have been developed that aid filtration by shunting aqueous to a site posterior to the limbus (Table 8-2) The shunts, or drainage devices, in current use generally have a tube placed in the anterior chamber or through the pars plana that flows to an extraocular reservoir, which is placed in the equatorial region on the sclera (Fig 8-13) They can be broadly categorized as resistance (valved) devices, also known as *flow-restricted,* or nonresistance (nonvalved) devices. The most popular nonresistance devices are the Molteno and Baerveldt designs. Popular resistance devices include the Krupin and Ahmed. The size of the plate varies and can influence IOP control and complications postoperatively. The anterior chamber tube shunt to an encircling band (ACTSEB) described by Schocket used an encircling element intended for scleral buckling with tubing attached to the encircling band. A variation on the ACTSEB can be used on eyes with a previously placed scleral buckle.

Weinreb RN, Mills RP, eds. *Glaucoma Surgery: Principles and Techniques.* 2nd ed. Ophthalmology Monograph 4. San Francisco: American Academy of Ophthalmology; 1998:65–85.

Table 8-2 Glaucoma Drainage Devices

	Molteno		Baerveldt		Krupin	Ahmed	
	Single plate	Double plate	250	350		Single plate	Double plate
Surface area	135 mm²	270 mm²	250 mm²	350 mm²	194 mm²	184 mm²	364 mm²
Height profile	2.16 mm	2.16 mm	0.84 mm	0.84 mm	2.54 mm	1.90 mm	1.90 mm
Plate material	Polypropylene	Polypropylene	Silicone	Silicone	Silicone	Polypropylene or silicone	
Tube	Open	Open	Open	Open	Valve	Valve	Valve

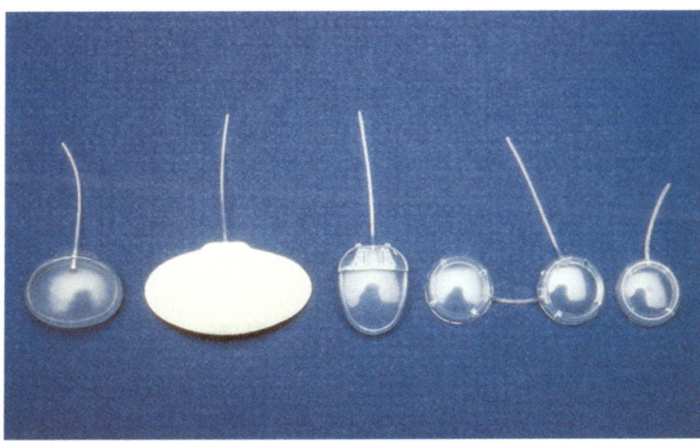

Figure 8-13 Glaucoma drainage devices, from left to right: Krupin, Baerveldt, Ahmed, double-plate Molteno, single-plate Molteno.

Indications

The devices mentioned and other, similar types of implants are generally reserved for difficult glaucoma cases in which conventional filtering surgery has failed or is likely to fail. One form of "failure" may be the inability of the patient to be a suitable candidate for trabeculectomy. A glaucoma tube shunt should be considered in the following clinical settings:

- *Trabeculectomy failure:* Failure of a trabeculectomy may lead to the need for further surgical intervention if IOP cannot be controlled medically.
- *Failed trabeculectomy with antifibrotics:* It may be appropriate to perform a repeat trabeculectomy in some clinical situations. However, when the factors that precipitated the initial failure cannot be modified, or when it is not technically possible to repeat the trabeculectomy, a glaucoma tube shunt may be the procedure of choice.
- *Active uveitis:* Although few randomized, prospective data are available comparing trabeculectomy with antifibrotics to a glaucoma tube shunt in the setting of active uveitis, the success of trabeculectomy in the setting of active inflammation is disappointingly low.
- *Neovascular glaucoma:* Eyes with neovascular glaucoma (NVG) are at high risk for failure of a trabeculectomy. In one prospective study, the 5-year success rate for trabeculectomy with 5-fluorouracil in NVG was 28%. When possible, retinal ablation is performed prior to glaucoma surgery in cases of NVG. When the IOP mandates urgent surgery, or when the NVG does not respond to retinal ablation, a glaucoma tube shunt is indicated.
- *Inadequate conjunctiva:* Following severe trauma or extensive surgery (eg, retinal detachment surgery), conjunctiva is often inadequate or has too much scarring for trabeculectomy to be successful. A glaucoma tube shunt can be placed, even in the presence of a scleral buckle. When vitrectomy has been performed, the tube can be placed through the pars plana.
- *Aphakia:* Aphakic patients may have extensive conjunctival scarring and a poor prognosis for the success of conventional filtration surgery.

Other factors should be considered when evaluating a patient for possible tube-shunt surgery:

- *Poor candidate for trabeculectomy:* In addition to the clinical settings just described, lack of an intact blood–aqueous barrier is a relative indication for a glaucoma tube shunt.
- *Potential for visual acuity:* It may not be appropriate to perform incisional surgery with a prolonged convalescence in an eye with little potential for useful vision. However, when the potential for useful vision remains, it is worth the risks and potentially complicated postoperative course of glaucoma tube-shunt surgery.
- *Need for lower IOP:* After a failed trabeculectomy, medical therapy should be resumed. If IOP is not controlled, additional surgery must be considered.

Contraindications

Tube-shunt surgery may have a complicated postoperative course. Thus, it is relatively contraindicated in patients unable to comply with self-care in the postoperative period. Borderline corneal endothelial function is a relative contraindication for anterior chamber placement of a tube.

Preoperative considerations

Preoperative evaluation should be similar to that for trabeculectomy. During the ophthalmic examination, the clinician should note the motility examination, the status of the conjunctiva, the health of the sclera at the anticipated tube and external reservoir sites, the location of PAS near possible tube insertion sites, and the location of vitreous in the eye.

Techniques

Although devices differ in design, the basic techniques for implantation are similar. The superotemporal quadrant is preferred over the superonasal quadrant, as surgical access is more easily achieved in the former. For the flow-restrictive devices, the tube must be primed prior to implantation of the device. The extraocular plate or valve mechanism is sutured between the vertical and horizontal rectus muscles posterior to the muscle insertions. The tube is then routed anteriorly to enter into the chamber angle or through the pars plana for posterior implantation in eyes that have had a vitrectomy. Typically, the tube is covered with tissue such as sclera, pericardium, or dura to help prevent erosion.

For the nonresistance devices, there are a number of techniques to restrict flow in the early postoperative period, such as putting a suture in the lumen of the tube or ligating the tube. This is not necessary with the resistance devices, but hypotony and a flat chamber can still occur despite the presence of a valve. Doses of antifibrotic agents similar to those used in trabeculectomy do not appear to improve the success of glaucoma tube-shunt surgery. For devices with 2 plates, the second plate and its interconnecting tube may be placed either over or under the superior rectus muscle; the distal plate is attached to the sclera in a manner similar to that in which the proximal plate is attached.

Postoperative management

The IOP in the early postoperative period can be variable. In nonresistance devices in which the tube has been occluded, early IOP spikes are best managed medically. After sufficient time has passed for a capsule to form around the extraocular reservoir, the occluding suture is released for the nonresistance devices. Topical corticosteroids, antibiotics, and cycloplegics are used as with trabeculectomy. Elevation of the IOP occurs around 2–8 weeks postoperatively, which probably represents encapsulation around the extraocular reservoir. Aqueous suppression can control the IOP, and this elevation usually improves or resolves spontaneously within 1–6 months.

Complications

Success rates have been encouraging, but the implant procedures share many of the complications associated with conventional filtering surgery. Unique problems related to the tubes and plates also arise. Early overfiltration in an eye with the tube in the anterior chamber results in a flat chamber and tube–cornea touch. This can compromise the cornea. Even when no touch occurs, however, an area of corneal decompensation can appear near the tube. Tube obstruction, tube migration, or tube erosion may require surgical revision. Eyes must be monitored for late complications such as tube erosion or migration. Motility disturbances may also occur. Table 8-3 lists several common complications, along with methods for avoiding or managing them.

Ciliary Body Ablation Procedures

Several surgical procedures reduce aqueous secretion by destroying a portion of the ciliary body. The secretory activity of ciliary body epithelium can be inhibited by treatment with cyclocryotherapy (Fig 8-14) and thermal lasers such as continuous-wave Nd:YAG, argon, and diode (Fig 8-15).

Table 8-3 Complications of Glaucoma Tube-Shunt Surgery and Prevention/ Management Options

Complication	Prevention/Management
Tube-cornea touch	Avoid by making the anterior chamber insertion parallel with the iris plane and using a tube occlusion technique to avoid a flat chamber. Pars plana insertion avoids this complication.
Flat chamber and hypotony	Flat chamber and hypotony caused by overfiltration are best avoided by using a resistance device, an occlusion technique, or viscoelastic agents. A flat chamber with tube–cornea touch and serous choroidal detachment should be managed by early drainage of choroidal effusion and re-formation of the anterior chamber. Viscoelastic can help maintain the chamber. A flat chamber resulting from a complication such as suprachoroidal hemorrhage must be managed based on the clinical setting.
Tube occlusion	Avoid by positioning tube away from uveal tissue (iris) or vitreous. A generous vitrectomy should be performed if needed. Although it is possible to use Nd:YAG laser to clear an occlusion, surgical intervention is often required.
Tube migration	Avoid by meticulous tube placement and coverage. Different materials used to cover the tube may vary in rate of degradation. It may be possible to reposition a tube with extraocular manipulation only. A new entry site can be fashioned without disturbing the capsule around the extraocular plate. Some surgeons suture the tube to the sclera with an S-curve in an effort to prevent extraocular scarring from causing tube migration.
Valve malfunction	Valves should be tested for patency prior to insertion of the tube. Several techniques have been described to unclog a valve.
Tube or plate exposure or erosion	Conjunctiva must not be under tension when covering the tube or plate. Most surgeons use a patch graft such as sclera or pericardium to cover the tube. Exposure increases the risk of endophthalmitis. In some settings the device should be removed if adequate coverage cannot be achieved.

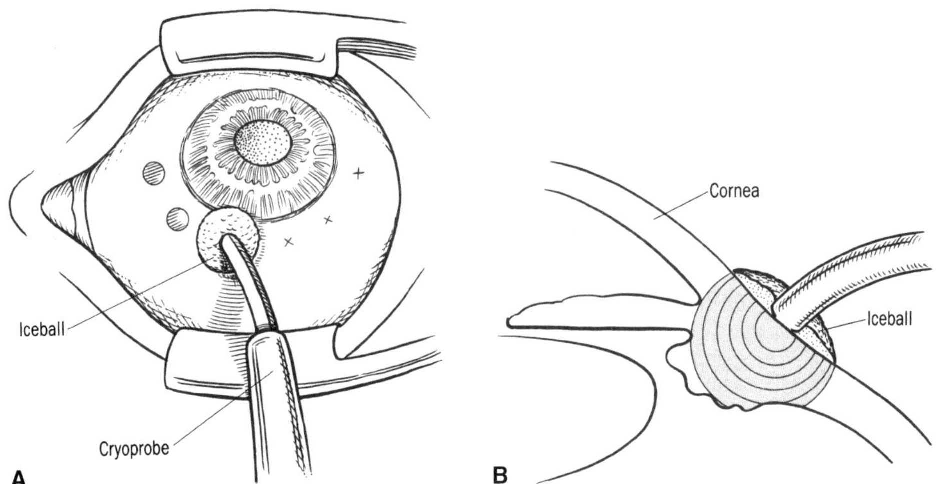

Figure 8-14 Cyclocryotherapy. **A,** The cryoprobe is placed with the tip approximately 2 mm posterior to the limbus. **B,** Cross-sectional view, showing iceball that has encompassed the ciliary body. *(Reproduced with permission from Weinreb RN, Mills RP, eds.* Glaucoma Surgery: Principles and Techniques. *2nd ed. Ophthalmology Monograph 4. San Francisco: American Academy of Ophthalmology; 1998:159.)*

Indications

Ciliary ablation is indicated to lower IOP in eyes that have poor visual potential or are poor candidates for incisional surgery. Surgery for blind eyes should be avoided, if possible, because of the small risk of sympathetic ophthalmia. Interventions such as retrobulbar alcohol injection, retrobulbar chlorpromazine injection, or enucleation can be considered for painful blind eyes. Ciliary body ablation is generally reserved for eyes that have been or are likely to be unresponsive to other modes of therapy.

Contraindications

Ciliary ablation is relatively contraindicated in eyes with good vision because of the risk of loss of visual acuity.

Preoperative evaluation

This step is the same as for incisional glaucoma surgery.

Methods and considerations

Cyclocryotherapy is no longer the most commonly used of these methods. *Transscleral Nd:YAG* and *transscleral diode laser cyclophotocoagulation* are better tolerated, causing less pain and inflammation than cyclocryotherapy. An *endoscopic laser delivery system* has been advocated for use with cataract surgery or in pediatric, pseudophakic, and aphakic eyes. Use of the argon laser aimed at the ciliary processes through a goniolens is possible in a small percentage of patients.

Postoperative management

Pain following these procedures may be substantial, and patients should be provided with adequate analgesics, including narcotics, during the immediate postoperative period.

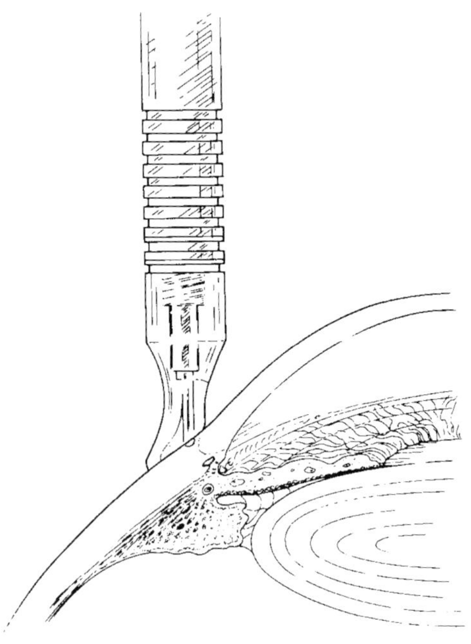

Figure 8-15 Cyclophotocoagulation. The diode laser handpiece attachment from one manufacturer is shown. After aligning the edge of the probe with the limbus, approximately 17–19 applications are placed 270° around the limbus, with a power of 1.5–2 W and a duration of approximately 2 seconds. *(Reproduced with permission from Weinreb RN, Mills RP, eds.* Glaucoma Surgery: Principles and Techniques. *2nd ed. Ophthalmology Monograph 4. San Francisco: American Academy of Ophthalmology; 1998:165.)*

Complications

Each of these procedures may result in prolonged hypotony, pain, inflammation, cystoid macular edema, hemorrhage, and even phthisis bulbi. Sympathetic ophthalmia is a rare but serious complication.

Pastor SA, Singh K, Lee DA, et al. Cyclophotocoagulation: a report by the American Academy of Ophthalmology. *Ophthalmology.* 2001;108:2130–2138.

Cyclodialysis

Cyclodialysis creates a direct communication between the anterior chamber and the suprachoroidal space. It can occur traumatically or surgically. Surgical cyclodialysis is rarely performed, but in the past may have been helpful in aphakic patients who did not respond to filtering surgery. In this procedure, a spatula is passed from the suprachoroidal space into the anterior chamber through a small scleral incision approximately 4 mm posterior to the limbus. Many complications can occur after the procedure, including bleeding, inflammation, and Descemet's detachment. Profound hypotony, or an equally significant rise in IOP should the cleft close, may also occur.

Nonpenetrating Glaucoma Surgery

Although the most widely accepted IOP-lowering incisional surgeries involve creating a direct communication between the anterior chamber and the subconjunctival space, nonpenetrating surgery has also been proposed. Nonpenetrating glaucoma procedures were initially described in the early 1970s. The goal was to achieve IOP lowering while avoiding some of the complications of standard trabeculectomy.

Recently, interest in nonpenetrating surgery has been revived. Several variations all involve a deep sclerectomy. These include deep sclerectomy, which may be performed with or without a collagen implant. Deep sclerectomy with injection of viscoelastic into Schlemm's canal has been described and named *viscocanalostomy.* Both nonpenetrating deep sclerectomy and viscocanalostomy involve creation of a superficial scleral flap and a deeper scleral dissection underneath to leave behind only a thin layer of sclera and Descemet's membrane.

At present, few long-term prospective, randomized data compare these new procedures with trabeculectomy. In theory, nonpenetrating surgery may avoid some of the complications associated with penetrating filtering surgery. However, the procedures are technically challenging, and initial results suggest that IOP reduction may be less than with trabeculectomy.

Netland PA, Ophthalmic Technology Assessment Committee, Glaucoma Panel, American Academy of Ophthalmology. Nonpenetrating glaucoma surgery. *Ophthalmology.* 2001;108: 416–421.

O'Brart DP, Rowlands E, Islam N, et al. A randomised, prospective study comparing trabeculectomy augmented with antimetabolites with a viscocanalostomy technique for the management of open angle glaucoma uncontrolled by medical therapy. *Br J Ophthalmol.* 2002;86:748–754.

Congenital/Infantile Glaucoma

For those glaucomas occurring within the first few years of life, initial surgical therapy is generally more effective than medical treatment. Goniotomy and trabeculotomy are the preferred procedures in congenital/infantile glaucoma. Goniotomy is possible only in an eye with a relatively clear cornea, whereas trabeculotomy can be performed whether the cornea is clear or cloudy. A standard trabeculotomy performed superiorly can be converted to trabeculectomy if needed. Published success rates are similar for trabeculotomy and goniotomy in eyes with clear corneas.

For an eye that has failed one of these procedures, debate continues whether the next procedure should be trabeculectomy with an antifibrotic agent or a glaucoma drainage device. Ciliary ablation is another procedure that can be considered in intractable cases. These procedures in infants are probably best performed by clinicians experienced in the surgical treatment of childhood glaucomas. BCSC Section 6, *Pediatric Ophthalmology and Strabismus,* discusses these issues in Chapter 21, Pediatric Glaucomas.

Goniotomy and Trabeculotomy

Indications

The presence of childhood glaucoma is an indication for surgery. The selection of procedure will, in part, depend on the training and experience of the surgeon.

Contraindications

Contraindications to surgery include an infant with unstable health, an infant with multiple anomalies with poor prognosis, and a grossly disorganized eye.

Preoperative evaluation

Thorough examination in the office is not always possible. Sometimes a bottle feeding will distract a young infant enough to allow tonometry and dilated examination. When this is not possible, examination under anesthesia is necessary. Surgery can be performed at the same or at a subsequent session. It is best not to dilate the eye expected to have angle surgery in order to better protect the lens during the procedure. BCSC Section 6 includes a chapter on examination techniques and tips written by pediatric ophthalmologists.

Technique

Most surgeons fill the anterior chamber with viscoelastic to prevent collapse and to tamponade bleeding. A disadvantage of viscoelastic use is that a postoperative IOP spike may occur if not all of the viscoelastic material is removed from the eye. With a *goniotomy,* a needle-knife is passed across the anterior chamber, and a superficial incision is made in the anterior aspect of the trabecular meshwork under gonioscopic control (Fig 8-16). A clear cornea is necessary to provide an adequate view of the chamber angle.

In a *trabeculotomy,* a fine wirelike instrument (trabeculotome) is inserted into Schlemm's canal from an external incision, and the trabecular meshwork is torn by rotating the trabeculotome into the anterior chamber (Fig 8-17). Schlemm's canal is more easily identified if a partial-thickness scleral flap is first elevated, similar to what occurs in a trabeculectomy. A gradual cutdown can then be made in order to better identify the canal. Alternative techniques have been developed in which a prolene or nylon suture is threaded through Schlemm's canal and the end is retrieved. The 2 ends of the suture are then pulled, and the suture ruptures the trabecular meshwork and passes into the anterior

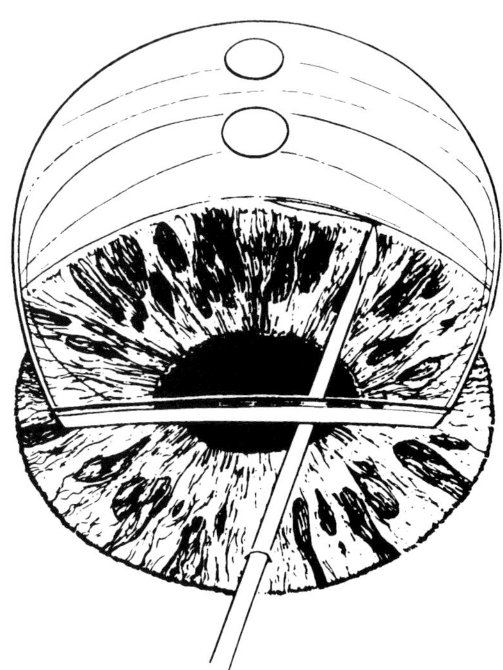

Figure 8-16 Goniotomy incision as seen through a surgical contact lens. *(Reproduced with permission from Shaffer RN.* Am J Ophthalmol. *1966;62:613–618. Copyright by the Ophthalmic Publishing Company.)*

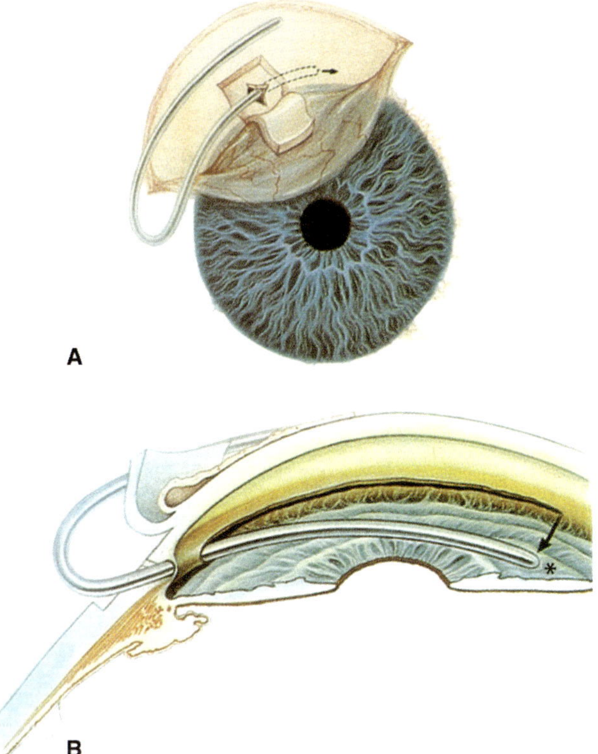

Figure 8-17 Trabeculotomy. **A,** Probe is gently passed along Schlemm's canal with little resistance for 6–10 mm. **B,** By rotating the probe internally *(arrow)*, the surgeon ruptures the trabeculum, and the probe appears in the anterior chamber with minimum bleeding. *(Reproduced and modified with permission from Kolker AE, Hetherington J, eds.* Becker-Shaffer's Diagnosis and Therapy of the Glaucomas. *5th ed. St Louis: Mosby; 1983.)*

chamber. The suture is then removed. This process may be performed over 180° or 360° of the angle. Trabeculotomy is particularly useful if the cornea is too cloudy to allow adequate visualization for goniotomy. However, the abnormal angle anatomy associated with congenital glaucomas sometimes precludes localization of Schlemm's canal.

Complications

Complications of both of these operations include hyphema, infection, lens damage, and uveitis. Descemet's membrane may be stripped during trabeculotomy. General anesthesia may cause serious complications in children, and bilateral procedures are indicated in some children because of anesthetic risks. There is a long-term risk of amblyopia, and the child must be followed closely over time. IOP elevation may recur at any time.

Beck AD, Lynch MG. Pediatric glaucoma. *Focal Points: Clinical Modules for Ophthalmologists.* San Francisco: American Academy of Ophthalmology. 1997, module 5.

Basic Texts

Glaucoma

Anderson DR, Patella VM. *Automated Static Perimetry.* 2nd ed. St Louis: Mosby; 1999.

Drance SM, Anderson DR, eds. *Automatic Perimetry in Glaucoma: A Practical Guide.* Orlando, FL: Grune & Stratton; 1985.

Epstein DL, Allingham RR, Schuman JS, eds. *Chandler and Grant's Glaucoma.* 4th ed. Baltimore: Williams & Willkins; 1997.

Harrington DO, Drake MV. *The Visual Fields: A Textbook and Atlas of Clinical Perimetry.* 6th ed. St Louis: Mosby; 1989.

Hart WM Jr, ed. *Adler's Physiology of the Eye: Clinical Application.* 9th ed. St Louis: Mosby; 1992.

Minckler DS, Van Buskirk EM, eds. Glaucoma. In: Wright KW, ed. *Color Atlas of Ophthalmic Surgery.* Philadelphia: Lippincott; 1992.

Ritch R, Shields MB, Krupin T, eds. *The Glaucomas.* 2nd ed. St Louis: Mosby; 1996.

Shields MB. *Textbook of Glaucoma.* 4th ed. Baltimore: Williams & Wilkins; 1997.

Stamper RL, Lieberman MF, Drake MV, eds. *Becker-Shaffer's Diagnosis and Therapy of the Glaucomas.* 7th ed. St Louis: Mosby; 1999.

Tasman W, Jaeger EA, eds. *Duane's Clinical Ophthalmology.* Philadelphia: Lippincott; 1998.

Thomas JV, Belcher CD III, Simmons RJ, eds. *Glaucoma Surgery.* St Louis: Mosby; 1992.

Zimmerman TJ, Kooner KS, Sharir M, Fechtner RD. *Textbook of Ocular Pharmacology.* Philadelphia: Lippincott; 1997.

Related Academy Materials

Focal Points: Clinical Modules for Ophthalmologists

Balyeat HD. Cataract surgery in the glaucoma patient, part 1: a cataract surgeon's perspective (Module 3, 1998).
Beck AD, Lynch MG. Pediatric glaucoma (Module 5, 1997).
Camras CB. Diagnosis and management of complications of glaucoma filtering surgery (Module 3, 1994).
Drake MV. A primer on automated perimetry (Module 8, 1993).
Greenfield DS. Dysfunctional glaucoma filtration blebs (Module 4, 2002).
Gross RL. Cyclodestructive procedures for glaucoma (Module 4, 1992).
Heuer D, Lloyd MA. Management of glaucomas with poor surgical prognoses (Module 1, 1995).
Jampel HD. Normal (low) tension glaucoma (Module 12, 1991).
Johnson CA, Spry PG. Advances in automated perimetry (Module 10, 2002).
Lieberman JM. Pigmentary glaucoma: new insights (Module 2, 1998).
Lundy DC. Ciliary block glaucoma (Module 3, 1999).
McGrath DJ, Ferguson JG Jr., Sanborn GE. Neovascular glaucoma (Module 7, 1997).
Mikelberg FS. Normal-tension glaucoma: the next generation of glaucoma management (Module 12, 2000).
Mitrev PV, Schuman JS. Lasers in glaucoma management (Module 9, 2001).
Moster MR, Azuara-Blanco A. Techniques of glaucoma filtration surgery (Module 6, 2000).
Panek WC. Role of laser treatment in glaucoma (Module 1, 1993).
Ritch R. Exfoliation syndrome (Module 9, 1994).
Rockwood EJ. Medical treatment of open-angle glaucoma (Module 10, 1993).
Samples JR. Management of glaucoma secondary to uveitis (Module 5, 1995).
Serle JB, Podos SM. New therapeutic options for the treatment of glaucoma (Module 5, 1999).
Sidoti PA, Heuer DK. Aqueous shunting procedures (Module 3, 2002).
Skuta GL. Cataract surgery in the glaucoma patient, part 2: a glaucoma surgeon's perspective (Module 4, 1998).
Wilson RM, Brandt JD. Update on Glaucoma Clinical Trials (Module 9, 2003).

Publications

Alward WL. *Color Atlas of Gonioscopy* (2000).
Lane SS, Skuta GL, eds. *ProVision: Preferred Responses in Ophthalmology. Series 3* (Self-Assessment Program, 2001).
Netland PA, Allen RC, eds. *Glaucoma Medical Therapy: Principles and Management* (Ophthalmology Monograph 13, 1999).

Skuta GL, ed. *ProVision: Preferred Responses in Ophthalmology. Series 2* (Self-Assessment Program, 2001).

Spencer WH, ed. *Robert N. Schaeffer, MD, at 90: An Oral History and Memoir* (2002).

Walsh TJ, ed. *Visual Fields: Examination and Interpretation.* 2nd ed. (Ophthalmology Monograph 3, 1996).

Weinreb RN, Mills RP, eds. *Glaucoma Surgery: Principles and Techniques.* 2nd ed. (Ophthalmology Monograph 4, 1998).

Wilson FM II, Gurland JE, eds. *Practical Ophthalmology: A Manual for Beginning Residents* (1996).

Slide-Script

Coleman A. *Glaucoma: Diagnosis and Management* (Eye Care Skills for the Primary Care Physician Series, 1999).

Multimedia

Eye Care Skills on CD-ROM (all seven titles from the Eye Care Skills for the Primary Care Physician Series) (2001).

ProVision Interactive: Clinical Case Studies. (Volume 2: Retina and Glaucoma on CD-ROM, 1997).

Sherwood MB, Brandt JD, Choplin NT, et al. LEO *Clinical Update Course on Glaucoma* (CD-ROM, 2001).

Continuing Ophthalmic Video Education

Lewis RA. *Goldmann Applanation Tonometry* (1988).

Ramanathan US, Choi JTL, Kumar V, et al. *Lamellar Scleral Patch Graft for the Repair of Leaking Trabeculectomy Bleb with Full-Thickness Scleral Deficits;* Prasad KK, Garudadri CS, Mandal AK, et al. *Gonioscopy: Learn and Teach;* Cohn HC. *The Evolution of Glaucoma Filtering Surgery* (2001).

Preferred Practice Patterns Committee, Glaucoma Panel. *Primary Open-Angle Glaucoma Suspect* (2002).

Preferred Practice Patterns Committee, Glaucoma Panel. *Primary Angle Closure* (2000).

Preferred Practice Patterns Committee, Glaucoma Panel. *Primary Open-Angle Glaucoma* (2003).

Ophthalmic Technology Assessments

Ophthalmic Technology Assessment Committee. *Automated Perimetry* (2002).

Ophthalmic Technology Assessment Committee. *Cyclophotocoagulation* (2001).

Ophthalmic Technology Assessment Committee. *Laser Peripheral Iridotomy for Pupillary-Block Glaucoma* (1994).

Ophthalmic Technology Assessment Committee. *Laser Trabeculoplasty for Primary Open-Angle Glaucoma* (1996).

Ophthalmic Technology Assessment Committee. *Nonpenetrating Glaucoma Surgery* (2001).

Ophthalmic Technology Assessment Committee. *Optic Nerve Head and Retinal Nerve Fiber Layer Analysis* (1999).

Complementary Therapy Assessments

Complementary Therapy Task Force. *Marijuana in the Treatment of Glaucoma* (2003).

LEO Specialty Clinical Update Online

Brandt JD, Pasquale, LR, eds. *Glaucoma,* Volume 1 (2004).

To order any of these materials, please call the Academy's Customer Service number at (415) 561-8540, or order online at www.aao.org.

Credit Reporting Form

Basic and Clinical Science Course, 2004–2005
Section 10

The American Academy of Ophthalmology is accredited by the Accreditation Council for Continuing Medical Education to provide continuing medical education for physicians.

The American Academy of Ophthalmology designates this educational activity for a maximum of 30 category 1 credits toward the AMA Physician's Recognition Award. Each physician should claim only those hours of credit that he/she actually spent in the activity.

The American Medical Association has determined that non-US licensed physicians who participate in this CME activity are eligible for AMA PRA category 1 credit.

If you wish to claim continuing medical education credit for your study of this section, you may claim your credit online or fill in the required forms and mail or fax them to the Academy.

To use the forms:

1. Complete the study questions and mark your answers on the Section Completion Form.
2. Complete the Section Evaluation.
3. Fill in and sign the statement below.
4. Return this page and the required forms by mail or fax to the CME Registrar (see below).

To claim credit online:

1. Log on to the Academy website (www.aao.org).
2. Go to Education Resource Center; click on CME Central.
3. Follow the instructions.

Important: These completed forms or the online claim must be received at the Academy within 3 years of purchase.

I hereby certify that I have spent _____ (up to 30) hours of study on the curriculum of this section and that I have completed the Study Questions.

Signature: ____
Date

Name: ____

Address: ____

City and State: ______________________________ Zip: __________

Telephone: (________) ____________________ Academy Member ID# ______________
area code

Please return completed forms to:
American Academy of Ophthalmology
P.O. Box 7424
San Francisco, CA 94120-7424
Attn: CME Registrar, Clinical Education

Or you may fax them to: 415-561-8557

2004–2005
Section Completion Form

Basic and Clinical Science Course

Answer Sheet for Section 10

Question	Answer	Question	Answer
1	a b c d e	23	a b c d e
2	a b c d	24	a b c d e
3	a b c d	25	a b c d e
4	a b c d e	26	a b c d e
5	a b c d e	27	a b c d e
6	a b c d e	28	a b c d e
7	a b c d	29	a b c d e
8	a b c d	30	a b c d e
9	a b c d	31	a b c d e
10	a b c d	32	a b c d
11	a b c d e	33	a b c d e
12	a b c d	34	a b c d e
13	a b c d e	35	a b c d e
14	a b c d	36	a b c d
15	a b c d e	37	a b c d e
16	a b c d e	38	a b c d
17	a b c d e	39	a b c d e
18	a b c d e	40	a b c d e
19	a b c d e	41	a b c d
20	a b c d e	42	a b c d
21	a b c d e	43	a b c d e
22	a b c d e		

Section Evaluation

Please complete this CME questionnaire.

1. To what degree will you use knowledge from BCSC Section 10 in your practice?
   - ☐ Regularly
   - ☐ Sometimes
   - ☐ Rarely

2. Please review the stated objectives for BCSC Section 10. How effective was the material at meeting those objectives?
   - ☐ All objectives were met.
   - ☐ Most objectives were met.
   - ☐ Some objectives were met.
   - ☐ Few or no objectives were met.

3. To what degree is BCSC Section 10 likely to have a positive impact on health outcomes of your patients?
   - ☐ Extremely likely
   - ☐ Highly likely
   - ☐ Somewhat likely
   - ☐ Not at all likely

4. After you review the stated objectives for BCSC Section 10, please let us know of any additional knowledge, skills, or information useful to your practice that were acquired but were not included in the objectives. [Optional]

5. Was BCSC Section 10 free of commercial bias?
   - ☐ Yes
   - ☐ No

6. If you selected "No" in the previous question, please comment. [Optional]

7. Please tell us what might improve the applicability of BCSC to your practice. [Optional]

Study Questions

Although a concerted effort has been made to avoid ambiguity and redundancy in these questions, the authors recognize that differences of opinion may occur regarding the "best" answer. The discussions are provided to demonstrate the rationale used to derive the answer. They may also be helpful in confirming that your approach to the problem was correct or, if necessary, in fixing the principle in your memory. Where relevant, additional references are given.

1. In normals, the average normal corneal thickness is
   a. 520 μm
   b. 540 μm
   c. 560 μm
   d. 580 μm
   e. 600 μm
2. In AGIS, the Advanced Glaucoma Intervention Study, patients had significantly better outcomes if their IOP was controlled
   a. below 18 mm Hg at all visits
   b. below 18 mm Hg at 50% of visits
   c. below 14 mm Hg at all visits
   d. below 14 mm Hg at 50% of visits
3. In the CNTG, Collaborative Normal-Tension Glaucoma Treatment Study, progression was reduced by nearly threefold by a reduction in IOP of
   a. 20%
   b. 30%
   c. 40%
   d. 50%
4. In the GLT, the Glaucoma Laser Trial, the group treated with laser, compared to the group treated with medical therapy, showed
   a. 20% lower IOP
   b. 20% less visual field loss
   c. nearly equivalent outcomes
   d. 10% greater IOP
   e. 10% greater visual field loss
5. A feature *not* associated with exfoliation syndrome is
   a. spontaneous lens dislocation
   b. earlier cataract formation
   c. higher incidence of vitreous loss during cataract surgery
   d. volatile IOPs
   e. deeper anterior chamber angles

6. In pigmentary dispersion syndrome with elevated IOP,
   a. laser iridotomy may help deepen the chamber
   b. laser trabeculoplasty requires greater energy settings
   c. African-American ancestry is more common
   d. myopic nerves may make detection of early glaucomatous change more difficult
   e. the risk of hyoptony maculopathy after filtration surgery with antimetabolites is reduced
7. All of the following statements about aqueous humor are true *except:*
   a. Aqueous humor is formed at a rate of approximately 2–3 μL/min.
   b. There is a 1% turnover in aqueous volume each minute.
   c. Normal aqueous humor has a high protein content.
   d. The composition of aqueous humor is altered as it flows from the posterior chamber through the pupil and into the anterior chamber.
8. Elevated episcleral venous pressure
   a. may be seen with facial hemangiomas
   b. can cause the collapse of Schlemm's canal and an increase in aqueous humor resistance
   c. causes a 1 mm Hg increase in intraocular pressure for every 1-mm increase in episcleral venous pressure in acute conditions
   d. all of the above
9. Screening for glaucoma based solely on IOP >21 mm Hg
   a. may miss up to half of the people with glaucoma in the screened population
   b. is a good strategy because glaucomatous damage is caused exclusively by pressures that are higher than 21 mm Hg
   c. is effective because IOPs in a population have a gaussian distribution
   d. is effective because a clear line exists between safe and unsafe IOP
10. The preferred therapy for infantile glaucoma is
    a. topical beta blockers
    b. topical bromonidine
    c. trabeculotomy or goniotomy
    d. oral acetazolamide
11. Sturge-Weber syndrome
    a. is usually bilateral
    b. is always inherited in an autosomal dominant pattern
    c. is more common in males
    d. is rarely associated with glaucoma
    e. may be associated with glaucoma in infants

12. Goldmann tonometry
    a. is not affected by alteration in scleral rigidity
    b. is unaffected by laser in situ keratomileusis (LASIK)
    c. may give an artificially high IOP measurement with increased central corneal thickness
    d. may give pressure measurements taken over a corneal scar that are falsely low
13. Elevated episcleral venous pressure may be associated with all the following *except:*
    a. Sturge-Weber syndrome
    b. facial cutaneous angiomas, such as nevus flammeus
    c. foreshortening of the conjunctival fornices
    d. thyroid ophthalmopathy
    e. dilation of episcleral vessels
14. Automated perimetry
    a. requires the pupil diameter to be at least 5 mm to obtain reliable results
    b. often employs "staircase" strategies to estimate the threshold sensitivity at individual locations
    c. is useful for the detection of glaucomatous vision loss but not for assessing progression of loss
    d. prevents lens rim artifacts, which are common with manual perimetry
15. With regard to neurofibromatosis:
    a. It may be associated with glaucoma.
    b. Anterior segment abnormalities and angle closure may develop.
    c. Plexiform neuromas may produce S-shaped upper eyelid deformities.
    d. Plexiform neuromas are a hallmark of type 1 variant neurofibromatosis.
    e. All of the above are true.
16. With regard to anterior chamber angle pigmentation, all of the following are true *except:*
    a. Pigmentation commonly increases with age.
    b. Decreased pigmentation is common following ocular trauma with hyphemas.
    c. Both exfoliation syndrome and pigment dispersion syndrome have increase angle pigmentation.
    d. Sampaolesi's line is a scalloped line of pigment deposition anterior to Schwalbe's line.
    e. Pigmentation of the angle is dynamic and changes over time.
17. Which of the following systemic disorders is not typically associated with glaucoma?
    a. tuberous asclerosis
    b. juvenile xanthogranuloma
    c. ocular dermal melanocytosis
    d. Fuchs endothelial dystrophy
    e. Bourneville syndrome

18. The anterior optic nerve
    a. has a diameter of of approximately 1.5 mm
    b. is commonly divided into 4 regions (nerve fiber layer, prelaminar, lamina, cribrosa and retrolaminar)
    c. receives its blood supply from both the central retinal artery and the posterior ciliary arteries
    d. is composed primarily of retinal ganglion cell axons, vascular tissues, glial tissues, and extracellular matrix
    e. all of the above
19. The prevalence of glaucoma is
    a. equal in blacks and whites
    b. 2 times more common in whites than blacks
    c. 8 to 10 times more common in whites than in blacks
    d. 3 to 6 times higher in blacks than in whites
    e. 2 times higher in blacks than in whites
20. The inheritance pattern of the 6 primary loci for adult-onset glaucoma is
    a. autosomal recessive
    b. autosomal dominant
    c. sex-linked
    d. more than one of the above
    e. none of the above
21. The percentage of primary congenital glaucoma that is now known to have a definite genetic component is
    a. 1%
    b. 10%
    c. 25%
    d. 50%
    e. 75%
22. Which of the following is *least* compelling as a risk factor for primary open-angle glaucoma (POAG)?
    a. IOP
    b. age
    c. race
    d. diabetes
    e. family history
23. The gene known to be associated with aniridia is
    a. *CYP1B1*
    b. *P1TX2*
    c. *FKHL7*
    d. *PAX6*
    e. *LMX1B*

24. Which of the following is *not true* regarding the gene known to cause *GLC1A*-associated glaucoma?
    a. It involves an abnormality of the TIGR/myocilin protein.
    b. It is associated with juvenile open-angle glaucoma.
    c. It is associated with adult open-angle glaucoma.
    d. It is found on chromosome 1.
    e. It is associated with a single, specific mutation.

25. Anterior chamber depth
    a. is less in women than in men
    b. increases with increasing age
    c. is increased by hyperopia
    d. is decreased in very high myopia
    e. rarely correlates with anterior chamber volume

26. Long-term (10-year) success after laser trabeculoplasty is achieved in what percentage of patients?
    a. 90%
    b. 70%
    c. 50%
    d. 30%
    e. none

27. Incisional surgery for glaucoma may be required in all of the following situations *except:*
    a. Maximal tolerated medical therapy fails to adequately reduce IOP.
    b. The patient is treated with multiple glaucoma medications and has had an adverse reaction to a glaucoma medication.
    c. Medical therapy necessary to control IOP is not well tolerated or places the patient at unacceptable risk.
    d. Glaucomatous optic neuropathy or visual field loss is progressing despite apparently "adequate" reduction of IOP with medical therapy.
    e. The patient cannot comply with the necessary medical regimen.

28. A single intraoperative application of mitomycin C has been associated with an increased risk of
    a. hyoptony
    b. bleb hyperemia
    c. bleb leaks and infections
    d. all of the above
    e. a and c only

29. Glaucoma drainage implants are indicated for all of the following conditions or situations *except:*
    a. elevated IOP despite maximal medical therapy
    b. a failed trabeculectomy
    c. conjunctival scarring
    d. poor prognosis for success of trabeculectomy
    e. ICE syndrome

30. Complications of cyclophotocoagulation include
    a. hypotony
    b. vision loss
    c. phthisis bulbi
    d. all of the above
    e. a and c only

31. The drawing shows a Zeiss gonioprism on a patient's right eye. The clock-hour of the angle that corresponds to the X is
    a. 11:00
    b. 1:00
    c. 4:00
    d. 7:00
    e. 6:00

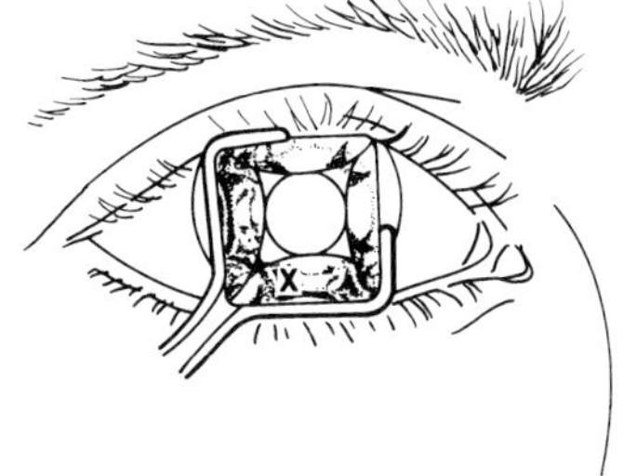

32. All of the following statements regarding Goldmann applanation tonometry are true *except:*
    a. The diameter of the applanated area is 3.06 mm.
    b. The tear film creates surface tension that increases the force of applanation.
    c. The cornea tends to resist deformation, which tends to balance out the surface tension effect of the tear film.
    d. The IOP tends to be overestimated in eyes with low scleral rigidity.

33. Each of the following conditions may produce nerve fiber bundle visual field defects similar to those seen in glaucoma *except:*
    a. chronic papilledema
    b. optic disc drusen
    c. AION
    d. occipital infarction
    e. branch retinal artery occlusion

34. All of the following are histologic changes in glaucoma *except:*
    a. posterior bowing of the lamina cribrosa
    b. thinning of the retinal nerve fiber layer
    c. loss of the outer nuclear layer of the retina
    d. loss of ganglion cells in the retina
    e. peripapillary atrophy

35. Secondary angle closure with pupillary block is the usual mechanism for glaucoma in each of the following conditions *except:*
    a. an intumescent lens
    b. iris neovascularization
    c. microspherophakia
    d. uveitis
    e. ectopia lentis

36. The iridocorneal endothelial (ICE) syndromes include all of the following *except:*
    a. Chandler syndrome
    b. Axenfeld-Rieger syndrome
    c. iris nevus syndrome
    d. essential iris atrophy

37. All of the following are true of ciliary block glaucoma, or malignant glaucoma, *except:*
    a. It responds to aqueous suppressants and hyperosmotic medical management in approximately 50% of cases.
    b. It results from posterior misdirection of aqueous into the vitreous cavity.
    c. It occurs only after incisional surgery and never following laser treatment.
    d. It occurs most commonly in eyes with a history of angle-closure glaucoma.
    e. It may occur in aphakic or pseudophakic eyes.

38. Which of the following causes of developmental glaucoma does *not* involve trabeculodysgenesis as a part of its pathophysiology?
    a. Sturge-Weber
    b. homocystinuria
    c. aniridia
    d. Peters anomaly

39. Which of the following beta blockers demonstrates the relative selectivity in the manner described?
    a. betaxolol: relatively selective for $beta_2$ receptors
    b. timolol: relatively selective for $beta_1$ receptors
    c. levobunolol: relatively selective for $beta_2$ receptors
    d. betaxolol: relatively selective for $beta_1$ receptors
    e. levobunolol: relatively selective for $beta_1$ receptors

40. All of the following statements concerning pilocarpine are true *except:*
    a. By relaxing tension on the zonular fibers, it may cause narrowing of the anterior chamber.
    b. It is a direct cholinergic agonist.
    c. It reduces IOP by increasing aqueous flow.
    d. It inhibits acetylcholinesterase.
    e. It is relatively contraindicated in the treatment of uveitic glaucoma.

41. The secondary angle-closure glaucoma in which peripheral anterior synechiae (PAS) extend anterior to Schwalbe's line is
    a. Axenfeld-Rieger syndrome
    b. neovascular glaucoma
    c. ICE syndrome
    d. Fuchs heterochromic iridocyclitis

42. The condition in which iris neovascularization is *not* associated with PAS and secondary angle closure is
    a. Fuchs heterochromic iridocyclitis
    b. ocular ischemic syndrome
    c. central retinal vein occlusion
    d. chronic retinal detachment

43. An 80-year-old white male presents with poor vision in his right eye with sudden onset of pain and conjunctival hyperemia. The examination reveals an IOP of 45 with a prominent cell and flare reaction without keratic precipitates, a dense cataract, and an open anterior chamber angle. The most likely diagnosis is
    a. phacolytic glaucoma
    b. phacoanaphylaxis
    c. ICE syndrome
    e. Fuchs heterochromic iridocyclitis

Answers

1. **b.** Average central corneal thickness ranges between 536 and 544 μm, depending on the type of pachymeter used.
2. **a.** AGIS found that patients with IOP consistently less than 18 mm Hg and an average IOP of 12.2 mm Hg had significantly better outcomes than patients with greater IOP fluctuations and higher average IOP.
3. **b.** The target pressure set in CNTG was 30%.
4. **c.** The GLT found that both arms of the study did equally well.
5. **e.** Patients with exfoliation syndrome tend to have narrow anterior chamber angles.
6. **d.** Patients with pigmentary dispersion syndrome are usually myopic with increased pigmentation of the trabecular meshwork. As a result, they require less energy with laser trabeculoplasty and have a higher incidence of hypotony maculopathy. Laser peripheral iridectomy may flatten the peripheral iris contour but will not deepen the anterior chamber in this condition.
7. **c.** Aqueous humor is essentially protein-free (1/200 to 1/500 of the protein found in plasma), which allows for optical clarity.
8. **d.** Each of the statements is correct.
9. **a.** Pooled data from large epidemiologic studies indicate that the mean IOP is approximately 16 mm Hg, with a standard deviation of 3 mm Hg. IOP, however, has a non-gaussian distribution with a skew toward higher pressures, especially in individuals over age 40. For the population as a whole, no clear line exists between safe and unsafe IOP. Screening for glaucoma based solely on IOP >21 mm Hg may miss up to half of the people with glaucoma in the screened population.
10. **c.** Medications have limited long-term value for congenital and infantile glaucoma in most cases, and the preferred therapy is surgical. The initial procedures of choice are goniotomy or trabeculotomy if the cornea is clear, and trabeculotomy ab externo if the cornea is hazy. Bromonidine should not be used in infants and topical beta blockers should be used cautiously.
11. **e.** Sturge-Weber syndrome is usually a unilateral condition. There is no race or gender predilection, and no inheritance pattern has been established. Glaucoma occurs in 30%–70% of patients. When glaucoma is seen in infants with this syndrome, it is thought to be due to congenital anterior chamber anomalies (similar to congenital glaucoma).
12. **c.** Increased central corneal thickness may give an artifically high IOP, and decreased central corneal thickness may give an artifically low IOP. IOP measured after PRK and laser in situ keratomileusis (LASIK) may be reduced because of changes in the corneal thickness induced by these procedures. Pressure measurements taken over a corneal scar will be falsely high secondary to increased corneal rigidity.
13. **c.** Foreshortening of the conjunctival fornices does not affect episcleral venous pressure.
14. **b.** Automated perimetry uses a variety of "staircase" strategies to estimate the threshold sensitivity. The strategy chosen will affect the speed and reproducibility of the visual field produced.

15. **e.** Each of the statements about neurofibromatosis is correct.

16. **b.** Ocular trauma with hyphemas usually will increase anterior chamber angle pigmentation.

17. **d.** Fuchs endothelial dystrophy is an ocular disorder that can, in very rare situations, cause a secondary angle-closure glaucoma.

18. **e.** Each of the statements is correct.

19. **d.** The prevalence of glaucoma in the black population is estimated to be 3 to 6 times higher than in the white population.

20. **b.** The 6 described POAG loci all appear to be inherited in an autosomal dominant pattern.

21. **e.** It is surprising that the 3 genes identified for primary congenital glaucoma are estimated to account for 75% of all known forms of the disease.

22. **d.** The data are the least compelling for diabetes being a risk factor for high-pressure POAG.

23. **d.** *CYP1B1* is responsible for primary congenital glaucoma. *PITX2* is associated with Rieger syndrome. *FKHL7* is associated with iridodysgenesis, and *LMX1B* is associated with nail-patella syndrome.

24. **e.** Over 40 mutations are known for *GLC1A*.

25. **a.** Anterior chamber depth decreases with increasing age and correlates with anterior chamber volume. Anterior chamber depth tends to be reduced in hyperopia and increased with myopia.

26. **d.** Although initial success rates are high after laser trabeculoplasty, the success rate declines over time to approximately 50% after 3–5 years and 30% after 10 years.

27. **b.** Many patients require more than one glaucoma medication to control their disease. Adverse reactions may occur with any glaucoma medication. These reactions resolve when the medication is discontinued. Usually an alternative medication or laser trabeculoplasty can be used to successfully treat the patient.

28. **e.** Use of mytomycin C during filtration surgery has been associated with persistent ocular hypotony, bleb leaks, and infections. The blebs are often less vascular than the surrounding tissues that are not treated with mitomycin C.

29. **a.** The usual primary glaucoma surgery is trabeculectomy. If patients have failed prior trabeculectomy, have inadequate conjunctiva (eg, due to extensive prior ocular surgery), or have a poor prognosis for successful trabeculectomy (eg, active uveitis, neovascular glaucoma, ICE syndrome), they may be candidates for drainage implant surgery.

30. **d.** Cyclophotocoagulation may be associated with visual loss, hypotony, pain, inflammation, cystoid macular edema, hemorrhage, and even phthisis bulbi. Sympathetic ophthalmia is a rare but serious complication.

31. **a.** With the Zeiss gonioprism, the superior angle is seen in the inferior mirror, but the nasal and temporal orientation is not changed.

32. **d.** The IOP in eyes with low scleral rigidity may be underestimated with applanation tonometry, although this effect is more pronounced when techniques of indentation tonometry are used.

33. **d.** All of the choices except occipital infarction may produce nerve fiber bundle defects that can mimic the visual field loss seen in glaucoma. Occipital infarction would typically produce a homonymous hemianopia.

34. **c.** Loss of the outer nuclear layer is not observed in glaucoma. Glaucoma results in loss of ganglion cells and their axons, which make up the retinal nerve fiber layer.

35. **b.** All of these conditions are associated with pupillary block except iris neovascularization.

36. **b.** Iris nevus syndrome, Chandler syndrome, and essential iris atrophy are the 3 characteristic syndromes that relate to the spectrum of findings that may be seen in the iridocorneal endothelial syndromes. Axenfeld-Rieger syndrome is a disorder of the iris stroma that may have other associated ocular and systemic abnormalities.

37. **c.** Ciliary block, or malignant, glaucoma is characterized by a shallow anterior chamber with elevated IOP as a result of posterior misdirection of aqueous. It occurs most commonly following intraocular surgery in eyes with a history of angle-closure glaucoma, but it may also follow laser iridectomy or other procedures. It has been reported in aphakic and pseudophakic eyes as well as phakic eyes.

38. **b.** Trabeculodysgenesis is probably the most common pathophysiologic mechanism behind the entire category of developmental glaucomas. It has never been reported in homocystinuria.

39. **d.** Because of its relative $beta_1$ selectivity, betaxolol has fewer pulmonary side effects. Timolol and levobunolol are nonselective beta blockers.

40. **d.** An indirect cholinergic agonist would inhibit cholinesterase. Pilocarpine is a direct-acting cholinergic agonist.

41. **c.** ICE syndrome has an abnormal corneal endothelium that allows for the PAS to extend anterior to Schwalbe's line. Neovascular glaucoma and Fuchs heterochromic iridocyclitis have a normal corneal endothelium. In Axenfeld-Rieger syndrome, Schwalbe's line is displaced anteriorly; however, the PAS are limited to this anterior displacement.

42. **a.** Fine neovascularization of the iris and anterior chamber angle occurs in Fuchs heterochromic iridocyclitis, but it is not associated with angle closure and PAS formation. The other three conditions can cause iris neovascularization associated with PAS and secondary angle-closure glaucoma.

43. **a.** This is the classic presentation of a patient with phacolytic glaucoma. Without keratic precipitates, both phacoanaphylaxis and Fuchs heterochromic iridocyclitis are unlikely. Fuchs heterochromic iridocyclitis is associated with cataract formation, primarily posterior subcapsular cataracts, but it tends to present in a much younger patient. ICE syndrome occurs in younger patients and causes a secondary angle-closure glaucoma.

Index

(*i* = image; *t* = table)

Acetazolamide, for glaucoma, 162*t*, 168
Achromatic automated perimetry, in glaucoma, 57
Adnexa(ae), ocular, in glaucoma evaluation, 32
Adrenergic agonists, for glaucoma, 160*t*–161*t*, 169–171, 170*i*
Advanced Glaucoma Intervention Study (AGIS), 90*t*
Age
  as factor in primary angle closure, 123
  as factor in primary angle-closure glaucoma, 11
  as factor in primary open-angle glaucoma, 7–8, 10, 86, 91*t*
Air-puff tonometers, 28–29
Alpha$_2$ agonists, in suppression of aqueous formation, 19
Alpha$_2$-adrenergic agonists, for glaucoma, 161*t*, 170–171
Angiomatosis, encephalofacial (Sturge-Weber syndrome), glaucoma associated with, 32
Angle closure
  chronic, 126–127
  creeping, 126
  definition of, 120
  intermittent, 125–126
  iris-induced, 122
  mechanisms of, 120, 121*t*
  primary, 122–128. *See also* Angle-closure glaucoma, primary
  with pupillary block, lens-induced, 128–132, 129*i*, 131*i*, 131*t*
  subacute, 125–126
  without pupillary block, 121–122, 121*t*
Angle-closure glaucoma, 119–146. *See also* Glaucoma
  categories of, 120
  childhood (congenital/infantile/juvenile), management of, 207–209, 208*i*, 209*i*
    goniotomy in, 207–209, 208*i*, 209*i*
    trabeculotomy in, 207–209, 208*i*, 209*i*
  classification of, 5, 6*t*, 8*i*
    mechanisms of outflow obstruction in, 9*t*
  definition of, 120
  described, 119–120
  genes in, 15
  history of, 119
  iris-induced, 122
  lens-induced, 122
  management of
    medical, 175–176
    surgical, 197–200, 198*i*
      cataract extraction in, 200
      chamber deepening in, 200
      goniosynechialysis in, 200
      incisional, 200
      laser gonioplasty in, 199–200
      laser iridectomy, 197–199, 198*i*
  pathogenesis of, 120–122, 121*i*, 121*t*
  pathophysiology of, 120–122, 121*i*, 121*t*
  phakic, 132
  prevalence of, 119
  primary, 122–128
    acute, 124–125
      characteristics of, 6*t*
    age and, 11, 123
    chronic, 126–127
      characteristics of, 6*t*
    definition of, 122
    epidemiology of, 10–12
    family history and, 123–124
    gender and, 11, 123
    hereditary factors in, 12
    intermittent, 125–126
    ocular biometrics and, 123
    race and, 11, 122–123
    refraction and, 12, 124
    with relative pupillary block, characteristics of, 6*t*
    risk factors for, 122–124
    subacute, 125–126
      characteristics of, 6*t*
  pseudophakic, 132
  pupillary block in, 120–121, 121*i*
  secondary
    central retinal vein occlusion and, 144
    drug-induced, 145–146
    epithelial downgrowth and, 141–143
    fibrous downgrowth and, 141–143
    flat anterior chamber and, 145
    inflammation and, 138–140, 139*i*
    nanophthalmos and, 145
    nonrhegmatogenous retinal detachment and, 141
    persistent hyperplastic primary vitreous and, 145
    with pupillary block, 128–132, 129*i*, 131*i*, 131*t*
      characteristics of, 6*t*
      ectopia lentis, 130, 131*i*, 131*t*
      lens-induced, 128–132, 129*i*–131*i*, 131*t*
      microspherophakia and, 130, 131*i*
    retinal surgery and, 143–144
    retinal vascular disease and, 143–144
    retinopathy of prematurity and, 145
    trauma and, 143
    tumors and, 138
    uveal effusions and, 141
    without pupillary block, 132–146
      characteristics of, 6*t*
  types of, 119–120
Angle-recession glaucoma, 113–114, 113*i*
Aniridia, 153–154
Anterior chamber
  examination of, in glaucoma, 34–36, 34*i*, 35*i*, 35*t*
  flat, secondary angle-closure glaucoma and, 145
Anterior chamber intraocular lens, 132
Antifibrotic agents, in trabeculectomy, 188, 190–192
Antisense oligonucleotides, for glaucoma, 177
Aphakic glaucoma, 132
Applanation tonometer (applanation tonometry), 25–28, 26*i*, 27*i*, 28*t*
  sources of error in, 28*t*
Apraclonidine, for glaucoma, 161*t*, 170–171

Aqueous humor
  composition of, 18–19
  formation of, 17–20, 19*i*
    process in, 18
  intraocular pressure and, 17–23
  outflow of, 20–22, 21*i*
    measurement of, tonography in, 22
    trabecular, 19*i*, 20–22
    uveoscleral, 22
  rate of, 20
  suppression of, 19–20
Aqueous misdirection (malignant/ciliary block glaucoma; posterior aqueous diversion syndrome), 140–141, 140*i*
Arcuate scotoma, 60, 62*i*
Armaly-Drance screening perimetry, 78, 79*i*
Arteriovenous fistulae, glaucoma associated with, 32
Artifact(s), in visual field testing, 70–71, 72*i*, 73*i*
Automated static perimetry. *See* Perimetry, automated static
Autoregulation, vascular, disturbances of, in glaucoma, 51
Axenfeld-Rieger syndrome, 152, 153*t*
  differential diagnosis of, 153*t*
  glaucoma associated with, 32

Background, wavelength of, perimetry affected by, 65
Baltimore Eye Survey, 86, 91*t*
Beta-adrenergic antagonists. *See* Beta-blockers
Beta-blockers
  for glaucoma, 159, 160*t*, 165–166
    side effects of, 160*t*, 165
  in suppression of aqueous formation, 19
Betaxolol, for glaucoma, 160*t*, 165
Bimatoprost, for glaucoma, 162*t*, 171–172
Biometrics, ocular, as factor in primary angle closure, 123
Biomicroscopy
  in glaucoma, 33–36, 34*i*, 35*i*, 35*t*
  slit-lamp, in optic disc evaluation, 51
Blunt trauma, gonioscopic findings due to, 44, 45*i*
Bourneville syndrome (tuberous sclerosis), glaucoma associated with, 32
Brimonidine, for glaucoma, 161*t*, 170–171
Brinzolamide, for glaucoma, 163*t*, 168–169
Buphthalmos (megaloglobus), in childhood glaucoma, 147

Carbechol, for glaucoma, 162*t*, 166
Carbonic anhydrase inhibitors
  for glaucoma, 162*t*–163*t*, 168–169
  in suppression of aqueous formation, 19
Cardiovascular disease, primary open-angle glaucoma and, 89
Carteolol, for glaucoma, 160*t*, 165
Cataract extraction, for angle-closure glaucoma, 200
Cataract surgery, filtering surgery with, for open-angle glaucoma, 195–197
Central corneal thickness, in applanation tonometry measurements, 27–28
Central neurofibromatosis, developmental glaucoma and, 156
Central retinal vein occlusion (CRVO)
  primary open-angle glaucoma and, 90
  secondary angle-closure glaucoma and, 144
Chamber angle
  anterior, 127
  narrow, 127
  occludable, 127
Chamber deepening, for angle-closure glaucoma, 200
Children, glaucoma in, 147–156. *See also* Glaucoma, childhood (congenital/infantile/juvenile)
Choroidal melanomas, open-angle glaucoma caused by, 106
Chromosome(s), human artificial, for glaucoma, 177
Ciliary block glaucoma. *See* Aqueous misdirection (malignant/ciliary block glaucoma; posterior aqueous diversion syndrome)
Ciliary body ablation procedures, in lowering intraocular pressure, 204–206, 204*t*, 205*i*, 206*i*
  complications of, 206
  contraindications to, 205
  indications for, 205
  methods in, 205
  postoperative management, 205
  preoperative evaluation for, 205
Ciliary processes, in aqueous humor formation, 17, 19*i*
Circle of Zinn-Haller, 48, 49
Cloverleaf field, 70, 71*i*
Cockayne syndrome, childhood glaucoma and, 155*t*
Collaborative Initial Glaucoma Treatment Study (CIGTS), 86, 89*t*, 158
Collaborative Normal-Tension Glaucoma Study (CNTGS), 92
Confocal scanning laser ophthalmoscopy, in optic nerve head evaluation, 55
Conjunctiva, examination of, in glaucoma, 33
Contrast sensitivity, in glaucoma, 59
Cornea
  examination of, in glaucoma, 33–34
  thickness of, primary open-angle glaucoma and, 10
Corrected loss variance, 69
Corrected pattern standard deviation, 69
Corticosteroid(s)
  glaucoma induced by, 116–117
  intraocular pressure affected by, 116–117
Cosopt, for glaucoma, 164*t*, 173
Cow's eye, 147
Cranial nerve II. *See* Optic nerve (cranial nerve II)
Creeping angle closure, 126
Cupping of optic disc
  glaucomatous, 51–53, 52*t*, 53*i*
    in infants and children, 49–50
    physiologic cupping *vs.*, 52, 52*t*
  physiologic, glaucomatous cupping *vs.*, 52, 52*t*
  vertical cup–disc ratio, 52
Cyclodialysis, 44
  in lowering intraocular pressure, 206
Cycloplegic drugs, intraocular pressure affected by, 117

Decibel, definition of, 60
Decosanoid(s), for glaucoma, 164*t*, 171–172
Depression, definition of, 60
Developmental glaucoma, 147

Diabetes mellitus
adult-onset, primary open-angle glaucoma and, 10–11
primary open-angle glaucoma and, 88–89
Diffusion, in aqueous humor formation, 18
Digital pressure, for intraocular pressure estimation, 29
Dipivefrin, for glaucoma, 161*t*, 169–170
Diurnal variation, in intraocular pressure, 25
Dorzolamide, for glaucoma, 163*t*, 168
Drug(s). *See also specific drug*
cycloplegic, intraocular pressure affected by, 117
glaucoma caused by, 116–117
secondary angle-closure glaucoma caused by, 145–146

Early Manifest Glaucoma Trial, 88*t*
Echothiophate iodide, for glaucoma, 166
Ectopia lentis, 130, 131*i*, 131*t*
causes of, 131*t*
secondary angle-closure glaucoma and, 130, 131*i*, 131*t*
Effusion(s), uveal, secondary angle-closure glaucoma and, 141
Electroretinography, in glaucoma, 59
Elevated intraocular pressure
corticosteroids causing, 116–117
in glaucoma, 3
open-angle glaucoma without, 92–96, 94*t*. *See also* Glaucoma, normal-tension
primary open angle glaucoma and, 10
Encephalofacial angiomatosis (Sturge-Weber syndrome), glaucoma associated with, 32
Encephalotrigeminal angiomatosis (Sturge-Weber syndrome), 154
Endoscopic laser delivery system, in lowering intraocular pressure, 205
Environmental factors, in glaucoma, 15
Epinephrine, for glaucoma, 160*t*, 165, 169, 170, 170*i*
Episclera, examination of, in glaucoma, 33
Episcleral venous pressure, 22–23
elevated, open-angle glaucoma caused by, 108–109, 108*t*, 109*i*
Epithelial downgrowth (ingrowth), secondary angle-closure glaucoma and, 141–143
Exfoliation syndrome (pseudoexfoliation), 42, 99–101, 99*i*, 100*i*
External adnexae. *See* Ocular adnexa
Extracapsular cataract extraction, 132

False-negative rate, in visual field testing with perimetry, 71
False-positive rate, in visual field testing with perimetry, 71, 73*i*
Family history
as factor in primary angle closure, 123–124
as factor in primary open-angle glaucoma, 10, 87
FASTPAC, 66
Fetal alcohol syndrome, childhood glaucoma and, 155*t*
Fibrous downgrowth (stromal ingrowth), secondary angle-closure glaucoma and, 141–143
Filtering surgery, cataract surgery with, for open-angle glaucoma, 195–197
Fistula(ae), arteriovenous, glaucoma associated with, 32
Fixation, perimetry affected by, 62–63
Flat anterior chamber, secondary angle-closure glaucoma and, 145
Flicker sensitivity, in glaucoma, 59
Fluorophotometry, aqueous formations measured by, 20
5-Fluorouracil, in trabeculectomy, 190–191
Focal abnormalities, of optic disc, examination of, 54–55
Forkhead transcription factor, *RIEG* gene and, 15
Frequency doubling, described, 58
Frequency-doubling technology (FDT) perimetry, 58–59, 71*i*
Fuchs heterochromic iridocyclitis, glaucoma and, 107–108, 108*i*
Fundus, examination of, in glaucoma, 36

Gender
as factor in primary angle closure, 123
as factor in primary angle-closure glaucoma, 11
Gene(s)
in angle-closure glaucoma, 15
in congenital glaucoma, 15
glaucoma
currently mapped, 12–13, 13*t*
open-angle, 14
RIEG, 15
Genetic factors, in glaucoma, 12–15, 14*t*
Genetic testing, for glaucoma, 15
Genetic therapy
evolution of, 13
for glaucoma, 176–177
Ghost cell glaucoma, 112–113, 112*i*
Glaucoma. *See also* Angle-closure glaucoma; Open-angle glaucoma
angle-closure, 119–146
angle-recession, 113–114, 113*i*
characteristics of, 6*t*, 8
childhood (congenital/infantile/juvenile), 147–156
anomalies associated with, 152–156, 153*t*, 155*t*
characteristics of, 6*t*
classification of, 147
clinical features of, 148–150, 149*i*
cupping in, 49–50
definitions of, 147
developmental
with associated ocular or systemic anomalies, 152–156, 153*t*, 155*t*
Axenfeld-Rieger syndrome, 152, 153*t*
neurofibromatosis, 154, 156
Peters anomaly, 152–153, 153*t*
Sturge-Weber syndrome, 154
differential diagnosis of, 150, 151*t*
epidemiology of, 147–148
follow-up of, 150–151
genes in, 15
genetics of, 147–148
pathophysiology of, 148
primary, characteristics of, 6*t*
prognosis of, 150–151
secondary, characteristics of, 6*t*
signs and symptoms of, diagnostic considerations for, 150, 151*t*

ciliary block. *See* Aqueous misdirection (malignant/ciliary block glaucoma; posterior aqueous diversion syndrome)
classification of, 4–7, 4*t*, 6*t*, 7*i*, 8*i*, 9*t*
  conceptual means of, 4, 4*t*
  mechanisms of outflow obstruction in, 9*t*
clinical evaluation of, 31–81
  anterior chamber, 34–36, 34*i*, 35*i*, 35*t*
  conjunctiva, 33
  cornea, 33–34
  episclera, 33
  external adnexae, 32–33
  fundus, 36
  general examination in, 31–36, 34*i*, 35*i*, 35*t*
  gonioscopy in, 34–44, 34*i*, 35*i*, 35*t*
  iris, 36
  lens, 36
  optic nerve, 44, 46–49, 46*i*, 47*i*. *See also* Optic nerve (cranial nerve II)
  optic neuropathy, 49–57, 50*i*, 52*t*, 53*i*, 54*i*. *See also* Optic neuropathy, glaucomatous
  patient history in, 31
  peripheral anterior synechiae, gonioscopy in, 39
  pupils, 33
  refraction in, 31–32
  sclera, 33
  tests in, 80, 81*i*
  visual field examination in, 57–81. *See also* Visual field, clinical evaluation of, in glaucoma
combined-mechanism, 5, 7
  classification of, 5, 7
congenital, primary, characteristics of, 6*t*
congenital anomalies–related, characteristics of, 6*t*
corticosteroid-induced, 116–117
defects due to, patterns of, 60, 61*i*–64*i*
definition of, 3
developmental, 147
environmental factors in, 15
epidemiologic aspects of, 7–12
genes in, currently mapped, 12–13, 13*t*
genetic factors in, 12–15, 14*t*
genetic testing for, 15
ghost cell, 112–113, 112*i*
hemolytic, 112–113
hereditary factors in, 12–15, 14*t*
introduction to, 3–15
lens particle, 104–105, 105*i*
lens-induced, 103–106, 104*i*, 104*t*, 105*i*
  angle-closure, 104*t*
  open-angle, 103–106, 104*i*, 104*t*, 105*i*
low-tension, 92–96, 94*t*. *See also* Glaucoma, normal-tension
malignant. *See* Aqueous misdirection (malignant/ciliary block glaucoma; posterior aqueous diversion syndrome)
management of
  goal in, 57, 157
  medical, 157–177
    adrenergic agonists in, 160*t*–161*t*, 169–171, 170*i*
    agents used in, 159–174, 160*t*–164*t*, 170*i*. *See also specific agent*
    $alpha_2$-adrenergic agonists in, 161*t*, 170–171
    beta blockers in, 159, 160*t*, 165–166
    carbonic anhydrase inhibitors in, 162*t*–163*t*, 168–169
    combined medications in, 164*t*, 173
    compliance in, 176
    future therapy in, 176–177
    general approach to, 174–177
    hyperosmotic agents in, 164*t*, 173–174
    hypotensive lipids in, 163*t*–164*t*, 171–172
    in nursing mothers, 176
    parasympathomimetic agents, 161*t*–162*t*, 166–168
    during pregnancy, 176
  progression of, 158–159
  risk-benefit assessment in, 158
  surgical, 179–209. *See also* Laser trabeculoplasty
    nonpenetrating, 206–207
neovascular, 132–136, 133*t*, 134*i*, 135*i*
nerve fiber bundle defect in, 60
normal-tension, 92–96, 94*t*. *See also* Open-angle glaucoma, without elevated intraocular pressure
  clinical features of, 92–93
  diagnostic evaluation of, 94–95
  differential diagnosis of, 93–94, 94*t*
  prognosis of, 95
  treatment of, 95–96
open-angle. *See* Open-angle glaucoma
ophthalmoscopic signs of, 52, 52*t*
optic nerve changes in, causes of, 4
optic neuropathy associated with, 49–57, 50*i*, 52*t*, 53*i*, 54*i*. *See also* Optic neuropathy, glaucomatous
peripapillary atrophy in, 55
phacolytic, 104, 104*i*, 104*t*, 105*i*
phacomorphic, 122, 128–129, 130*i*, 131*i*
pigmentary, 101–103, 101*i*–103*i*
primary
  definition of, 5
  described, 5
secondary
  characteristics of, 6*t*
  definition of, 5
  described, 5
  developmental glaucoma and, 156
traumatic, 113–114, 113*i*
visual field changes in, causes of, 4
Glaucoma hemisphere test, 70, 71*i*
Glaucoma Laser Trial (GLT), 158
Glaucoma Laser Trial (GLT) Research Group, 180
Glaucoma suspect, 96–98, 97*i*
  characteristics of, 6*t*
  definition of, 96
Glaucoma tube shunt, 201–204. *See also* Tube-shunt surgery, in lowering intraocular pressure
Glaucomatocyclitic crisis (Posner-Schlossman syndrome), 107
Glaucomatous cupping. *See* Cupping of optic disc, glaucomatous
Glaukomflecken, 124
Glycerin, for glaucoma, 164*t*, 173–174
Goldmann applanation tonometer, 25–28, 26*i*, 27*i*, 28*t*
Goldmann equation, 17
Goldmann lens, 38
Goldmann perimeter. *See* Armaly-Drance screening perimetry

Goldmann-type lens, 39
Goniolens, 38–39
Gonioplasty, laser, for angle-closure glaucoma, 199–200
Gonioscopy
in blunt trauma evaluation, 44, 45*i*
described, 36–37, 37*i*
direct, 37–39, 37*i*
in glaucoma evaluation, 34–36, 34*i*, 35*i*, 35*t*, 36–44
indirect, 37–39, 37*i*
Koeppe-type lenses in, 38
normal angle landmarks in, 39–44, 41*i*–43*i*
in pigmentary dispersion syndrome, 101, 102*i*
Goniosynechialysis, for angle-closure glaucoma, 200
Goniotomy, trabeculotomy and, for childhood glaucoma, 207–209, 208*i*, 209*i*
complications of, 209
contraindications to, 207
indications for, 207
preoperative evaluation for, 208
technique for, 208–209, 208*i*, 209*i*

Hallermann-Streiff syndrome (dysphalic mandibulo-oculofacial syndrome, François dyscephalic syndrome), childhood glaucoma and, 155*t*
Hemolytic glaucoma, 112–113
Hemorrhage(s), splinter, in glaucoma, 53–54, 54*i*
Hereditary factors
in glaucoma, 12–15, 14*t*
in primary angle-closure glaucoma, 12
High-pass resolution perimetry, 58
Human artificial chromosomes (HACs), for glaucoma, 177
Humphrey Field Analyzer (HFA), 65
Humphrey Field Analyzer (HFA) II (700 series), 70, 71*i*
Humphrey STATPAC 2 program, 69, 69*i*
Hyperosmotic agents, for glaucoma, 164*t*, 173–174
Hypertension, ocular, 96
Hyphema, glaucoma and, 110–112, 111*i*
Hypotensive lipids, for glaucoma, 163*t*–164*t*, 171–172

ICE syndrome. *See* Iridocorneal endothelial (ICE) syndrome
Incisional surgery
for angle-closure glaucoma, 200
for open-angle glaucoma, 183–194, 187*i*–191*i*, 193*i*, 193*t*
antifibrotic agents in, 188, 190–192
complications of, 192–194, 193*i*, 193*t*
contraindications to, 185
flap management in, 192
indications for, 184
postoperative considerations in, 192
preoperative evaluation for, 185–186
trabeculectomy technique, 186–188, 187*i*–191*i*
Incorrect corrective lens, in visual field testing, 70
Indirect ophthalmoscope, in optic disc evaluation, 51
Infantile glaucoma, 147
primary, 147
secondary, 147
Infection control, in clinical tonometry, 29
Inflammation (ocular)
secondary angle-closure glaucoma caused by, 138–140, 139*i*
secondary open-angle glaucoma and, 106–108, 108*i*
Intraocular pressure (IOP)
aqueous humor dynamics and, 23–30
calculation of, 18*t*
clinical measurement of, 25–29, 26*i*, 27*i*, 28*t*
digital pressure in estimation of, 29
distribution in population, 23–24, 23*i*
diurnal variation in, 25
elevated. *See* Elevated intraocular pressure
factors influencing, 3–4, 3*i*, 24–25, 24*t*
increased. *See* Elevated intraocular pressure
lowering of, in glaucoma management, 157
normal range for, 3
in primary open-angle glaucoma, 83–84
Intraocular tumors, open-angle glaucoma caused by, 106
Iridectomy
laser, for angle-closure glaucoma, 197–199, 198*i*. *See also* Laser iridectomy, for angle-closure glaucoma
peripheral, for angle-closure glaucoma, 200
Iridocorneal endothelial (ICE) syndrome
glaucoma in, 136–138, 136*i*, 137*i*
variants of, 136
Iridocyclitis, Fuchs heterochromic, glaucoma and, 107–108, 108*i*
Iridoplasty, peripheral, for angle-closure glaucoma, 199–200
Iris
examination of, in glaucoma, 36
neovascularization of, disorders predisposing to, 132, 133*t*, 134*i*, 135*i*
plateau, 128, 129*i*, 130*i*
Ischemic theory, of glaucomatous optic nerve damage, 51
Isopter, definition of, 60

Juvenile open-angle glaucoma, 6*t*
Juvenile xanthogranuloma, glaucoma associated with, 32

Keratoplasty, penetrating, secondary glaucoma and, 116, 116*t*
Kinetic perimetry, in glaucoma, 57, 58*i*
Kinetic testing, definition of, 59
Klippel-Trénaunay-Weber syndrome, glaucoma associated with, 32
Koeppe-type lenses, for gonioscopy, 38
Krukenberg spindle, in pigmentary dispersion syndrome, 101, 101*i*

Laminar cribosa, of optic nerve head, 48
Laminar region, of optic nerve, 48, 49
Laser gonioplasty, for angle-closure glaucoma, 199–200
Laser iridectomy, for angle-closure glaucoma, 197–198, 198*i*
complications of, 199
contraindications to, 198
indications for, 197
postoperative care, 199
preoperative consideration in, 198
technique for, 198–199
Laser trabeculoplasty
for open-angle glaucoma, 180–183, 181*i*

complications of, 182–183
contraindications to, 181
indications for, 180
long-term follow-up after, 183
mechanism for, 180
preoperative evaluation for, 181
results of, 183
technique of, 181–182, 181*i*
selective, for open-angle glaucoma, 182
Latanoprost, for glaucoma, 162*t*, 171–172
Latency period, perimetry effects of, 65
Learning effect, in automated perimetry, 74, 75*i*
Lens, examination of, in glaucoma, 36
Lens particle glaucoma, 104–105, 105*i*
Lens rim, in visual field testing, 70, 72*i*
Lens-induced angle closure, 128–132, 129*i*–131*i*, 131*t*
Lens-induced angle-closure glaucoma, 128–132, 129*i*, 131*i*, 131*t*
Lens-induced glaucoma, 103–106, 104*i*, 104*t*, 105*i*
angle-closure, 104*t*, 122
open-angle, 103–106, 104*i*, 104*t*, 105*i*
Levobunolol, for glaucoma, 160*t*, 165
Lipid(s), hypotensive, for glaucoma, 163*t*–164*t*, 171–172
Lowe (oculocerebrorenal) syndrome, childhood glaucoma and, 155*t*
Low-tension glaucoma, 92–96, 94*t*. *See also* Glaucoma, normal-tension
Luminance
background, perimetry affected by, 63
stimulus, perimetry affected by, 63

M cells (magnocellular neurons), in optic nerve, 44, 46
Magnocellular neurons (M cells), in optic nerve, 44, 46
Malignant glaucoma. *See* Aqueous misdirection (malignant/ciliary block glaucoma; posterior aqueous diversion syndrome)
Mannitol, for glaucoma, 164*t*, 173–174
Manual perimetry, 78–79, 79*i*, 80*i*
Marfan syndrome, lens subluxation in, 122
Mechanical theory, of glaucomatous optic nerve damage, 50–51
Megaloglobus, in childhood glaucoma, 147
Melanocytosis, oculodermal (nevus of Ota), glaucoma associated with, 32
Melanoma(s), choroidal, open-angle glaucoma caused by, 106
Methazolamide, for glaucoma, 163*t*, 168
Metipranolol, for glaucoma, 160*t*, 165
Microspherophakia, pupillary block and angle-closure glaucoma caused by, 130, 131*i*
Miotic agents, for glaucoma, 166–167
Mitomycin C, in trabeculectomy, 191–192
Mobile lens syndrome, 122
Myopia, primary open-angle glaucoma and, 88

Nanophthalmos, secondary angle-closure glaucoma and, 145
Neovascular glaucoma, 132–136, 133*t*, 134*i*, 135*i*
Nerve fiber(s), diffuse loss of, examination of, 55
Nerve fiber bundle defect, in glaucoma, 60
Nerve fiber layer
in glaucoma, quantitative measurement of, 55–56
of retina, in glaucoma evaluation, 47–48
Neural rim, 51, 53*i*
Neurofibromatosis (von Recklinghausen disease)
developmental glaucoma and, 154, 156
glaucoma associated with, 32
Neurofibromatosis, central, developmental glaucoma and, 156
Neuron(s). *See specific type, eg,* Magnocellular neurons (M cells)
Neuropathy(ies), optic, in glaucoma, 3
Neuroretinal rim, 51, 53*i*
Nevus flammeus, 154
Nevus of Ota (oculodermal melanocytosis), glaucoma associated with, 32
Noncontact (air-puff) tonometers, 28–29
Nonrhegmatogenous retinal detachment, secondary angle-closure glaucoma and, 141
Normality, of field, in perimetry interpretation, 68–69, 69*i*
Normal-tension glaucoma. *See* Glaucoma, normal-tension
Nursing mothers, glaucoma medications in, 176

Octopus 1-2-3, 70, 71*i*
Octopus perimeters, 65, 70, 71*i*
Ocular adnexa, in glaucoma evaluation, 32
Ocular biometrics, as factor in primary angle closure, 123
Ocular hypertension. *See* Hypertension, ocular
Ocular Hypertension Treatment Study (OHTS), 28, 86, 87*t*, 97–98, 157
Oculodentodigital dysplasia (Meyer-Schwickerath and Weyers syndrome), childhood glaucoma and, 155*t*
Oculodermal melanocytosis (nevus of Ota), glaucoma associated with, 32
Oligonucleotide(s), antisense, for glaucoma, 177
Open-angle glaucoma, 83–117. *See also* Glaucoma
classification of, 5, 6*t*, 7*i*
mechanisms of outflow obstruction in, 9*t*
genes in, 14
management of
medical, 174–175
surgical, 180–197, 181*i*, 187*i*–191*i*, 193*i*, 193*t*, 195*i*. *See also specific procedure*
cataract and filtering surgery combined, 195–197
full-thickness sclerectomy in, 194–195, 195*i*
incisional, 183–194, 187*i*–191*i*, 193*i*, 193*t*
laser trabeculoplasty in, 180–183, 181*i*
peripheral anterior synechiae in, 5, 7
primary, 82–93
adult-onset diabetes and, 10–11
age and, 86, 91*t*
age-related, 7–8
cardiovascular disease and, 89
central retinal vein occlusion and, 90
characteristics of, 6*t*
clinical features of, 83–87, 85*t*, 91*t*
clinical trials of, 85*t*, 87*t*–90*t*
demographics in, 10
described, 83
diabetes mellitus and, 88–89
disorders associated with, 87–90

epidemiology of, 7–11
family history and, 87
intraocular pressure in, 83–84
myopia and, 88
optic disc appearance in, 84–86, 85*t*, 87*t*–90*t*
prevalence of, 7–8
prognosis of, 91–92
race and, 86, 91*t*
risk factors for, 7, 10–11, 86–87, 91*t*
visual field loss in, 84–86, 85*t*, 87*t*–90*t*
secondary, 99–117
characteristics of, 6*t*
drug use in, 116–117
episcleral venous pressure elevation and, 108–109, 108*t*, 109*i*
hyphema and, 110–112, 111*i*
intraocular tumors causing, 106
lens-induced, 103–106, 104*i*, 104*t*, 105*i*
ocular inflammation and, 106–108, 108*i*
penetrating keratoplasty and, 116, 116*t*
pigmentary, 101–103, 101*i*–103*i*
trauma causing
accidental, 109–114, 110*i*–113*i*
surgical, 114–115, 115*i*
without elevated intraocular pressure, 92–96, 94*t*. *See also* Glaucoma, normal-tension
Ophthalmopathy, thyroid, glaucoma associated with, 32
Ophthalmoscope(s), indirect, in optic disc evaluation, 51
Ophthalmoscopy, confocal scanning laser, in optic nerve head evaluation, 55
Optic disc (optic nerve head)
clinical evaluation of, 51–57, 52*t*, 53*i*, 54*i*
cupping of, in glaucoma. *See* Cupping of optic disc, in glaucoma
evaluation of
in glaucoma, 51
quantitative measurement in, 55–56
hemorrhaging of, in glaucoma, 53–54, 54*i*
laminar cribosa of, 48
nerve fiber layer of
examination of, 54
diffuse loss in, 55
focal abnormalities of, 54–55
perimetry changes correlated with, 78
in primary open-angle glaucoma, appearance of, 84–86, 85*t*, 87*t*–90*t*
Optic disc pit, acquired, 52
formation of, 52–53, 53*i*
Optic nerve (cranial nerve II)
anatomy of, 44, 46–49, 46*i*, 47*i*
anterior
arterial supply of, 48
vascular anatomy of, 48
vasculature of, 47, 47*i*
anterior zone of, 47–48
clinical evaluation of, findings in, recording of, 56–57
damage to, in glaucoma, theories of, 50–51
described, 44
distribution of nerve fibers in, 46, 46*i*
examination of, in glaucoma, 44, 46–49, 46*i*, 47*i*
in glaucoma, 4
laminar region of, 48, 49
pathology of, 44, 46–49, 46*i*, 47*i*
prelaminar region of, 48, 49
retinal ganglion cells in, 44, 46
retrolaminar region of, 49
superficial nerve fiber layer of, 48–49
Optic nerve head (optic disc). *See* Optic disc (optic nerve head)
Optic neuropathy
described, 51
glaucomatous, 3, 49–57, 50*i*, 52*t*, 53*i*, 54*i*
theories of damage and, 50–51
Optical coherence tomography (OCT), in optic nerve head evaluation, 56
Orbital varices, glaucoma associated with, 32

P cells (parvocellular neurons), 44, 46
Paracentral scotoma, 60, 61
Parasympathomimetic agents, for glaucoma, 161*t*–162*t*, 166–168
Parvocellular neurons (P cells), 44, 46
Patient refraction, perimetry affected by, 65
Penetrating keratoplasty, secondary glaucoma and, 116, 116*t*
Perimetry
achromatic automated, in glaucoma, 57
Armaly-Drance screening, 78, 79*i*
automated
short-wavelength, 58
static, 59
automated static, 65–68, 66*i*, 68*i*
artifacts seen on, 70–71, 72*i*, 73*i*
in glaucoma, 57
learning effect and, 74, 75*i*
screening tests, 67
testing strategy in, categories of, 65–67
definitions of terms used in, 59–60
described, 57
frequency-doubling technology, 58–59
full-threshold, 66–67
in glaucoma, purposes of, 57
high-pass resolution, 58
interpretation in
artifacts and, 70–71, 72*i*, 73*i*
optic disc correlation and, 78
progression and, 74–78, 76*i*, 77*i*
series of fields, 72, 74–78, 75*i*
single field, 68–71, 69*i*, 71*i*–73*i*
comparison of techniques, 70
normality *vs.* abnormality, 68–69, 69*i*
quality in, 68
kinetic, 57, 58*i*
manual, 78–79, 79*i*, 80*i*
manual kinetic, 59
standard automated, in glaucoma, 57
static, 59
suprathreshold, 65–66
Swedish interactive thresholding algorithm testing, 67
threshold, 66, 67–68, 68*i*
threshold-related, 66, 66*i*
types of, 59–60

variables in, 60–65, 72*i*
background luminance, 63
background wavelength, 65
fixation, 62–63
patient, 60
patient refraction, 65
perimetrist, 61
presentation time, 64–65
pupil size, 65
stimulus luminance, 63
stimulus movement speed, 65
stimulus size, 64
stimulus wavelength, 65
Peripapillary atrophy, examination of, 55
Peripheral anterior synechiae (PAS)
identification of, in glaucoma, gonioscopy in, 39
in open-angle glaucoma, 5, 7
Peripheral iridectomy, for angle-closure glaucoma, 200
Peripheral iridoplasty, for angle-closure glaucoma, 199–200
Peripheral neurofibromatosis, developmental glaucoma and, 154, 156
Persistent hyperplastic primary vitreous (PHPV), secondary angle-closure glaucoma and, 145
Peters anomaly, 152–153, 153*t*
Phacoanaphylaxis. *See* Phacoantigenic endophthalmitis/uveitis
Phacoantigenic endophthalmitis/uveitis (lens-induced granulomatous/phacoanaphylactic endophthalmitis; phacoanaphylaxis), 105–106
Phacolytic glaucoma, 104, 104*i*, 104*t*, 105*i*
Phacomorphic glaucoma, 122, 128–129, 130*i*, 131*i*
Pigment dispersion syndrome, 101–103, 101*i*–103*i*
Pigmentary glaucoma, 101–103, 101*i*–103*i*
Pigmentation, of trabecular meshwork, 41–42
Pilocarpine, for glaucoma, 161*t*–162*t*, 166–167, 167
Plateau iris, 128, 129*i*, 130*i*
Plateau iris configuration, 128
Plateau iris syndrome, 128, 130*i*
characteristics of, 6*t*
Pneumatic tonometer (pneumatonometer), 28–29
Pneumatonometer(s), 28–29
Polarimetry, scanning laser, in retinal nerve fiber evaluation, 55–56
Portable electronic applanation devices, 28–29
Port-wine stain, 154
Posner-Schlossman syndrome (glaucomatocyclitic crisis), 107
Posterior aqueous diversion syndrome. *See* Aqueous misdirection (malignant/ciliary block glaucoma; posterior aqueous diversion syndrome)
Posttraumatic angle recession, 42–43, 43*i*
Prader-Willi syndrome, childhood glaucoma and, 155*t*
Pregnancy, glaucoma medications during, 176
Prelaminar region, of optic nerve, 48, 49
Presentation time, perimetry affected by, 64–65
Pressure, episcleral venous, 22–23
Pressure-independent outflow, 22
Primary angle-closure glaucoma. *See* Angle-closure glaucoma, primary
Primary congenital glaucoma, 147
Primary open-angle glaucoma. *See* Open-angle glaucoma, primary
Prostaglandin analogs, for glaucoma, 163*t*, 171–172
Prostamide(s), for glaucoma, 163*t*, 171–172
Pseudoexfoliation (exfoliation syndrome), 42, 99–101, 99*i*, 100*i*
Pseudophakic angle-closure glaucoma, 132
Pupil(s), examination of, in glaucoma, 33
Pupil size, perimetry affected by, 65
Pupillary block
angle closure without, 121–122, 121*t*
in angle-closure glaucoma, 120–121, 121*i*
secondary angle closure with, 128–132, 129*i*, 131*i*, 131*t*
secondary angle-closure glaucoma without, 132–146

Quality, of field, in perimetry interpretation, 68

Race
as factor in primary angle closure, 122–123
as factor in primary angle-closure glaucoma, 11
as factor in primary open-angle glaucoma, 10, 86, 91*t*
Refraction
as factor in primary angle closure, 124
as factor in primary angle-closure glaucoma, 12
in glaucoma evaluation, 31–32
patient, perimetry affected by, 65
Retina, nerve fiber layer of, examination of, in glaucoma, 47–48
Retinal detachment
nonrhegmatogenous, secondary angle-closure glaucoma and, 141
surgery for, secondary angle-closure glaucoma and, 143–144
Retinal disease, vascular, secondary angle-closure glaucoma and, 143–144
Retinal ganglion cells, in optic nerve, 44, 46
Retinal nerve fiber(s), distribution of, 46, 46*i*
Retinal nerve fiber layer, in glaucoma evaluation, 47–48
Retinal vein occlusion, central, primary open-angle glaucoma and, 90
Retinopathy of prematurity, secondary angle-closure glaucoma and, 145
Retrolaminar region, of optic nerve, 49
Ribozyme(s), for glaucoma, 177
RIEG gene, 15
Rieger anomaly, *RIEG* gene and, 15
Rieger syndrome, 152, 153*t*
Rubinstein-Taybi (broad-thumb) syndrome, childhood glaucoma and, 155*t*

Sampaolesi's line, 42
Scanning laser polarimeter, in optic nerve head evaluation, 55–56
Schiøtz tonometry, 29
Schlemm's canal
aqueous outflow through, 17, 20–22, 21*i*
gonioscopic visualization of, 40, 41*i*
Schwalbe's line, as angle landmark, in gonioscopic assessment and documentation, 39
Schwartz-Matsuo syndrome, 116
Schwartz's syndrome, 116
Sclera, examination of, in glaucoma, 33

Sclerectomy, full-thickness, for open-angle glaucoma, 194–195, 195*i*
Sclerosis(es), tuberous (Bourneville syndrome), glaucoma associated with, 32
Scotoma(ta)
  arcuate, 60, 62*i*
  definition of, 60
  paracentral, 60, 61
Secondary infantile glaucoma, 147
Secondary open-angle glaucoma. *See* Open-angle glaucoma, secondary
Secretion, active, in aqueous humor formation, 18–19
Selective laser trabeculoplasty, for open-angle glaucoma, 182
Sensitivity
  contrast, in glaucoma, 59
  flicker, in glaucoma, 59
Shaffer system, for gonioscopic grading, 40
Short-wavelength automated perimetry (SWAP), 58, 70, 71*i*
Shunt(s), glaucoma tube, 201–204. *See also* Tube-shunt surgery, in lowering intraocular pressure
Slit-lamp examination. *See* Biomicroscopy, slit-lamp
Spaeth gonioscopic grading system, 40, 41*i*
Standard automated perimetry (SAP), in glaucoma, 57
Static testing, in glaucoma, 59
STATPAC procedure, 70, 71*i*
Stickler syndrome, childhood glaucoma and, 155*t*
Stimulus(i)
  size of, perimetry affected by, 64
  wavelength of, perimetry affected by, 65
Stimulus luminance, perimetry affected by, 63
Stimulus movement, speed of, perimetry affected by, 65
Sturge-Weber syndrome (encephalofacial angiomatosis; encephalotrigeminal angiomatosis), glaucoma associated with, 32
Superior vena cava syndrome, glaucoma associated with, 32
Suprathreshold, definition of, 59
Suprathreshold testing (perimetry), 65–66
Swedish interactive thresholding algorithm (SITA) testing (perimetry), 67

Tendency-oriented perimeter (TOP) algorithm, 67
Threshold (perimetry), 66, 67–68, 68*i*
Threshold, definition of, 59
Threshold-related strategy (perimetry), 66, 66*i*
Thyroid ophthalmopathy, glaucoma associated with, 32
Timolol, for glaucoma, 160*t*, 165
Tomography, optical coherence, in retinal nerve fiber evaluation, 56
Tonography, in aqueous outflow measurement, 22
Tonometer(s)
  applanation. *See* Applanation tonometer (applanation tonometry)
  noncontact (air-puff), 28–29
  pneumatic, 28–29
Tonometry
  applanation. *See* Applanation tonometer (applanation tonometry)
  infection control in, 29
  Schiøtz, 29
  sources of error in, 28*t*
Trabecular meshwork, pigmentation of, 41–42
Trabecular outflow, 19*i*, 20–22
Trabeculectomy technique, for open-angle glaucoma, 186–188, 187*i*–191*i*
Trabeculoplasty, laser, for open-angle glaucoma, 180–183, 181*i*. *See also* Laser trabeculoplasty, for open-angle glaucoma
Trabeculotomy, goniotomy and, for childhood glaucoma, 207–209, 208*i*, 209*i*. *See also* Goniotomy, trabeculotomy and, for childhood glaucoma
Transscleral diode laser cyclophotocoagulation, in lowering intraocular pressure, 205
Transscleral Nd:YAG, in lowering intraocular pressure, 205
Trauma(s)
  angle-recession glaucoma and, 113–114, 113*i*
  blunt
    gonioscopic findings due to, 44, 45*i*
    secondary open-angle glaucoma due to, 109–114, 110*i*–113*i*
  corneal blood staining following, 110, 110*i*
  penetrating, secondary open-angle glaucoma due to, 109–114, 110*i*–113*i*
  secondary angle-closure glaucoma and, 143
  surgical, secondary open-angle glaucoma due to, 114–115, 115*i*
Travoprost, for glaucoma, 162*t*, 171–172
Trisomy 13 (Patau syndrome), childhood glaucoma and, 155*t*
Trisomy 18 (Edwards syndrome, trisomy E syndrome), childhood glaucoma and, 155*t*
Trisomy 21 (Down syndrome, trisomy G syndrome), childhood glaucoma and, 155*t*
Tuberous sclerosis (Bourneville syndrome), glaucoma associated with, 32
Tube-shunt surgery, in lowering intraocular pressure, 201–204
  complications of, 203–204, 204*t*
  contraindications to, 203
  described, 201
  devices in, 201, 201*i*, 201*t*
  indications for, 202
  postoperative management, 203
  preoperative considerations for, 203
  techniques for, 203
Tumor(s)
  intraocular, open-angle glaucoma caused by, 106
  secondary angle-closure glaucoma caused by, 138
Turner (XO/XX) syndrome, childhood glaucoma and, 155*t*

Ultrafiltration, in aqueous humor formation, 18
Unoprostone, for glaucoma, 164*t*, 172
Uveal effusions, secondary angle-closure glaucoma and, 141
Uveitis-hyphema-glaucoma (UGH) syndrome, 115, 115*i*
Uveoscleral outflow, 22

Van Herick method, 34
Varice(s), orbital, glaucoma associated with, 32
Visual field
  clinical evaluation of, in glaucoma, 57–81

contrast sensitivity in, 59
decibel in, 60
depression in, 60
electroretinography in, 59
flicker sensitivity in, 59
isopter in, 60
kinetic testing in, 59
static testing in, 59
suprathreshold in, 59
tests in. *See* Perimetry
threshold in, 59
visually evoked cortical potentials in, 59
definition of, 57
described, 57
Visual field changes, in glaucoma, 4
Visual field defects, glaucomatous, 60, 61*i*–64*i*
Visual field loss, in primary open-angle glaucoma, 84–86, 85*t*, 87*t*–90*t*
Visually evoked cortical potentials (VECPs), in glaucoma, 59
von Recklinghausen disease (neurofibromatosis)
developmental glaucoma and, 154, 156
glaucoma associated with, 32

Xanthogranuloma(s), juvenile, glaucoma associated with, 32

Zeiss-type lens, 39
Zellweger (cerebrohepatorenal) syndrome, childhood glaucoma and, 155*t*